Everywoman's
MEDICAL
HANDBOOK

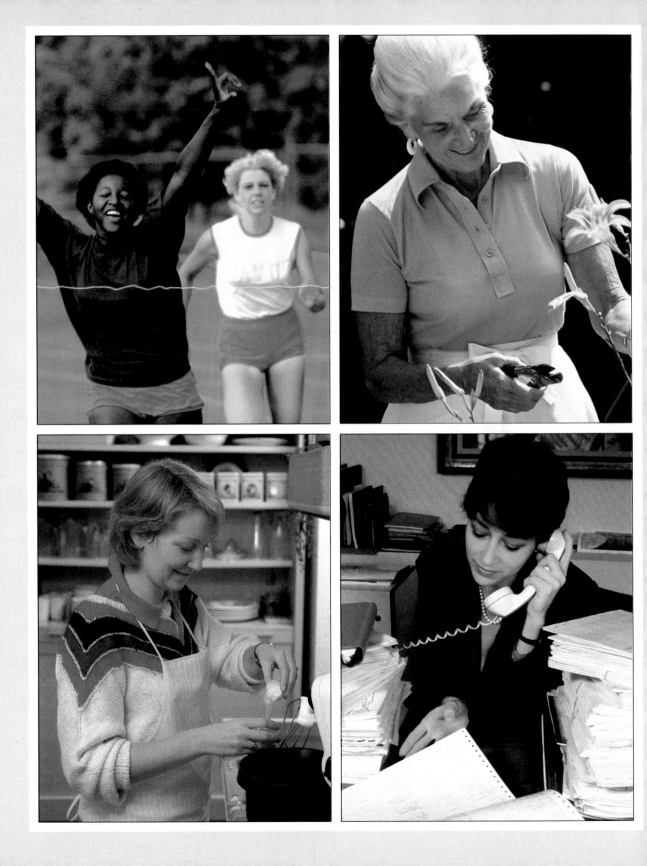

Dr MIRIAM STOPPARD
Everywoman's
MEDICAL
HANDBOOK

BALLANTINE BOOKS · NEW YORK

For Gemma, Mary, Nicole and Vicki

Editor
Charyn Jones

Managing Editor
Amy Carroll

Art editor
Julia Harris

Designer
Sarah Ponder

Copyright © 1988 by Dorling Kindersley Ltd.

Text Copyright © 1988 by Miriam Stoppard

All rights reserved under International and Pan-American Copyright Conventions. Published in the United States by Ballantine Books, a division of Random House, Inc., New York and distributed in Canada by Random House of Canada Limited, Toronto.

Originally published in Great Britain by Dorling Kindersley Publishers Limited, London in 1988.

Library of Congress Cataloging-in-Publication Data

Stoppard, Miriam.
    Everywoman's medical handbook.
    Includes index.
1. Women–Health and hygiene. 2. Women–Diseases.
3. Women–Physiology. I. Title,
RA778.S828 1989   613'.0424   88-47681

ISBN 0-345-35721-3

Manufactured in the United States of America

First Amercian Edition: April 1989

10 9 8 7 6 5 4 3 2 1

The recommendations and information in this book are appropriate in most cases. For specific information concerning your personal medical condition, however, it is suggested that you consult a physician. The names of organizations appearing in the book are given for informational purposes only. Their inclusion implies neither approval nor disapproval by Miriam Stoppard.

INTRODUCTION

Every author aspires to writing the "definitive book"
but few have the opportunity and the assistance to achieve this
goal. With this book, I feel we've come close.
We live in an age where more and more women see as their
unalienable right the freedom to take part in the
health decisions which affect their lives. Many of these
decisions involve doctors, and without information a woman
goes unarmed and vulnerable into the doctor's surgery.
Only with good, accurate information can she hope to be an
equal participant in medical discussions.
I want this book to succeed in helping women to achieve peer
status with their doctors, thereby enabling them to take
responsibility for their own health and their own lives.
The book aims to be exhaustive, not only from the
point of view of including as many common and
important female medical conditions as possible, but also in
preparing a woman for all eventualities once her case
comes under scrutiny from the medics. If you are aware of how
doctors are thinking, what their priorities are and the likely
steps they will take to achieve a firm diagnosis and correct
treatment, then you will be less fearful, able to cope better
with difficulties and remain calm and rational even if the news
is depressing. One of the most uplifting sensations is the
awareness that you are in control of your life; lack of
control is one of the most depressing experiences. This book
aims to help you to gain control of a crucial aspect of your
life – your health. If you feel in control of your body, its health
and maintenance, you are well on the way to finding
tranquillity and happiness.

CONTENTS

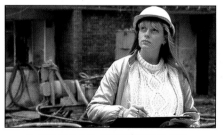

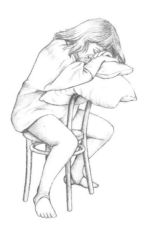
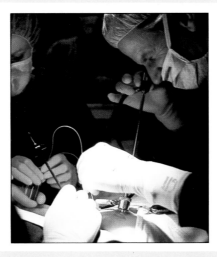
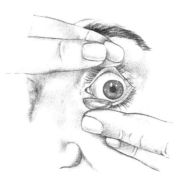

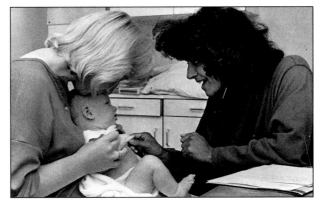

HOW TO USE THIS BOOK

This book deals with all aspects of a woman's health. Good health care is only a small part of the content; the main emphasis is on things that can go wrong and how they are diagnosed and treated.

At first glance it will become apparent that more than just women's "complaints" are covered. In fact, among the diseases, disorders and conditions that I have included are those that only or predominantly affect women, those that affect women differently than men, those that are of more concern to women today than previously, (e.g. AIDS and heart disease), and any about which I believe women are particularly concerned.

This book has three major sections. The first section, The Healthy Female Body, is an illustrated guide to your body and how it works. Here you will also find advice on keeping fit and avoiding those things that can be dangerous to your health. Knowing how your body works when you're well should be helpful when something goes wrong with it. Then you turn to the A-Z section.

Signpost entries such as Menstrual Problems can point the way when you are not quite certain what's wrong but know the general area. These deal with the problems that affect parts of the body and also serve to bring the strands of a major area of health concern such as cancer or sexually transmitted diseases into one entry to give an overview and an understanding of the implications of the problem. These articles have wide gray borders. As a means of cross referencing, the name of the entry you should refer to has been printed in italics.

Also in the A-Z section are those tests and procedures used to diagnose and treat many of the conditions in the book. (These include non-invasive tests such as colposcopy and surgical treatments such as hysterectomy.) By reviewing the reasons for doing them and finding out what is likely to happen, you will know what to expect if you have one.

When you know exactly what is wrong, disorders, diseases and conditions are listed in alphabetical order. These range from acne to wrinkles and each topic contains questions and answers to help you understand the causes, symptoms, treatment and prevention (if applicable). All entries have cross-references to other pertinent articles. Common symptoms are also covered, such as backache and diarrhea. These are in chart form to help you make a diagnosis.

While the book is comprehensive, not every subject merits its own entry and some items are linked with other related subjects – e.g. fibrositis is covered in osteoarthritis. Therefore, it's a good idea if you cannot find what you need by leafing through the alphabetical listings to refer to the index at the back of the book.

The final section of the book, Women and the Medical Profession, tells you how to deal with the medical profession and how to help yourself be in control of your own treatment and condition.

The Healthy Female Body

THE FEMALE BODY

The female body is beautifully adapted to perform all the major biological functions of a woman's life. We start being female at the moment of conception when the X ovum unites with an X sperm. This conjunction begins to affect our anatomy and hormonal patterns from the moment of fertilization.

After just a few weeks of development, an embryo can be seen to be female: the ovaries already contain a lifetime's complement of ova, many in excess of those shed monthly from the menarche to the menopause. The labia, clitoris, vagina and primitive uterus are all present long before we are born.

The potent female hormones determine a cycle of monthly fertility making us the most fertile species on earth, the ovaries ovulate on alternate months. The uterus has two fallopian tubes with connecting tunnels and is a unique muscle. It is capable of exerting an extremely great force over a relatively short distance.

Any mothering instincts, partly engendered by our hormones, ensure that our children are suckled, cared for and loved in the early years of their development. The maternal instinct can serve us well all our lives. It makes us particularly suited to the caring professions of social work, teaching, medicine and counseling because we often see our roles as conciliatory and not deferential; we tend to be peace loving and good arbitrators.

The combination of hormones and biology determines what we are as women. The way we are perceived is another matter. Our bodies are often centers of attention, whether for suckling babies, or ardent lovers, or as the objects of desire in magazines and advertising. It is important that we realize that in certain crucial and inerasable ways we are definitely female with all that means to us as individuals, and we should not allow ourselves to be molded or controlled by others and made to feel inadequate.

Our femaleness is a positive strength. We must accept our femaleness and make it a cause for celebration and pride. The concept of femaleness has room for all variations and permutations; of course there is no such thing as a model or average woman. Individuality is one of our greatest possessions and strengths – if we are proud of being female, we will be proud of it in any form. This means the rejection of all stereotyping and fashionable trends.

MILESTONES IN DEVELOPMENT

From babyhood the differences in body shape between boys and girls are noticeable. Girls tend to have more rounded buttocks and their angled thigh bones make an obvious difference in shape.

At about the age of 9 or 10 the pelvic bones begin to grow and more fat is deposited on the thighs, hips and breasts. By about 12 years, the nipples have budded and pubic hair is sprouting.

By the age of about 18, bone growth is completed and a girl has reached her adult height.

The next time of change is a period of transition known as the climacteric. With menopause, periods stop and the hormones that maintain our fertility level off.

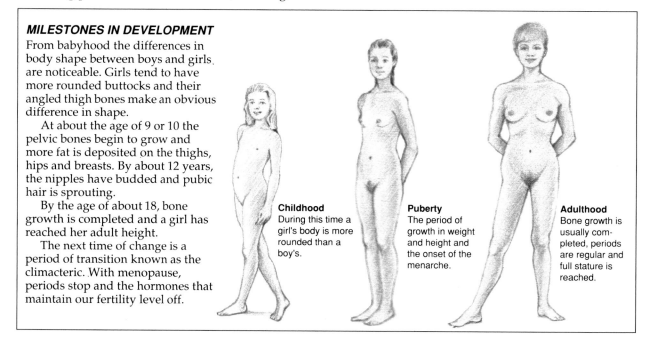

Childhood
During this time a girl's body is more rounded than a boy's.

Puberty
The period of growth in weight and height and the onset of the menarche.

Adulthood
Bone growth is usually completed, periods are regular and full stature is reached.

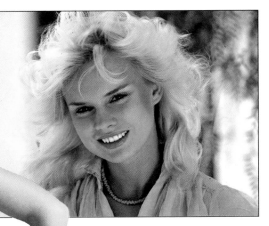

Images of women

Despite attempts by advertisers to present an unreal feminine ideal – the housewife who cares only for her white washing; the "dumb" blonde, or the weak, feeble creature who needs her suitcase carried – women all over the world emerge as distinct and different.

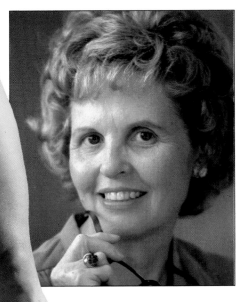

THE MUSCLES AND SKELETON

The skeleton is the basic scaffolding of the body. The muscles which clothe it make us mobile and give many of our joints a wide range of complex movements. The male and female skeletons differ only slightly; men's bones are slightly longer and heavier, their shoulders are broader and rib cages longer. The main difference is the pelvis. The female skeleton develops with wide pelvic bones in order to permit the passage of a baby, and this confers on us another female characteristic, our thigh bones are angled from this wide pelvis inwards towards the knees giving many women the appearance of being knock-kneed. This female blueprint determines that a girl will walk with shorter steps and more precise movements.

The bones must be strong enough to carry weight, and resistant enough not to break under severe stress. Their health can only be achieved and maintained by a diet that contains minerals and vitamins. If diet is neglected, deficiencies may cause the leg bones to soften and bow.

During certain times in a woman's life the bones become more vulnerable. During pregnancy, if the diet is deficient in bone minerals, the baby will feed off you like a parasite and lower your own body stores. At menopause, with the decrease of the female hormones, the health of the bones may deteriorate and soften, a condition known as osteoporosis. If for any reason you suffer from amenorrhea, you may experience premature osteoporosis. Therefore, it is vital that your diet is particularly rich in Vitamin D and calcium. Calcium cannot be efficiently absorbed by the body without Vitamin D but the best source of Vitamin D is sunshine, so getting out in the sun and eating calcium-rich dairy foods, leafy vegetables, legumes and nuts should fulfill your needs.

After the age of 65, when the protective factor of your hormones is lost, you may need hormone therapy to protect the health of your bones and reduce the other troublesome symptoms of menopause.

TAKING CARE OF YOUR BACK

Because of carrying and lifting that occur in the course of our everyday lives, backache is a common complaint. This is made worse during pregnancy when ligaments between and surrounding joints soften, making the joints less stable and likely to strain.

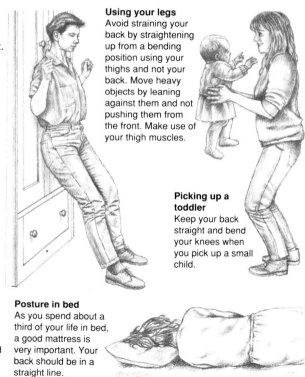

Using your legs
Avoid straining your back by straightening up from a bending position using your thighs and not your back. Move heavy objects by leaning against them and not pushing them from the front. Make use of your thigh muscles.

Picking up a toddler
Keep your back straight and bend your knees when you pick up a small child.

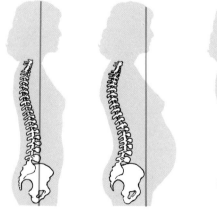
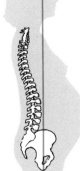

Correcting bad posture
There are many ways you can protect your back. Good posture is the first essential. By correcting your balance and concentrating on a straight back, you will avoid aches and pains and improve your breathing and digestion, too.

Posture in bed
As you spend about a third of your life in bed, a good mattress is very important. Your back should be in a straight line.

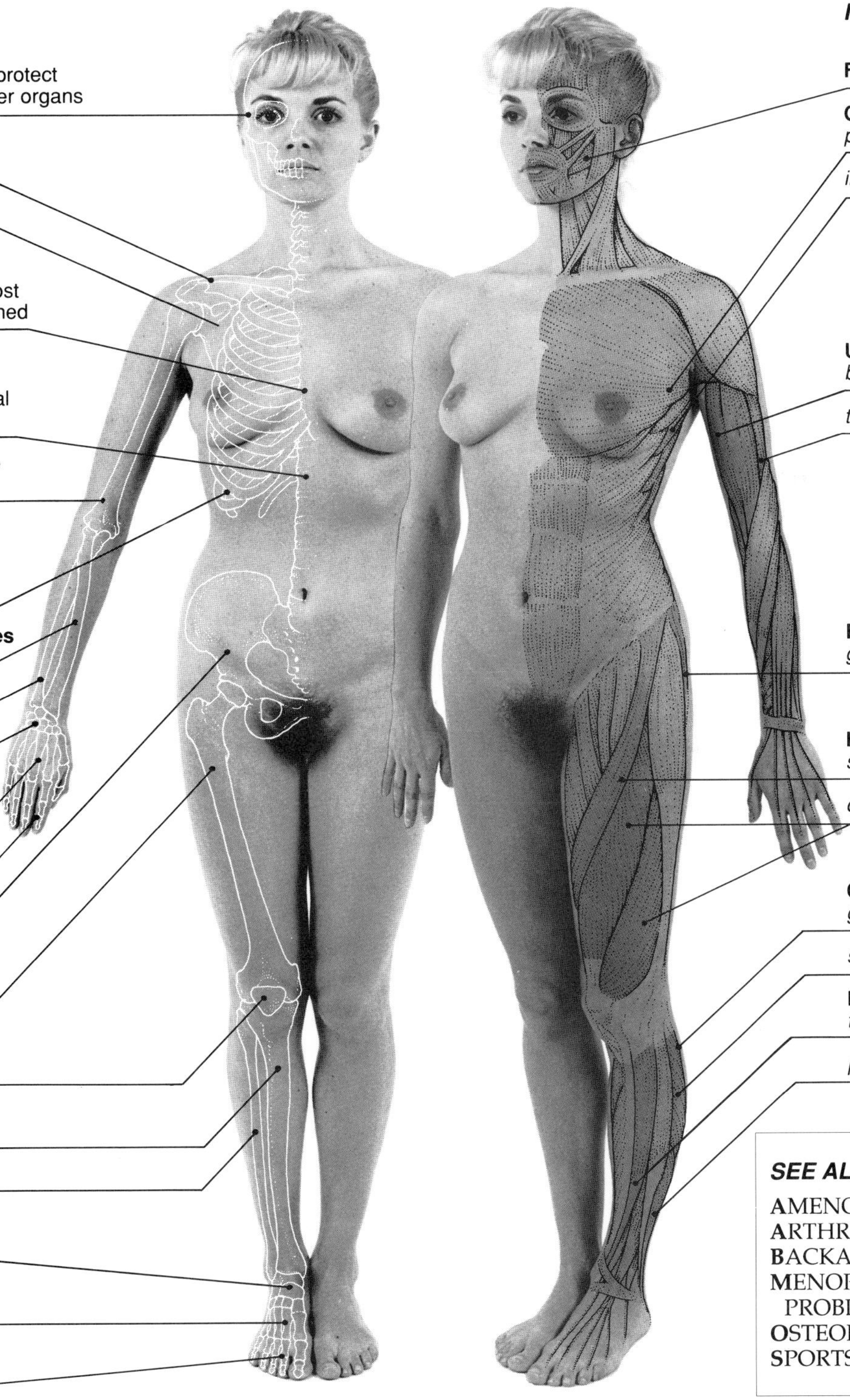

BONES

Skull
a solid casing to protect the brain and other organs

Collar bone
clavicle

Shoulder blade

Breastbone
sternum - central bone to which most of the ribs are joined

Spinal column
surrounds and protects the spinal cord

Upper arm bone
humerus

Ribs
the cage that houses the vital organs

Lower arm bones
radius

ulna

Wrist bones
carpals

Hand bones
metacarpals

Finger bones
phalanges

Pelvis

Thigh bone
femur

Knee cap
patella

Leg bones
tibia

fibula

Ankle bones
tarsals

Foot bones
metatarsals

Toe bones
phalanges

MUSCLES

Facial muscles

Chest muscles
pectoralis major

intercostal muscles

Upper arm muscles
biceps

triceps

Buttock muscles
gluteus maximus

Hamstrings
sartorius

quadriceps

Calf muscles
gastrocnemius

soleus

Leg muscles
tibialis anterior

peroneal muscles

SEE ALSO:

AMENORRHEA
ARTHRITIS
BACKACHE
MENOPAUSAL
   PROBLEMS
OSTEOPOROSIS
SPORTS INJURIES

THE SKIN

The skin is the largest organ in the body; its blood supply is so rich that if all the blood vessels dilate, more than half the blood in the body is drained away from the rest of the body – hence the feeling of faintness after a hot bath.

The skin is elastic, protecting, supple and it helps control the amount of water in the body, the excretion of waste products and body temperature. It is worth looking after.

We tend to concentrate on those parts of the skin that are exposed. For example, we take infinite care of our faces and little of the soles of our feet. Our feet are in fact more important to us than our faces. Despite the attention we lavish on our face and hands, they are constantly exposed to the elements, differences in temperature, dry central heating and sunshine. The hands are also exposed to household detergents and water.

What is the skin?

The skin has two layers – the epidermis or outer layer and an inner layer, the dermis. The epidermis, like the hair and nails, is dead and millions of cells are shed every day. The skin grows from within outwards, the developing layer being very close to the junction of the dermis and the epidermis. New cells bud off and migrate towards the surface, dying as they do so. Many modern cosmetics are aimed at this actively growing layer but whether any of them reach the cells and have any effect is extremely doubtful because the skin forms an efficient barrier against the entry of many chemicals. The only real mode of entry into the deeper layers is through the hair follicles, sebaceous glands and sweat ducts.

Care of the skin

What the skin needs is protection from the sun and moisture. A wide variety of products containing sunscreens and sunblocks are available and much research in the cosmetic industry is spent on trying to find a moisturizer that works.

It is extremely difficult to moisturize the skin. The thin type of moisturizer which disappears into your skin immediately has an effect which lasts no longer than 30 minutes. Much better is the moisturizer which is fashioned to simulate the effect of natural sebum. Sebum acts as a barrier all over the surface of the skin. This kind of moisturizer, which prevents moisture loss, lasts about four or five hours. However, cosmetics which mimic natural sebum seem to be missing some unknown ingredient because none is as efficient as sebum.

Unfortunately for the cosmetics industry, none of their claims is proven. Myths include the efficacy of natural products in cosmetics such as avocado oil, queen bee jelly and placental extracts. However, none of these has been shown to be any more effective than baby lotion or pure lanolin.

So how should you look after your skin? First, always use sunscreen/sunblock products when out of doors for prolonged periods. Handling, massage and gentle circular motions will keep the skin well nourished if done against the force of gravity and line of natural wrinkling. So taking off and putting on makeup is beneficial as a massage and skin conditioner. Skin without make up but with lots of moisturizer is probably happy skin. I do believe that makeup is good for you though. It acts as a protection against the effects of weather, central heating, dust and chemicals in the air. It also acts as a barrier to water loss and it is a great boost to morale.

The daily routine of skin care should involve cleansing, toning and moisturizing. Doing this every day is good for your skin. Paradoxically most water is drying to the skin and so is soap which defats the surface making it dry and scaly. Take showers whenever you can and avoid long soaks in the bath. Keep soaping to a minimum, especially of the face, and put oil in your baths to clothe your skin in an emollient film. After you have bathed, use body lotions, especially if you have black skin.

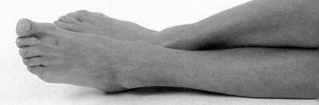

Heels and soles
With a pumice stone remove hard skin after a bath when it is softened. Use hard-skin removing cream to keep your feet soft.

Knees
Wear pads to prevent rough skin and calluses if you do a lot of kneeling, say while gardening.

SKIN STRUCTURE

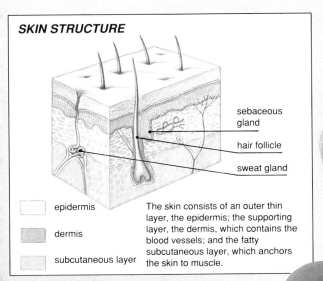

sebaceous gland

hair follicle

sweat gland

epidermis

dermis

subcutaneous layer

The skin consists of an outer thin layer, the epidermis; the supporting layer, the dermis, which contains the blood vessels; and the fatty subcutaneous layer, which anchors the skin to muscle.

Face
Cleanse and moisturize regularly. Don't hesitate to use makeup. It acts as a barrier against moisture loss.

Neck
Moisturize as often as you can; always use upward stroking movements to counteract the downward drag of gravity.

Underarms
Wash morning and night and use a combined anti-perspirant/deodorant to help cut down odor.

Abdomen
Stretch marks from weight gain are due to collagen breakdown and cannot be removed by oils or creams.

Vaginal area
Don't use vaginal deodorants; they may cause irritation and detract from your natural odor which is a sexual attractant.

Elbows
Moisturize as often as you can to make the skin softer.

Hands
Moisturize with a hand or barrier cream whenever you can, especially during winter and after washing up.

SEE ALSO:

ACNE

BODY ODOR

FACIAL TREATMENTS

RASHES

SKIN CANCER

SKIN PROBLEMS

WRINKLES

TEETH, HAIR AND NAILS

It may seem odd to think of teeth, hair and nails together because they differ so greatly in appearance and structure. However, they are derived from exactly the same cell of the embryo and so from the physiological point of view, it is quite logical to discuss them together.

Hair

The sort of hair you have is determined by your ancestry although you can change it with chemicals and hairdressing. Hair develops from a papilla below the surface of the scalp, but once it emerges on the outside of your head, it is dead. It follows, therefore, that it is impossible to affect the health of your hair by applying anything to it, despite what the advertisements proclaim. The only way to nourish your hair is with a good diet to feed the hair root well.

So there is no reason why your hair should not be bouncing with good health and be beautiful in appearance. Hair technology means that even after chemical onslaughts like bleaching and perming, hair can be conditioned back to good health. When a shaft of hair is plucked, or falls out at the natural end of its growing stage, the papilla is still there to provide another one. The growth cycle of our hair is staggered so that it doesn't all fall out at once.

Hair is formed from rather simple chemical chains. Perming, for example, removes some chemicals from the hair making it flexible, and then implants other chemicals into the hair to fix it into the desired shape – usually curls. This process doesn't exactly damage the hair but it does change the chemical nature and with it the appearance and behavior.

Hormonal changes at puberty can cause normal hair to become oily and difficult to handle. This will occur again at menopause when you may notice hair loss as the hormone levels change. The tiny organ at the root of the hair ceases to deposit pigment as you get older and this results in white or grey hairs. When this occurs also depends on heredity.

Nails

Nails are made up of the same substance as hair and they protect the sensitive ends of the fingers from injury. They, too, are dead when they emerge from the cuticle. But while growing, they can be affected by ill health. Detergents and solvents weaken and cause nails to become brittle. You should wear protective gloves whenever you use

---

CARE OF THE HANDS

Personally I do not think that a manicure is a luxury. It is essential care for your nails. You should look after your nails once a week - shaping them, keeping the cuticles trim and soft. If they are weak, put some kind of strengthener on them to prevent them cracking and splitting. There are many clever commercial products which contain fibers or hardeners. They are hardly visible and can increase your nails' strength by 100%.

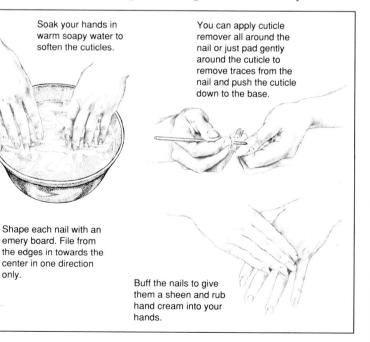

Soak your hands in warm soapy water to soften the cuticles.

You can apply cuticle remover all around the nail or just pad gently around the cuticle to remove traces from the nail and push the cuticle down to the base.

Shape each nail with an emery board. File from the edges in towards the center in one direction only.

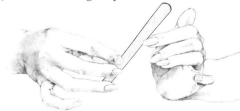

Buff the nails to give them a sheen and rub hand cream into your hands.

water or any of these household products. Toenails need careful attention, too. Cut them after a bath or shower when they are soft and cut them straight across; cutting them down at the sides encourages ingrowing toenails.

Teeth

The health of the teeth relies on calcium and fluoride. Research demonstrates unequivocally that fluoride maintains teeth and protects them. This applies to everyone, not just children. A fluoride coating on the surface of the teeth helps prevent tooth decay.

Caring for your teeth has obvious advantages for your whole life. You should approach this as a preventative measure to avoid tooth decay and gum disease. Unhealthy gums are more central to the problem because they may cause the teeth to loosen and eventually fall out.

To care for your gums you need to brush regularly. This is necessary to remove food particles and to prevent the build up of plaque. Dental floss gets rid of plaque too. If plaque forms under the gum margins, it irritates the gums which become swollen, soft and bleed easily. They are then prey to bacteria. Once an infection has taken hold it is very difficult to eradicate. The gums of pregnant women are naturally softer, predisposing them to infection.

The health of your teeth relies on a good diet, good personal dental habits and regular visits to your dentist. Decay will then be stopped before it has inflicted damage sufficient enough to necessitate removal of teeth.

CARE OF THE TEETH

- Brush your teeth twice a day, making sure you go to bed with clean teeth.
- Buy a new brush every two months.

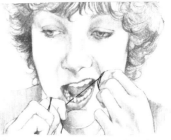

- Use floss once a day but be careful not to damage the delicate gum margins.
- Visit a dentist at least twice a year.

THE SENSES

We have five senses: sight, smell, taste, hearing and touch. All work in a similar way. At the site where the sense is appreciated, there are small receptor organs formed from the ends of microscopic nerve fibers. These pick up a sensation and pass the message along sensory nerves to the brain. In the nerve ending, the sensation is transformed into electrical energy which passes up to the brain almost instantaneously. Within the sensory cortex of the brain, electricity is converted back to the original sensation and we feel, see, hear, taste or smell it. This whole process takes less than a second. For example, if your fingers touch a piece of ice, coldness is picked up by a temperature receptor organ in the skin. The variation in the other senses exists only in the type of receptor.

Sight
The eyes lie well protected within the skull bones. At the back of the eye are rods and cones, the light-sensitive nerve cells lying in the retina. Light and color falling onto the retina forms an upside-down image of what you are looking at. This leads to chemical changes in the rods and cones which are transmitted via the optic nerve to the brain. To see properly, the brain has to unscramble the confusion and interpret the picture for you. The brain also has to co-ordinate the two views that the right and left eyes receive.

object

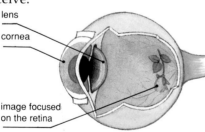

lens

cornea

image focused on the retina

Touch
The skin provides us with essential information about our surroundings. Particularly in sensitive areas such as the tips of the fingers, the mouth and the genital organs, there are millions of touch receptors. The skin on the back, however, has relatively few nerve endings.

Hearing
Sound waves are channeled into the ear canal and onto the ear drum by the pinna (the ear lobes). This starts the drum vibrating. These vibrations are transmitted to the hearing part of the inner ear, the cochlea, across a chain of small bones. There is another source of sound through the vibrations of the skull bones. This is how we hear our voices.

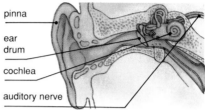

pinna

ear drum

cochlea

auditory nerve

The cochlea is lined with tiny hairs which transform the vibrations into electrical impulses that pass up the auditory nerve to the brain where they are turned back into sound.

Smell
The nose is lined with a hairy mucous membrane. The receptor organs pick up their sensations in moist droplets from the atmosphere or from dry chemicals dissolved in the mucus secretions.

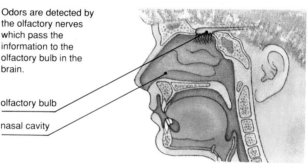

Odors are detected by the olfactory nerves which pass the information to the olfactory bulb in the brain.

olfactory bulb

nasal cavity

Taste
On the upper surface of the tongue and within the mouth there are receptors of taste which can pick up four main groups of flavors.

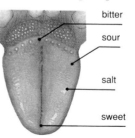

bitter

sour

salt

sweet

Saliva begins to be produced when you are about to eat and while you are eating and the solution of the flavor with the saliva is picked up by these receptors.

THE ENDOCRINE SYSTEM

The endocrine system is a collection of interrelated glands that produce hormones. Hormones are chemicals that travel through the blood to exert an effect on distant parts of the body. The master gland of this system is the brain's pituitary gland which manufactures specific releasing hormones which trigger the flow of hormones from other glands. For example, follicle-stimulating hormone (FSH) is secreted by the pituitary into the bloodstream. When it reaches the ovary, it causes the growth of an ovarian follicle and its egg which brings about the secretion of estrogen and progesterone to prepare the breasts and uterus for a possible pregnancy.

Many of the glands work through a negative feedback system. The brain secretes FSH at the beginning of the menstrual cycle when estrogen levels are low. The ovary responds with the production of estrogen. The brain senses the rising levels of estrogen and shuts off FSH secretion.The entire system works so delicately that a fine balance of hormones and releasing hormones is maintained throughout the body.

As well as the pituitary, the system also includes the thyroid and parathyroid glands, the adrenal glands, the pancreas, the gonads (ovaries and testes), and in pregnant women, the placenta. The amount of hormone secreted can be affected by a number of factors including illness, stress, age and a change in another chemical in the body. The various glands have specific functions that are outlined below.

Adrenal glands are divided into two organs. One produces adrenaline and noradrenaline to regulate the heart rate and blood pressure. The other produces the steroid hormones. One group balances the concentrations of chemicals such as sodium in the body. Another group helps convert carbohydrates into energy; one such hormone is hydrocortisone. The third group consists of the sex hormones, estrogen, progesterone (and androgens in a man). These are the hormones that affect our sexual development and characteristics.

The pancreas produces insulin which helps our bodies maintain blood sugar and metabolize carbohydrate. If this is not made by the pancreas, or in too small quantity, diabetes results. Glucagon is another hormone secreted by the pancreas which stimulates the liver to produce insulin.

The ovaries produce sex hormones and release them throughout the menstrual cycle to affect the breasts, the endometrium, cervical mucus and the retention of water by the body.

The pituitary gland is the size of a peanut and consists of two parts – the anterior and posterior lobes. The anterior lobe produces growth hormone, and prolactin which stimulates milk production.

The posterior lobe produces antidiuretic hormone (ADH) which regulates the volume of urine, and oxytocin which stimulates uterine contractions and the release of milk from the breasts during lactation. The pituitary also sends messages to other glands to stimulate them to produce hormones of their own.

The thyroid gland produces thyroid hormone which affects the heart and metabolic rate.

The parathyroid glands are four tiny glands producing parathyroid which affects bones through its control over the metabolism of calcium and phosphorus. It acts with Vitamin D to help strengthen our teeth, bones and clot our blood.

SEE ALSO:

DIABETES MELLITUS
HORMONE
  REPLACEMENT
  THERAPY
MENSTRUAL
  PROBLEMS

BLOOD

The circulatory system is the transport system of the body. Through the various components, food, oxygen, water and all other essentials are carried to the tissue cells and waste products are carried away. It consists of three parts: blood is the fluid in which materials are carried to and from the tissues; the heart is the driving force that propels the blood; and the blood vessels are the routes by which the blood travels to and through the tissues and back to the heart.

Healthy women have three to five liters (approximately six to ten pints) of blood circulating in their bodies according to their size. Blood is composed of a straw-colored liquid, the plasma, in which are suspended blood cells, the latter being divided into two types – the red blood cells and the white blood cells. Serum is the clear fluid content of the blood that is left after clotting agents and blood cells are removed. It is this substance that is usually required for blood tests.

Blood forms about 5% of the body weight. It is a thick red fluid, bright red in the arteries where it is oxygenated, and a dark purplish-red in the veins where it is de-oxygenated, having given up some of its oxygen to the tissues.

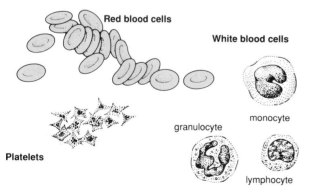

Red blood cells

White blood cells

Platelets

granulocyte

monocyte

lymphocyte

Plasma
The fluid part of the blood, plasma, consists of water (which is about 90% of the whole), mineral salts (chlorides, phosphates, carbonates, sodium, potassium and calcium, the chief salt being sodium chloride), plasma proteins (albumin, globulin, fibrinogen and prothrombin), foodstuffs in their simplest form (glucose, amino acids, fatty acids, glycerol and vitamins), gases in solution (oxygen, carbon dioxide and nitrogen), waste products from the tissues (urea, uric acid and creatinine), antibodies and antitoxins, which protect the body against bacterial infection, hormones from the various endocrine glands around the body, and enzymes.

Red blood cells
The red cells are minute disc-shaped bodies, concave on either side. There are about five million to every cubic millimeter of blood and they contain a special protein called hemoglobin. Hemoglobin contains iron and this iron is essential to normal health. Hemoglobin has a great attraction for oxygen. As the red cells pass through the lungs, hemoglobin combines with oxygen from the air, forming oxy-hemoglobin and becomes bright red in color. As the red blood cells pass through the tissues, oxygen is given off and hemoglobin becomes a dull color making the blood a dark, purplish-red.

The function of red cells is to carry oxygen to the tissues from the lungs and to carry away some carbon dioxide. This is their sole function and their efficiency depends on the amount and type of hemoglobin they contain. If there is a lack of hemoglobin, either because the red cells are reduced in number or because each one does not contain the normal quantity or quality of hemoglobin, the person will suffer from anemia.

Red cells are produced in the red bone marrow found in the long bones of the extremities such as the femur in the thigh, and in flat, irregular bones such as the pelvic girdle.

For the healthy growth of red blood cells, protein, iron, Vitamin B_{12}, Vitamin B_6, Vitamin C, thyroxine, traces of copper and manganese are all needed. If any of these substances is absent or deficient, anemia will result. In sickle cell anemia, red blood cells become sensitive to low oxygen levels when they become "sickle" in shape and rupture. Sickle cell anemia is genetically inherited and is carried as a recessive trait.

White blood cells
The white cells are larger than the red cells, but they are less numerous. There are only 7 to 10 thousand per cubic millimeter of blood, though the number may increase three-fold when an infection is present. The white blood cells are divided into

three different types. Polymorphonuclear leukocytes, also known as granulocytes because they have granules inside the cells, make up about 75% of the total white cells and are manufactured in the bone marrow. They survive for only 21 days and are then destroyed. There are three kinds of granulocytes: eosinophils, basophils (which are also known as mast cells) and neutrophils. Neutrophils are the most numerous and have the ability to engulf, ingest and destroy bacteria and cell debris. This process is known as phagocytosis and the cells are sometimes known as phagocytes.

The second type of white blood cells are lymphocytes which make up about 20% of the total white cell count. They are manufactured in the lymph nodes and in the lymphatic tissue. They are concerned with the production of antibodies against invasion by microbes – part of the body's defense system. The third type, known as monocytes, make up about 5% of the total white cell count. They are the largest of all the white blood cells and are phagocytic.

Platelets

Platelets or thrombocytes are even smaller than red blood cells and are also made in the bone marrow. They are necessary for blood clotting. There are about 250,000 per cubic millimeter of blood. They are vital clotting agents.

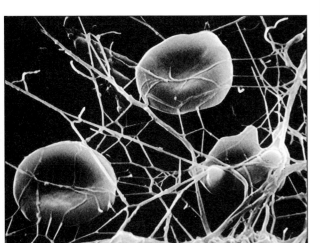

ABNORMAL HEMOGLOBIN

If the hemoglobin in the blood is abnormal, this can result in incurable anemic diseases. Sickle-cell disease is an inherited condition where the red blood cells become sickle-shaped because of their abnormally low oxygen levels. They then fail to flow smoothly through the capillaries. The condition almost exclusively affects people of African descent. It is a recessive trait, in that both parents carry the abnormal gene while they are themselves healthy. The risk to any child they may have is 1 in 4.

The anemia develops in the first six months of life, and the symptoms are mild jaundice and pain in the limbs and body wherever the blockage of the blood vessels occurs. The sufferers often have acute crisis attacks that are brought on by infection.

Thalassemia is another inherited blood disorder where normal blood pigment is not formed in the red blood cells. Severe anemia results, requiring blood transfusions, although this true form is uncommon. It is more common to inherit the condition from one parent when it is known as thalassemia trait. The condition is most common among people of Eastern and Mediterranean origin.

Genetic counseling and tests allow those carrying these abnormal genes to decide whether to have children or not, depending on the risk.

Sickle shaped red blood cells
When deprived of oxygen, the defective hemoglobin in the red blood cells precipitates out, forming elongated crystals that distort the shape of the cell. These cells are more rapidly removed from the blood, thereby leading to the anemia typical of sickle cell disease.

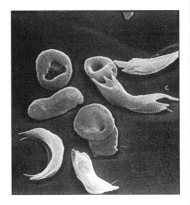

The clotting process
In order for the blood to clot, it requires a protein, fibrinogen. Platelets collect and stick together wherever a blood vessel suffers damage. When they disintegrate, they eventually produce fibrinogen which converts into fibrin, a substance that unites the blood cells so any accidental breach is closed.

SEE ALSO:

AIDS
ANEMIA
CANCER
CHROMOSOMAL
 PROBLEMS

HEART AND CIRCULATION

A female's circulation is different from that of a male in that it can support another being when necessary through the life-support system of the placenta (see index).

The circulatory system is made up of two parts. One part is the systemic circulation which supplies blood to the body, except the lungs; the other part is circulation of blood to the lungs to be reoxygenated. It is called pulmonary circulation.

From the left side of the heart, the aorta sends reoxygenated blood out through arteries to replenish the muscles and tissues of the body. These major arteries, which are deep in the body so they cannot be easily severed (the wrists are an exception), divide into arterioles and then into tiny capillaries. The capillaries have thin walls which allow oxygen and nutrients to pass from the blood into the tissues. Waste passes in the opposite direction. Used blood returns with the waste through venules and veins back to the right side of the heart for reoxygenation in the lungs.

The blood in the arteries flows under high pressure until it reaches the veins. To prevent the blood flowing back down the veins, because on its return journey it is at low pressure, the veins have valves. If these fail, varicose veins in the legs can result.

THE HEART

The heart has four chambers: two upper chambers (atria) and two lower ones (ventricles). The flow is controlled by four valves. Blood enters the heart from the body at the right atrium and thence to the right ventricle through the tricuspid valve. The pulmonary arteries send the blood to the lungs for reoxygenation, then the pulmonary veins conduct it back to the left atrium. The mitral valve controls the flow to the left ventricle from where the aorta sends blood out to the body. This goes on while simultaneously fresh blood is passing out to the body and spent blood is being sent for reoxygenation.

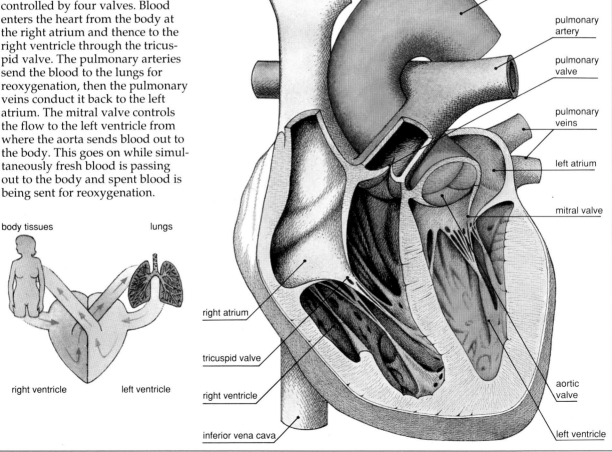

body tissues

lungs

right ventricle

left ventricle

superior vena cava

aorta

pulmonary artery

pulmonary valve

pulmonary veins

left atrium

mitral valve

right atrium

tricuspid valve

right ventricle

aortic valve

inferior vena cava

left ventricle

Circulation

The circulation system takes blood to all parts of the body. The aorta is about 2.5cm (1 in) thick but the capillaries, at the other end of the scale, are tiny. In the illustration (left), red represents the systemic circulation, the fresh blood, and blue the pulmonary circulation, that is stale or deoxygenated blood.

carotid artery

jugular vein

aorta

heart

inferior vena cava

descending aorta

brachial artery

iliac artery

iliac vein

femoral artery

femoral vein

CHANGES DURING PREGNANCY

The female heart has to enlarge and increase its workload during pregnancy because the volume of blood increases by about 1.5 liters (3 pints). The heart pumps out more blood per minute than ever it does during the rest of a woman's life and yet maintains blood pressure at a normal level. To accomplish this, the heart has to increase its stroke volume (the amount of blood pumped at every beat) by as much as 40%. No man's heart is ever called upon to do this.

Hemoglobin levels

Blood contains a pigment, hemoglobin, which gives the red cells their color. Hemoglobin carries oxygen around the body, so that the more hemoglobin the blood contains, the more oxygen can be carried to the various tissues in the body such as the muscles and, in a pregnant woman, the placenta. Due to the loss of blood every month during menstruation, many women are deficient in hemoglobin, for which iron is an essential ingredient. If our diets are not rich enough in iron or we have heavy menstrual periods regularly, and never catch up, anemia results.

Diet and exercise

We were never meant to be sedentary animals and the health of our heart and lungs depends on taking some exercise. This needs to be vigorous enough to cause sweating and panting but within the guidelines determined by fitness testing. The most effective way is to use the leg muscles which are big and require the most oxygen. Walking, jogging, swimming, cycling and tennis are good if you practice them regularly.

It has been proven that our present day Western diet has a detrimental effect on our hearts because we consume large amounts of fat. The excessive intake of fats (especially those of animal origin) coupled with the body's own production of blood fats (the most important of which are cholesterol and triglycerides), leads to a higher incidence of heart disease in industrialized countries such as the United States and Britain. In countries where dairy products and animal fats are not eaten as much, like Japan, cholesterol levels are lower and coronary disease rarer.

THE BODY'S DEFENSES

Just as blood passes through the capillaries, fluid oozes out through the porous walls of the tissues and circulates through them, bathing every cell. This fluid is called lymph or tissue fluid. It fills in the spaces between the cells which form the different tissues.

It is a clear, watery, straw-colored fluid similar to the plasma of the blood from which it is derived. While blood circulates only through the blood vessels, tissue fluid circulates through the actual tissue and carries food, oxygen and water from the bloodstream to each individual cell. It also carries away waste products such as carbon dioxide, urea and water, returning them to the blood. Lymph is the conduit between the tissue cells and the blood.

The lymphatic system consists of lymphatic vessels made up of lymphatic capillaries, and lymph nodes or glands which lie along these lymph vessels. The lymphatic capillaries arise in cell spaces like fine, hair-like vessels with porous walls. They gather up excess fluid from the tissues and unite to form lymphatic vessels. The walls of the lymphatic capillaries are so permeable that substances of greater size can pass through their walls than through the walls of blood vessels.

The lymphatic vessels are thin-walled collapsible tubes similar in structure to the veins but they carry lymph instead of blood. They are finer and more numerous than the veins and like them are provided with valves which prevent the lymph moving in the wrong direction. Lymphatic vessels are found in most tissues, except the central nervous system. They lie close to veins and arteries and pass through one or more lymph nodes.

The lymphatic nodes or glands are small bodies varying in size from a pin-head to an almond. Lymphatic vessels bring lymph to them, and once inside the node, enter and divide up, discharging the lymph into the node itself. The lymph is then gathered again into fresh lymphatic vessels which carry it on and ultimately empty it into a lymphatic duct and then to the heart via a main vein, the superior vena cava.

The role of the lymph nodes

The lymph nodes filter the lymph of bacteria and other harmful substances; therefore when tissues are infected they may become swollen and tender.

They produce the particular cells involved in body defence, the lymphocytes (types of white blood cell), which when mature are poured into the vascular circulation. The lymph nodes help the absorption of digested food, especially fat, in the abdomen. The nodes also filter off any malignant cells which may enter the lymphatic circulation; a swelling in the armpit may signify a possible breast cancer. Finally, the lymphocytes produce antibodies and antitoxins to control and prevent infection.

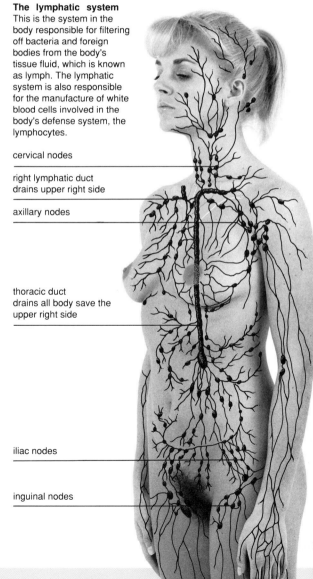

The lymphatic system
This is the system in the body responsible for filtering off bacteria and foreign bodies from the body's tissue fluid, which is known as lymph. The lymphatic system is also responsible for the manufacture of white blood cells involved in the body's defense system, the lymphocytes.

cervical nodes

right lymphatic duct drains upper right side

axillary nodes

thoracic duct drains all body save the upper right side

iliac nodes

inguinal nodes

The nodes are massed together in various groups throughout the body. The groups in the neck and under the chin (cervical nodes) filter the lymph from the head, tongue and floor of the mouth. The group in the armpit (axillary nodes) filters the lymph from the upper limb and the chest wall. A group in the groin (inguinal nodes) filters the lymph from the lower limb and lower abdominal wall, and groups in the chest and abdomen (mediastinal and abdominal nodes) filter the lymph from the internal organs.

After filtration by the nodes, the lymph is emptied first into the lymphatic vessels and then into the two lymphatic ducts – the thoracic duct and the right lymphatic duct. The ducts join one of the main veins returning to the heart. Lymph is thereby put back into the bloodstream from which the fluid in the tissues is constantly renewed.

How does it work?

The lymphatic circulation is maintained partly by suction and partly by pressure. Suction is the more important factor. The lymphatics empty into the large veins approaching the heart and here, due to heart action, suction is created as the heart expands, drawing lymph towards it. Inspiration also creates suction. Pressure is exerted on the lymphatics by the contraction of muscles and this outside pressure drives lymph onwards because the valves prevent a backward flow.

If there is obstruction to the flow of the lymph through the lymphatic system, edema results. This is a swelling of the tissues due to excess fluid collecting in them. It can occur after radical mastectomy when the lymph nodes are cleared from the armpit. This obstructs the free circulation of lymph back from the arm towards the heart and gives rise to the swollen, white, painful arm.

The defense system

The lymphatic system, particularly the lymph nodes, forms a crucial part of the body's defense system. The lymph nodes manufacture a variety of lymphocytes, one of them, the T helper lymphocyte, is at least partly responsible for two crucial aspects of the body defenses. In the first place it is involved in the allergic response to foreign proteins, producing antibodies which neutralize the

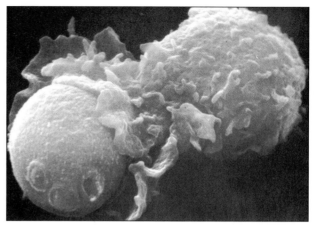

The action of lymphocytes
This scanning electron micrograph shows a cultured lymphocyte in the act of destroying (phagocytosing) a yeast cell.

Other lymphocytes do not act directly but produce further substances, known as antibodies, that help in the destruction of organisms foreign to the body.

foreign proteins and prevent the body from being damaged by them. In this way we are protected from infections as foreign organisms invade the body. It is also the mechanism which defends the body after vaccination and immunization. The basic antigen-antibody reaction which is involved in allergic diseases is partly maintained by the T helper lymphocytes. If their integrity is damaged, the body's defense system is seriously undermined. This can occur in AIDS, resulting in overwhelming lung infections and malignant tumors in the form of Kaposi's sarcoma in the skin as well as a wide variety of other infections and cancers.

The cells in the lymph nodes are also responsible for manufacturing some of the antibodies to bacteria and viruses and destroy them whenever they enter the body. Antitoxins, specific antidotes to poisonous substances, are also manufactured in the lymph nodes thereby shielding the body from chemicals which could destroy it.

SEE ALSO:	
AIDS	**F**LUID RETENTION
AUTOIMMUNE	**M**ASTECTOMY
DISEASE	**R**HEUMATOID
BREAST CANCER	ARTHRITIS
CANCER	**S**YSTEMIC LUPUS

THE BRAIN AND NERVOUS SYSTEM

The brain and nerve tracts of the spinal cord make up the nervous system that controls our bodies. The brain keeps our hearts beating, monitors our blood pressure and crucial factors like blood sugar levels and body temperature. It keeps us breathing without us ever being aware of the effort. It is also the seat of emotions and the intellect. The brain is extremely complex in nature. What makes us different from most other animals is the size of the cerebral hemisphere which contain the vital "gray" matter that bestow on us all our skills including our capacity with words and the complicated mechanisms of reading and writing. The brain, through our senses, makes us uniquely aware of our surroundings and therefore able to adjust and adapt to the environment. It has an enormous capacity for work, needing only small periods of sleep to recharge its batteries.

The brain maintains control over the rest of the body by connections through the spine and nerves. The body of the embryo is derived from segments and each segment has a motor and a sensory nerve on both sides. Sensory nerves carry information to the brain, which then sifts this information, makes a decision and acts by sending messages down to the muscles, bones and joints via the motor nerves. The result is that parts of the body move, and the action is completed.

There is also an auxiliary nervous system called the autonomic nervous system which oversees those parts of the body we are unaware of such as the stomach, intestines, lungs and heart. The brain, via these two nervous sytems, one "external" and one "internal", maintains the body in equilibrium,

HOW THE BRAIN WORKS

All the functions of brain are inter-linked in such a complex way, that they should not be seen in isolation. The brain is divided into the forebrain, midbrain and hindbrain. The fore-brain contains the cerebral hemis-pheres with four lobes in each hemisphere – the occipital, parietal, temporal and frontal. The mid-brain contains the pituitary, thalamus and hypothala-mus and the hindbrain contains the brain stem and cerebellum.

Color image of the brain
The colored body scan shows a section through a normal adult brain. The cerebral hemi-spheres appear red and yellow, the cerebellum at bottom right appears yellow and feathery, and the cerebro-spinal fluid appears dark blue.

The occipital lobes control vision.

The parietal lobes have some con-trol over touch and balance.

The cerebellum helps us to maintain balance, posture and co-ordinates our movements.

The temporal lobes control hearing.

The brain stem controls the vege-tative functions such as heart, breathing, body temperature. The nerve fibers run through the stem to receptor organs and they regulate our sensory responses.

The frontal lobes are responsible in part for taste, smell, voluntary movements such as language and emotions.

In the middle of the brain lie the pituitary which controls other hormone-secreting glands in the body thus affecting sexual characteristics, reproduction, kidney function and growth of long bones, and the hypothalamus which controls hunger, sex drive and mood.

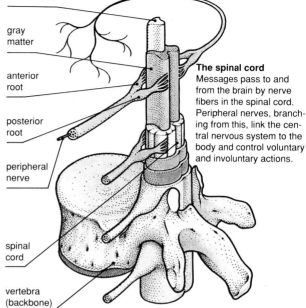

The spinal cord
Messages pass to and from the brain by nerve fibers in the spinal cord. Peripheral nerves, branching from this, link the central nervous system to the body and control voluntary and involuntary actions.

Labels: white matter; gray matter; anterior root; posterior root; peripheral nerve; spinal cord; vertebra (backbone)

both within itself and with the outside world.

The complexity of the brain is difficult to imagine. It is constantly receiving sets of messages from many different sites. One is from receptor organs in the skin, eyes, nose, ears and mouth, pertaining to our senses; another is from the joints and muscles so that we can walk, run, perform athletic feats, stay upright and not topple over; another set of messages from the balancing organ in the inner ear relates the body to space. It tells us if we are upright or upside down, swaying to one side or the other so that the body, through the muscles and limbs, can correct its position.

Of all the messages coming from the various parts of the body, those from the eyes override almost all other sets of messages. This is why a small baby will refuse to crawl across the floor over a visual cliff even though the "cliff" is only painted on the flat surface. It is also why we are aware that messages from our eyes do not fit in with what is happening around us when we say that we "can't believe our eyes."

Reflexes

Quite independent of this interconnected system is a mechanism which is protective and sometimes life saving. Excluding the brain altogether, it is called a reflex. For example, a protective reflex operates when we put our hand on something very hot. The heat receptors carry this message only as far as the spinal cord and once interpreted there, a message immediately goes down a motor nerve to the arm muscles making us withdraw our hand without us even having felt the heat or thought of removing the hand. We experience the sensation of heat or burning only after removing the hand because the sensation of pain takes longer to interpret in the brain than the reflex message going to the hand through the spinal cord.

Other reflex actions occur within the internal organs without us being conscious of them. One is the gastro-colic reflex. When food is taken into the mouth and reaches the stomach, the intestine is stimulated to make room for the next meal. This is why babies very often pass a stool immediately after food and why as adults we often need to open our bowels after a meal. Heeding the gastro-colic reflex is one of the ways of preventing constipation. If the gastro-colic reflex is ignored then the bowel becomes lazy.

SEE ALSO:

AUTOIMMUNE DISEASE	FAINTING AND DIZZINESS
BODY SCAN	HEART DISEASE
DEPRESSION	

THE RESPIRATORY SYSTEM

Oxygen is essential to life. It is the fuel we need for all the metabolic processes that occur in our bodies. We die very quickly without it. The lungs are the means by which oxygen is taken into the body, dispersed in the blood, and circulated to where it is needed. The lungs also act in the reverse way. Carbon dioxide, a waste product from these metabolic processes, is carried by the blood back into the lungs where it is lost from the blood and breathed out. This means that with a healthy circulation to the lungs, our blood can absorb enough oxygen and get rid of enough carbon dioxide to cope with the greatest physical stress and the greatest needs.

Respiration is therefore more than just breathing. The lungs are crucial to life, not only because they transport oxygen in and carbon dioxide out; they also help to maintain the acid base balance which is vital to most metabolic processes, and by blowing off more or less carbon dioxide, they can correct the acidity or alkalinity in the blood. A build up of carbon dioxide causes an increase in the acidity balance in the blood, thus altering the rate of breathing. The lungs therefore are excretory organs, acting in concert with the kidneys and the skin to maintain a homeostatic internal environment. They have a natural elasticity or recoil which allows them to expand, sometimes as much as 12cm (5in) during deep breathing, and to contract automatically at the end of the breath. They act like bellows and are helped by the muscles of the chest wall between the ribs and the diaphragm.

All the muscles of respiration are under central control by the brain and nerves from the autonomic nervous system.

Damage to the lungs
Smoking does damage in the short term, inflicting winter coughs, colds and bronchitis, and to your baby during pregnancy. It also carries with it the legacy of chronic chest disease which may eventually go on to emphysema. This breaks down the delicate structure of the lungs, distorting the alveoli, scarring the elastic lung tissue and making breathing inefficient. In the long term, emphysema can cause distressing shortness of breath and in some people the inability to walk even short distances.

BREATHING IN PREGNANCY
Women experience difficulty breathing in pregnancy because of the growing baby in the uterus. The pressure of the expanding uterus on the diaphragm makes inhalation difficult and exhalation is no longer as efficient. By the third trimester you can easily become breathless just walking up a flight of stairs. Towards the end of the pregnancy when the baby's head or bottom presses up under the ribs on the right hand side, breathing can become painful because the muscles of the abdomen and the ribs are subjected to repeated pressure. The pressure is nearly always worst when you are lying down, so use two or three pillows to keep you semi-upright.

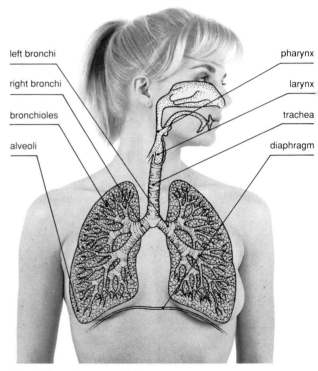

left bronchi
right bronchi
bronchioles
alveoli
pharynx
larynx
trachea
diaphragm

To make breathing more efficient, the anatomical structure of the lungs is arranged so that each tiny air passage ends with small alveoli, grape-like swellings arranged in bunches so that the surface area for gaseous exchange is greatly increased. In fact, by this simple anatomical trick, the surface area of the lungs is maximized to the size of a tennis court.

SEE ALSO:
CANCER
COUGH
FAINTING AND
   DIZZINESS
LUNG CANCER
PALPITATIONS

THE DIGESTIVE SYSTEM

Food is first chopped up into small pieces by the mastication process in the mouth, using the teeth, hard palate and the tongue. Digestion starts in the mouth with a digestive enzyme found in the saliva which begins the conversion of carbohydrates. Food passes down through the esophagus by contractions of the esophagus wall into the stomach where it is mixed with quite strong acids, one of which, pepsin, begins to act on the proteins. The stomach is a grinding and storage organ, being able to store the food from a whole meal so that its contents are well mixed with acid and enzymes.

In very small quantities, usually within an hour or two of the meal being taken, the well-mixed food is squirted out into the small intestine at the duodenum where the environment changes from acid to alkaline. More enzymes are added to the mixture so that digestion can proceed further. It is in the duodenum that bile from the gall bladder is added to aid digestion of fatty foods. The pancreas also secretes vital enzymes.

If the contents of the stomach are extremely acidic, they may irritate and inflame the lining of the duodenum. This may eventually give rise to ulceration. From this process you can see why alkaline substances relieve the discomfort from a duodenual ulcer.

It is further down in the small intestine where digestion is completed and food is broken down into very small molecules which can pass through into the blood stream.

The large intestine is mainly for the absorption of water and the retrieval of some important chemicals. If you have diarrhea and the contents move very fast through your bowel, then water cannot be absorbed by your body and this is why the stools in diarrhea are watery and slimy. Under normal circumstances, however, most water will be absorbed back into the body. When the feces enter the rectum, the last of the water is absorbed and the stools can become quite dry. If the stools stay several hours in the rectum without being passed, they will actually become very dry and hard, what most people call constipation.

The digestive system starts at the mouth and ends at the anus. If you think of it as a simple tube running through the body you can see that it is really a space enclosed by the body on all sides. It does not excrete waste. Excretion is the waste products from metabolic processes within the body but as food is always "outside" of the body, the feces are not true body waste substances.

SEE ALSO:

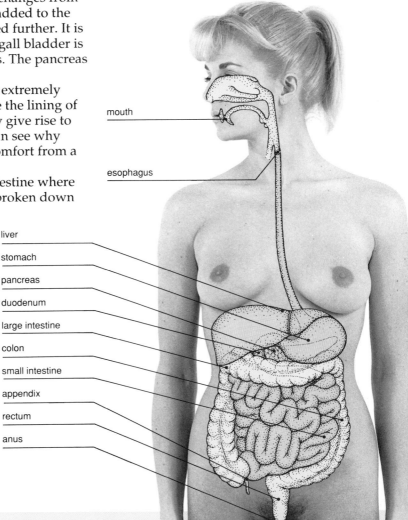

mouth

esophagus

liver

stomach

pancreas

duodenum

large intestine

colon

small intestine

appendix

rectum

anus

MENSTRUATION AND REPRODUCTION

Menarche literally means the beginning of menstruation. The age of the menarche varies throughout the world. In general, Eastern and Semitic races start menstruating earlier, at around 10 years of age. The average among Western nations is about 12. At the turn of the century it was several months older than this and it was thought that the onset of menstruation might continue to get earlier and earlier, but over the last decade the average age of onset has stabilized around the middle of the twelfth year.

The advent of the menarche means that a girl is entering her fertile life. Cyclical female hormone production has started and ovulation each month is a possibility. Very few girls ovulate consistently in the first years of menstruation. Ovulation is usually sporadic and does not stabilize until the age of about 16 or 17. The production of the cyclical female hormones is not smooth either and may result in peaks and troughs explaining why a girl can become moody, a loner, depressed, rebellious, confused and mixed up. The cycle of female hormones also leads to maturation of a girl's body and the appearance of secondary sexual characteristics. It is therefore the most important physiological event of the early teenage years.

Hormonal effects
The production of hormones results in various changes in your organs. In the first half of the cycle, estrogen has an almost youthful effect. It keeps the hair in good condition, it makes the skin bloom, it raises our mood so that we feel that we can tackle anything. It also affects the quality of the vaginal discharge prior to ovulation. The discharge is thin, clear and runny and has very little smell.

After ovulation, progesterone shows its effects. The vaginal secretions become thicker, opaque, more rubbery and definitely have a fishy odor. The breasts enlarge, become heavy, tender and they may assume the consistency of orange pips. Towards menstruation the nipples may tingle and feel sore. These are quite normal effects and subside on or before menstruation beginning. Progesterone has an androgenic effect and can cause acne-like spots on the face. Few of us escape menstruation without one or two of these. Don't squeeze them; they are due to hormones and will disappear when menstruation starts.

Menstrual hygiene
Menstruation is no longer the taboo subject it once was. When I was young it was said that young

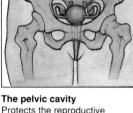

The pelvic cavity
Protects the reproductive organs and is large enough to accommodate an enlarged uterus at pregnancy.

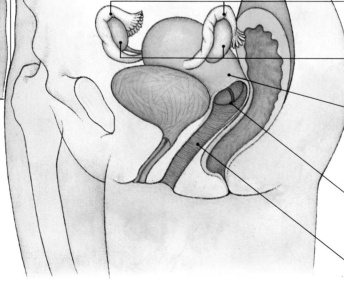

Fallopian tubes
Each one leads from an ovary to the uterus.

Ovaries
They contain a life's supply of eggs.

The uterus
A muscular organ about the size of a pear.

The cervix
The neck of the uterus has a small opening where menstrual blood can pass out during menstruation and sperm can enter at intercourse.

The vagina
An elastic tube running from the vulva to the cervix.

THE MENSTRUAL CYCLE

This lasts on average about 28 days but may be as long as 33 or as short as 26. Once menstruation is established, however, there is usually a fixed number of days for each individual. The first day of the cycle is counted from the day that bleeding begins.

Days 1 – 13

At the beginning of the cycle there are no female hormones – estrogen or progesterone – circulating in the body. Then the pituitary gland in the brain secretes follicle stimulating-hormone (FSH). It stimulates the ovary to start to grow egg follicles which, in their turn, secrete estrogen. The estrogen level rises, encouraging the lining of the uterus – the endometrium – to thicken and prepare for a possible pregnancy.

Day 14 Ovulation

When estrogen levels reach their peak, this stimulates production of yet more FSH and another hormone, luteinizing hormone (LH). This causes the follicle to burst, releasing the egg. This is ovulation.

Days 15 – 28

The egg starts to move down the fallopian tube and the follicle matures into a corpus luteum which secretes large amounts of progesterone in the second half of the month. Three days prior to menstruation, the corpus luteum ages and dies and progesterone levels fall. The unfertilized egg and the endometrium are discharged through the cervix. Menstruation has begun.

girls shouldn't wash their hair or bathe during menstruation because the blood might go to their brains. This is nonsense and the general rule should be to bathe as often as you wish while menstruating. Ordinary soap and water is best.

Some girls prefer sanitary napkins and these are ideal until you are about 17 or 18 when you might want to start experimenting with tampons, which are more comfortable, hygienic and discreet. Quite a good way to start is to try with a friend. I remember doing so with one of my college friends as we stood in adjacent toilets and gave running commentaries on our progress. Don't forget about them; they should be changed every four hours.

MENSTRUATION AND AIDS

The AIDS virus reaches a high concentration in the blood of those infected by it. It follows that a woman suffering from AIDS could pass the virus in her menstrual flow. AIDS sufferers and people carrying the AIDS antibodies should refrain therefore from sexual intercourse during menstruation. In fact, it is risky for an infected partner to engage in intercourse whether menstruating or not.

The irony is that many races historically considered women to be unclean when they were menstruating. These religious and cultural teachings are not necessarily adhered to as many couples do enjoy sexual intercourse during menstruation. We now have a modern reason for considering abstinence.

SEE ALSO:

ACNE
AMENORRHEA
DYSMENHORREA
MENORRHAGIA
MENSTRUAL
  PROBLEMS

PREMENSTRUAL
  SYNDROME
VAGINAL
  DISCHARGE

CONCEPTION AND FERTILITY

Fertility is the ability to have a baby and conception is the first step to pregnancy. During sexual intercourse, millions of sperm are released into the vagina. If ovulation has occurred, the mucus at the cervix is thinner so that the sperm can swim up the vagina through the cervix. Only about 2000 sperm reach the uterus and the fallopian tube, and only one of the chemically-attracted sperms attaches to the surface of the comparatively enormous ovum and penetrates its outer shell. The rest lose their attraction, drop off and die. Fertilization then takes place mainly due to the strength, determination and staying power of the sperm.

Conception is usually quite a dramatic event for a woman's body. The ovary does not cease hormone production as it does when conception has not occurred. It continues to increase the levels of female hormones to prepare the lining of the uterus and support the pregnancy until the placenta can take over. This may produce symptoms of morning sickness, giddiness, fainting, soreness and tingling in the breasts, a metallic taste in the mouth and the desire to pass urine frequently.

Fertility

Fertility depends on several factors but the most crucial is that even a woman who is ovulating is only fertile for two or three days each month. Infertility or sub fertility (where the barriers to conception can be overcome by some means, medical or psychological) is not usually the fault of one person within a partnership. Two people with marginal fertility may fail to conceive together but in another liaison, their new partners' fertilities can compensate for theirs and they can conceive.

The age of the woman is a significant factor in fertility. A woman's fertility reaches a peak at about 24 years of age, exactly the same as a man's. There is a definite decline after 30, and it is rare, though not impossible, for a woman to conceive after 50. Ovulation becomes less frequent with age, and the second half of the cycle becomes irregular in the pre-menopausal years. So even with fertilization, the uterine environment may be less favorable and the ovum has less chance of survival. All forms of sexual activity decline in men from their early twenties but the decline is not as steep as with women. Fertility has been recorded at 94 years of age in men.

Timing of intercourse

The single most crucial factor to ensure fertilization is to have intercourse within a day or so of ovulation occurring. This can be calculated from

HOW GENES DETERMINE SEX

An ovum contains half the future fetus' genetic material. When an ovum is fertilized, it receives the other half from the sperm. The father's major contribution is the sex of the child. Both X or female sperm, and Y or male sperm are produced. Ova are always X. If an X sperm unites with the ovum, the child will be female; if a Y sperm unites with the ovum, the child will be male. Besides the pair of sex chromosomes, there are 22 other pairs of chromosomes which contain genetic material such as hair and eye color. The tendency to inherit certain diseases and conditions such as color blindness is also carried in the genes.

These physical characteristics and diseases are inherited in dominant or recessive form. The dominant form will always determine the characteristic; for example, blue as an eye color is recessive and will not appear if either the sperm or ovum carries the dominant characteristic for brown eyes. That is why two brown-eyed people usually have brown-eyed children unless there is a recessive blue-eyed gene in both. A recessive gene may stay hidden for generations.

At the moment of conception, gender is determined. If the sperm carries an X chromosome, the baby will be a girl; if a Y chromosome, the baby will be a boy. The ovum carries only the X chromosome.

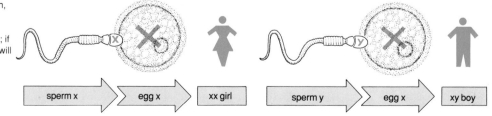

| sperm x | → | egg x | → | xx girl | | sperm y | → | egg x | → | xy boy |

When the follicle bursts releasing the egg at ovulation – usually about 14 days after the first day of bleeding – it is caught in the end of the fallopian tube and propelled towards the uterus by muscular contractions.

If intercourse takes place, the fastest, strongest and healthiest sperm will swim up the tube. An ovum can live for up to 36 hours and sperm for around 24 hours. This means that the fertile period could be in the region of 3 days.

Immediately after fertilization, the fertilized ovum starts dividing up until it has formed a ball of cells. This is called a blastocyst.

The blastocyst continues to travel down the fallopian tube to the uterus.

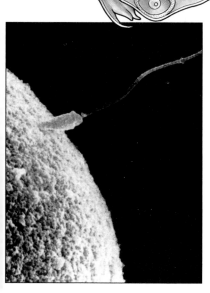

Seven days after fertilization, the blastocyst reaches the uterus where it usually implants in the roof of the upper third of the uterine wall. Conception has occurred.

Because the ovum is chemically attractive to all sperm, the strongest will fertilize the ovum and the rest will die.

your menstrual cycle, temperature charts and the appearance of your vaginal secretions.

It isn't true that conception is more likely if you have intercourse very frequently. The opposite is true. The more often a man ejaculates, the fewer sperm are contained in his ejaculate. It is a good idea to abstain for a few days prior to ovulation to build up the numbers of sperm.

SEE ALSO:

CHROMOSOMAL
  PROBLEMS
DOWN'S SYNDROME
GENETIC
  COUNSELING
INFERTILITY

MENSTRUAL
  PROBLEMS
MORNING SICKNESS
PREGNANCY
  PROBLEMS
PREGNANCY TESTING

SEX AND SEXUALITY

While we associate certain areas of the body with erogenous stimulation – the breasts, the nipples, the mouth, palms of the hands, all around and inside the genital area – almost any area of a woman's body is an erogenous zone if it is caressed and kissed by someone to whom the woman is attracted or finds exciting. It is up to individual couples to explore mutual pleasuring and to a woman to help her partner to discover what gives her pleasure.

While the first signs of her sexuality, her primary sexual characteristics, appear in a baby girl at birth, the onset of menstruation is the time when other obvious physical changes occur. These are known as secondary sexual characteristics.

Primary sexual characteristics

These are the sex organs situated in the pelvis, including the uterus, fallopian tubes, ovaries, cervix and vagina. They have very nearly matured by the time menstruation starts. Lower down there are the external sex organs sited around the vaginal opening, an area known as the vulva.

When a girl is physiologically mature, this is signalled by a discharge in the vagina originating in the cervix. At the entrance to the vagina lies the clitoris, the seat of most female sexual pleasure. From puberty onwards, the clitoris can become enlarged when aroused; this can happen quite spontaneously or due to friction during gymnastics, horseriding or even from tight clothes. At this time the clitoris becomes proud and free of its protective hood in preparation for further sexual stimulation.

Secondary sexual characteristics

These give the female body its contours. There is a gradual narrowing of the waist, widening of the hips and the appearance of a pad of fat on the inner and outer sides of the thighs and around the upper arms. The breasts, the other external sex organs, enlarge to full roundness and hair appears in the armpits and in the pubic region. These pads of fat are specially laid down as energy stores for lactation; an amazing piece of future planning by our bodies. Women who don't breastfeed may therefore run the risk of keeping plumper upper arms and thighs than those who do.

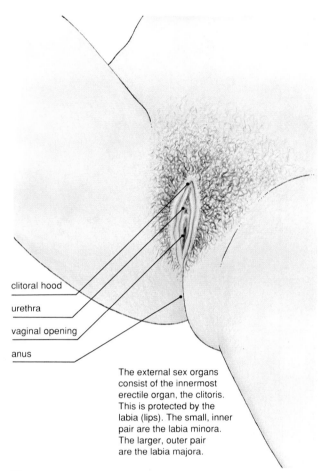

clitoral hood

urethra

vaginal opening

anus

The external sex organs consist of the innermost erectile organ, the clitoris. This is protected by the labia (lips). The small, inner pair are the labia minora. The larger, outer pair are the labia majora.

Erogenous zones

Although almost any part of the body is erogenous if stroked and touched by someone you care about or are attracted to, certain areas are inherently more sensitive than others. These areas are known as the primary erogenous zones, and include the internal and external genitals, the lips, the buttocks, breasts and nipples.

The reason these areas have become considered erogenous zones is that they have a rich supply of sensory nerve endings and are particularly sensitive to stimulation by touch. When the primary erogenous zones are touched certain physical changes take place. There is an increase in blood supply to the area, which then leads to swelling, pinkness and increased sensitivity. There is also an increase in breathing rate, the pulse rate, blood pressure and sweating.

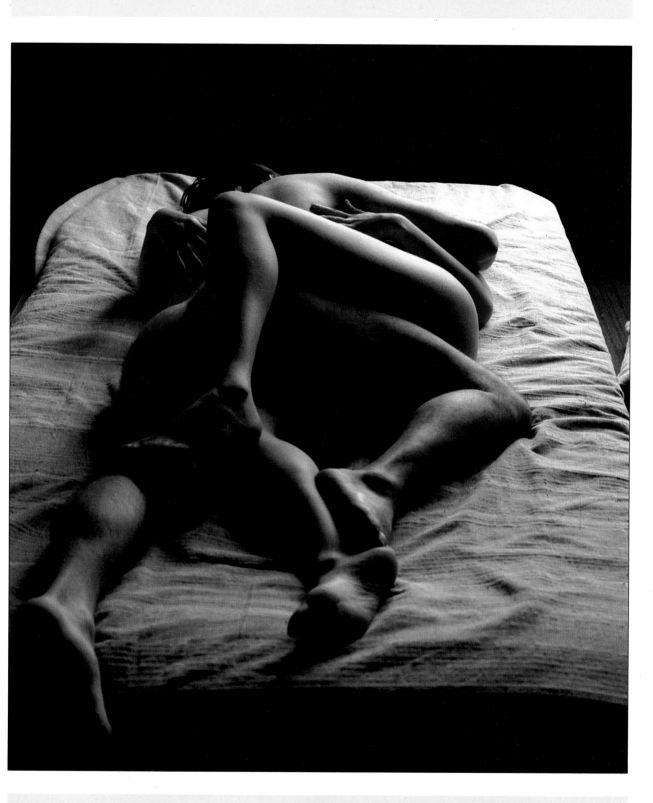

SEX AND SEXUALITY

Sexual awakening

Most girls start to explore themselves intimately around the age of 11 or 12, even if it is only by looking and touching. Around 14 or 15 they may share experiences with girlfriends. At this time masturbation is one way to achieve sexual satisfaction and it is important that girls try it. It is almost the only way that you can come to know yourself sexually, and your desires and preferences.

At the same time many girls find that they are experiencing sexual fantasies stimulated by reading, writing, films, boys or even teachers to whom they feel attracted. This is not a bad thing; certainly a girl should be able to choose to do whatever she finds heightens her sexual pleasure and she should try to continue this throughout her life. Many women, because of the intrusions of childbearing, careers and over extension of their energies, forget how to appreciate what their bodies feel and much of the enjoyment from sex can be lost if we don't listen to and enjoy our bodies. Fantasizing is one way of doing this.

Sexual arousal

Libido is the word used to describe the instinct that accompanies sexual arousal. Foreplay is a crucial part of sexual arousal and often a more important part of sex for women than men. Women and men are aroused with different stimuli. While men are more likely to find looking at the female body, and talking and thinking about sex erotic, women tend to need direct and continuous physical stimulation in order to become fully aroused. Hence the importance of erogenous zones (see above). When a woman is aroused by touch or anticipation, the sensation affects all parts of the body. The heartbeat increases so the pulse becomes rapid, breathing is faster, and the increased blood flow to all parts of the body causes the skin to turn pink and sweat. Blood flows to the breasts, nipples and the genitals where the vaginal secretions increase and two tiny organs, Bartholin's glands, which lie near the vaginal opening, start to secrete mucus too. These secretions, together with the enlargement of the labia, allow the penis a smooth, soft entrance to the vagina.

The next phase is sometimes referred to as the plateau phase because the congestion in the pelvic organs remains at a peak until climax or orgasm. The orgasm is impossible to describe as it is different for everyone. The body may stiffen and the muscles contract and many women call out involuntarily. The uterus contracts and the clitoris retracts under its hood. The orgasm is controlled by a reflex. Your brain may, however, override this reflex and you'll fail to achieve orgasm if, for example, you feel inhibited by your physical surroundings, someone in the next room or feelings of insecurity about the person you are having intercourse with.

The final or resolution phase is one of relaxation. It takes several minutes for the congestion caused by the increased blood flow to disappear when you'll feel loving and peaceful.

Of course sexual intercourse is different for everyone, and there is no such thing as a right way to do it; it depends entirely upon what gives you pleasure and whether both partners enjoy the experience. Oral sex, cuddling and caressing one another, and massage alone can be enjoyable too. There are, however, some physical and emotional reasons why you may fail to enjoy sex or achieve sexual satisfaction.

Orgasm

The fact that orgasm has come to be called the big "O" by many women means, I think, that our ideas about orgasm are a long way from being well thought out. Female orgasm used hardly to be discussed at all until it became a major plank of the women's liberation movement. While I support every woman's right to experience an orgasm and to go on experiencing it if this is her desire, there should be no pressure upon other women who don't experience orgasm, since this can lead to guilt and feelings of inadequacy. About 10% of women never experience orgasm at all, even with masturbation. This, in part, may be because they are women who find intimacy, cuddling and caressing as satisfying as anything else in sexual relationships, or they may lack a strong libido. Other women may not achieve orgasm because their partners are inexpert. Many men believe that women achieve orgasm through the friction of the penis in the vagina. This is not so; most women need clitoral stimulation to achieve orgasm.

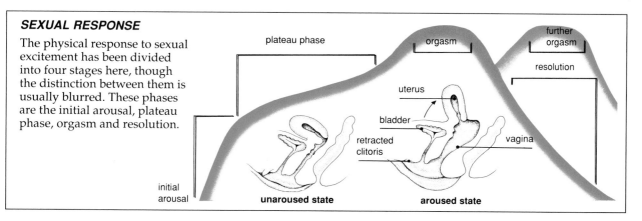

SEXUAL RESPONSE

The physical response to sexual excitement has been divided into four stages here, though the distinction between them is usually blurred. These phases are the initial arousal, plateau phase, orgasm and resolution.

plateau phase

orgasm

further orgasm

resolution

uterus

bladder

retracted clitoris

vagina

initial arousal

unaroused state

aroused state

In order to reach some satisfaction from her sexual relationships a woman should explore her needs and desires and communicate them to her partner. Atavistic ideas about the correctness of oral sex, different sexual positions, or sexual orientation shouldn't deter you if you find them satisfying. Nothing is wrong if both partners enjoy it and neither of you is doing anything you don't want to do. For most women the sex drive and the desire for sexual happiness is very important. It is foolish to ignore it or say that things should be otherwise.

Enriching your sex life
Most couples don't have major physical or emotional problems with sex, they just experience nagging doubts about their ability to excite their partner, or they feel bored and in a rut. A large part of being a good sexual partner is improving your techniques so that both of you experience mutual affection and lasting sexual pleasure. This isn't just a matter of technical ability. You could alternate who takes the initiative, for example; couples often get into a routine which, by its very existence, leads to sex becoming boring. Imagination is therefore a factor.

Don't be dismayed if you've never tried something before. Oral sex, where you use your mouth and tongue, is something many women regard as too intimate an act. Don't imagine that you smell or taste bad; your vaginal secretions, provided that you keep clean and don't use deodorants, are a normal natural odor of sexual arousal.

Many women dislike the idea of taking semen into their mouths. It is a harmless fluid. You could ask your partner to alert you to when he is about to ejaculate. Oral sex between longterm sexual partners is quite safe, but should be avoided if there is any indication of a herpes infection or any other sexually transmitted disease.

Overcoming your inhibitions
Besides the real emotional worries, such as fear of pregnancy and anxiety about your sexual performance, there are other areas where there may be problems. The solution is to discuss these worries with your partner and together try to sort them out. Maybe you are a spectator during intercourse, never getting involved, lying back and thinking about other things. Sex therapists use programs for improving responsiveness to help you focus on your sensations and your partner's body.

Many women, who, for years may have faked orgasms, need to be slightly selfish and focus on their own pleasure in the pursuit of sexual fulfilment. Any woman who feels inhibited, guilty or indifferent about sex needs to become more of a hedonist to pursue positively her sexual identity.

SEE ALSO:

AIDS
BODY ODORS
CONTRACEPTION
CYSTITIS
GENITAL HERPES
GONORRHEA

SEX THERAPY
SEXUAL PROBLEMS
VAGINAL DISCHARGE
VAGINISMUS
VAGINITIS

PREGNANCY

Pregnancy is divided up into three three-month periods called trimesters. This isn't simply for convenience, it is because certain well-circum-scribed events occur in these three separate periods. If complications are going to occur, they tend to be confined to one or other of the three trimesters, and doctors perform tests at the optimum time. However, because pregnancy is above all a continuous process, you need not take too much notice of these artificial timescales.

The statistics that relate to how a woman's body adjusts to a pregnancy are staggering. Your body will make any change or sacrifice necessary for the healthy growth of your baby. These changes nearly all occur in the first trimester and are designed to anticipate the possible demands of the embryo, and to provide stores of fat and minerals which can be converted later to milk for breastfeeding.

The first signs

After your missed period, one of the first changes you will notice is in your breasts. The veins become more obvious and the breasts increase in size and feel heavy, sore and tingling as the milk-producing glands develop. Your nipples will be particularly sensitive and darken in color.

Because of the hormonal changes, you will find yourself needing to urinate more often. Your waist will thicken slightly, but your lower abdomen hardly swells. These changes are more rapid and noticeable with subsequent pregnancies. Another effect of the pregnancy hormones is to make you more tranquil and sleepy. However, you will also feel tired and lethargic all the time, both through interrupted sleep and the hormonal changes.

The development of the fetus

The first trimester is when the embryo develops rapidly and by the end of 14 weeks since the first day of your last period, the fetus is recognizably human. All the organs, limbs and bones are developed; after this time the fetus only has to grow larger and mature. For this reason, the first trimester is the time when drugs or infections can have a damaging effect on development.

By the end of the first month the fetal heart is

THE BABY'S LIFE SUPPORT

The amniotic space and the placenta make up the baby's life-support system. The placenta can be considered as a blood-filled space. On one side, where it is attached to the uterine wall, it carries oxygen, protein, vitamins and carbohydrates from the mother to the baby. From the baby's side, where it is attached to the baby via the umbilical cord, it carries waste products including carbon dioxide back to the mother. However, despite this central organ, the blood of the fetus and the mother do not mix. The circulations are independent of one another. Some leakage may occur at birth but this is only a problem if there is a blood type (especially Rhesus type) incompatibility.

The umbilical cord is made up of three blood vessels; two for carrying blood to the placenta for cleansing and purification, and one for carrying the oxygenated blood and nutrients to the baby.
The fetus is contained within the membranes and floats in amniotic fluid from about week 4. The fluid protects and supports the baby and takes in its urine.

During the first trimester, the placenta has been growing until it is about the same weight and size as the baby. By week 12, the placenta is the sole organ of the baby's nutrition.

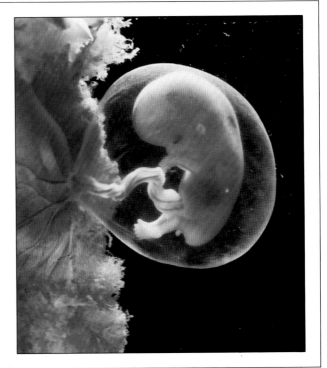

beating. The head, brain and spinal column have started to form and limb buds can be seen. The embryo is still fish-like in that the eyes are prominent. There are no external ears, but the mouth is recognizable and nostrils are present. The lungs are formed, but solid, and the genitals of both sexes have formed.

The end of the first trimester

By now you will notice some weight gain. The wall of the uterus is four times thicker and beginning to soften, so your abdomen will be visibly enlarged. The individual muscle fibers of the uterus increase in length 40 times. (During the second trimester they will stretch and thin out so the uterus rises out of the pelvis.)

Your heart will have increased its output by one third because the volume of circulating blood has increased by about 1.5 liters (3 pints). The extra blood is required by the uterus. All this means the kidneys and heart have to work harder. Fat stores for lactation are built up on your thighs and arms.

Week 8
It will be 8 weeks since the first day of your last period, you should go to your doctor.
You may be suffering from nausea and notice a change in your tastes.

Week 14
You should start to feel better and be thinking about the type of birth you want.
Begin an exercise program and review your diet now the nausea isn't so troubling.
Buy good supporting bras for your heavier breasts.

The fetus is 25mm (1 in) long with all internal organs in place. The heart is now beating frequently. Stomach is formed and limb buds are visible. The jaw is being formed and a face is developing.

The fetus is 75mm (3 in) in length and weighs about 30g (1 oz). It is completely formed. Its growth phase now starts. Your baby's heartbeat can be heard with a fetal stethoscope and gender is distinguishable.

During the second and third trimesters, you will gain weight steadily so that when the baby is born you will weigh between 9 and 13kg (20/28 lbs) more than your pre-pregnant weight. The most rapid weight gain is in the second trimester. The uterus, placenta, baby and increased fluids account for half of this, and that is all lost at the birth.

Our attitude to weight gain has changed markedly in the last ten years. Research has shown that babies born to women who gained more than average were healthier than those who gained less than average. At one time, if you gained more than was thought healthy for your height and frame, you were castigated and told to control your diet and get more exercise. The general rule now is that you should eat well to satisfaction – there are obvious limiting factors with the uterus crowding your stomach anyway – and not eat for two. Weight gain only becomes a risk factor when it is accompanied by a rise in blood pressure and swelling of your hands and feet. It may then be a symptom of pre-eclampsia.

Week 20
You and your partner can feel your baby moving. You are noticeably pregnant and will need to wear loose-fitting, comfortable clothes.
You may notice pigmentation changes besides those on your nipples.
Chloasma will be worse if you expose your face to the sun.

The fetus is approximately 25cm (10in) long and weighs about 340g (¾lbs). The muscular development and the fully formed arms and legs mean you can clearly feel as the baby twists and turns within the amniotic sac. Fine hairy lanugo is found on the back and limbs.

Week 28
As your uterus grows, the skin over your abdomen stretches and you may notice stretchmarks.
You will be feeling tired again and the minor problems of pregnancy such as indigestion, backache and constipation may return after a relatively easy few months.

The baby is 37cm (14 in) long, weighing 900g (2 lbs). Fat is beginning to accumulate and as the lungs are reaching maturity, the baby could survive if born now. Vernix covers the baby's body so it doesn't become soggy in the amniotic fluid.

Emotional changes

As you prepare for the birth, stop working and think about the future, you may find your nesting instinct becomes strong and you set about getting clothes and nursery equipment ready. At the same time there are definite anxieties about the baby and whether it will be healthy and "normal."

During pregnancy, you and your partner will have been attending prenatal classes and become familiar with the procedures for childbirth. You should have found out about the various positions for delivery, pain relief and monitoring techniques used by your medical advisers. Make sure that any points about which you feel strongly are fully explained to the people who will attend you.

> **SEE ALSO:**
>
> LABOR
> PREGNANCY
>   PROBLEMS
> PRENATAL CARE
>
> RHESUS
>   INCOMPATIBILITY
> TOXEMIA OF
>   PREGNANCY

Week 34
The baby should have turned head down by now. If it hasn't, you may be offered external version or be prepared for a breech birth.
If this is your first baby the head will engage in the pelvis ready for delivery and this eases pressure on your diaphragm but increases pain in the pelvic and back region.
Your navel will bulge out.

Week 40
This is known as term. Because the baby fills the uterus, the movements are very strong.
Frequency of urination and tiredness will make you look forward to the birth. The stronger Braxton Hicks contractions may trick you into imagining that every twinge is imminent labor.

The baby is 43cm (17in) long and weighs 2.3kg (5lbs 1 oz); it is getting plumper all the time. The eyes are blue and fingernails reach to the end of the fingers.

The baby will be at its birth weight; the average is 3.4kg (7lbs), although this varies widely. It has increased in weight 600 times since conception. The average length is 51cm (20 in). The vernix only remains in the skin folds of the arms and legs.

CHILDBIRTH

Childbirth is an event like no other in a woman's life. You owe it to yourself, your partner and your baby to read up about it as much as you can, to find out what your options are, decide which ones you would like to adopt and inform your medical advisers of these decisions.

No one knows quite how labor starts but we do know that the baby almost certainly controls it. Just prior to the onset of labor, at a signal from the baby, the placenta produces a hormone which sets labor in motion. The uterus responds by starting to contract regularly and with increasing force. The uterus is primed and ready for action. Throughout your pregnancy it has been having trial runs of weak, short contractions which can be felt by you. These are known as Braxton Hicks contractions. Once labor is fully established, the contractions are strong and regular, about 15–20 minutes apart. They may be painful and last 40 seconds or more.

A normal labor which is allowed to proceed

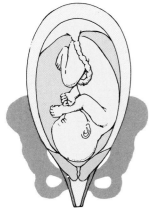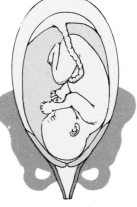

Effacement and dilatation
With uterine contractions, the cervix is slowly stretched to allow the baby to pass through. This occurs gradually so that the muscles of the cervix aren't torn – this would lead to problems in subsequent pregnancies and to prolapse. Contractions in the upper segment of the uterus pull the cervix into the lower segment to eliminate the cervical canal.

without intervention lasts six to 12 hours. Many women find the birth of a second baby easier and smoother, less painful and less exhausting. We know roughly that it takes 150 contractions to expel your first baby; about 75 for the second and 50 for the third and fourth. For about one in ten women, however, labor lasts more than 24 hours. A factor which needs to be taken into account

when considering these figures is that for your first baby you are understandably apprehensive and tense; for subsequent babies you may ignore the early contractions and be more relaxed and less fearful. Fear increases the pain in childbirth. If you relax, a large part of the pain will be controllable.

Major decisions you need to make
There are two main questions you need to ask yourself. Where do I want to have my baby? and What type of labor do I want? The first question relates to whether you want to have the baby at home, in the hospital or in a birth center. The further you get away from hospital, the more informal, friendly and comfortable you will find your childbirth. Home, surrounded by your family, is a relaxed option but it is quite difficult to arrange. It will be more likely for second and subsequent children. Birth centers and small maternity homes retain a lot of the family atmosphere. Hospitals vary according to where you live; large teaching hospitals can be technology-mad, formal and impersonal.

For every woman who wants to have her baby without anesthesia or painkillers, there is one who finds comfort, consolation and reassurance in a high-tech birth with fetal monitoring of the baby and a variety of anesthetics on offer. Doctors and nurses are always there in case of an emergency. On the other hand, natural childbirth is very attractive with you being fully conscious to experience the labor and delivery and in a fit state to take initiative. By being fully informed, you give yourself the best possible chance to avoid fear and tension and enjoy yourself. Natural childbirth does depend on attending the prenatal classes and learning the relaxation techniques.

Whatever you choose, there is no compunction to accept painkillers or monitoring if they are offered and if the pain is worse than you expected, you can opt for painkillers at any moment. Keep an open mind based on your research and feelings.

What is labor?
For the purposes of description, labor is divided into three stages. Before it actually starts, there may be some backache in the lower part of the back. The first sign is usually powerful, regular

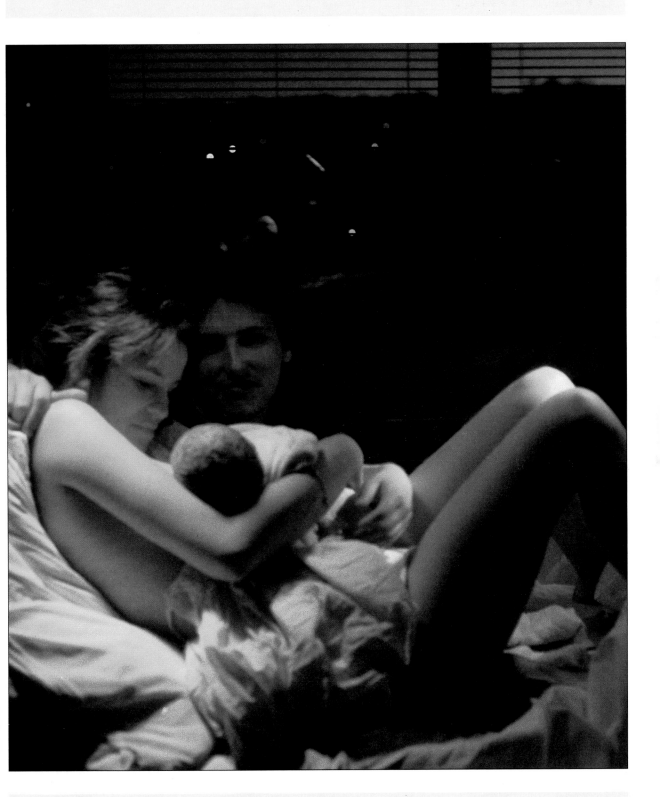

contractions of the uterus or a gush of water as the membranes break. Sometimes this isn't the gush you expect, but a slow leakage or it could be a show of blood stained mucus which is the plug that has blocked the cervix during pregnancy.

The first stage of labor is by far the longest and it continues from the onset to the time when your cervix effaces and dilates to allow the baby's head to pass through the birth canal. The first stage contractions stretch the normally tough, fibrous cervix upwards and outwards and around the baby's head. When the cervical canal is eliminated (effaced), further contractions dilate the cervix to accomodate the widest measurement of the baby's body – the head. This normally takes several hours. It is monitored by the physician or nurse, who measures the dilatation with an internal examination and may comment that you are three fingers or three centimeters dilated. Ten centimeters is full dilatation when only a thin rim of the cervix can be felt.

Transition is between full dilatation and the second stage with the delivery of the baby. During this stage the contractions may be accompanied by shivering, nausea and vomiting. The transition is particularly difficult if you are not fully dilated and yet feel the need to bear down. Breathing techniques and different positions can help overcome this urge until the cervix is fully dilated and the baby can safely pass through without damage to your cervix.

The second stage is the birth of your baby when gradually its head is pushed through the cervix and down the vagina until the head appears at the opening of the vagina. The contractions are now strong but you will use them to bear down and help to push the baby out. At last you are doing something.

In the last five years or so we have learned that the old-fashioned idea of remaining mobile during labor and adopting an upright or semi-upright posture for the birth greatly helps the force of gravity. The first stage occurs more quickly, the birth is quicker and smoother and forceps and episiotomy are rarely needed because the vaginal tissues are given the chance to stretch. The lithotomy position where you are lying on your back is no doubt more convenient for the doctor,

but it is like pushing the baby uphill.

As the baby is born, she tilts her head upwards so that the first part to be delivered is the brow, then the nose, face and chin. The physician will check that the cord is not around the neck and then ask you to bear down again because it is with the next contraction that the baby slithers out.

The third stage is the birth of the placenta.

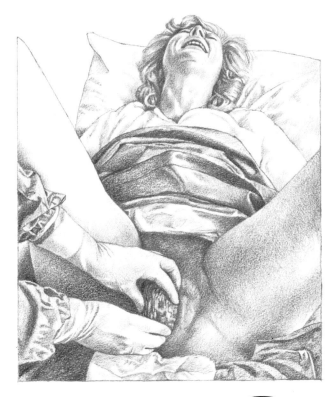

At the crowning of the head, the largest part of the baby, the vaginal tissues are stretched so thin that the nerves are blocked and there is no real pain. The head is born facing downwards but it turns so that the body can be more easily delivered.

This is normally speeded up with an injection of Pitocin in your thigh. The uterus will contract again after about four minutes. To help expulsion of the placenta, the physician may pull gently on the umbilical cord, while pressing your abdomen upwards and backwards. When the placenta enters the vagina, you will again feel the desire to bear down and the placenta will be delivered.

SEE ALSO:

BREECH BIRTH
CERVIX PROBLEMS
EPISIOTOMY
FORCEPS DELIVERY
INDUCTION
LABOR
MULTIPLE PREGNANCY
PERINEAL TEAR
PROLAPSE
VACUUM EXTRACTION

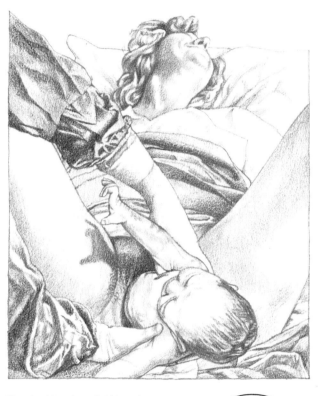

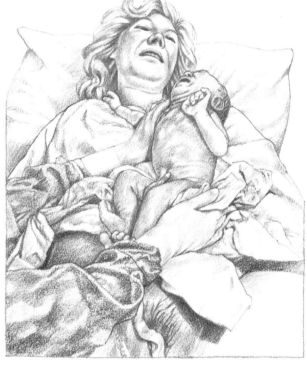

The physician clears fluid from the baby's air passages with a catheter and suction, and then one more contraction is usually enough to deliver the body. The baby may cry out which is a sign that breathing is normal. The baby is then handed to the mother.

There will be a 15-minute delay while the uterus rests before contracting again to expel the placenta. It is important that no part of the placenta is retained in the uterus.

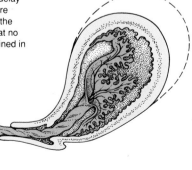

BREASTS AND BREASTFEEDING

Most of us have ambivalent attitudes towards our breasts. On the one hand, we are aware that they are biological equipment for feeding babies, with a strict functional purpose. On the other hand, even as girls growing up, we cannot escape the sexual connotations of the breast in our society and its role as an organ of sexual stimulation.

Factors determining size and shape

Breasts come in all shapes and sizes, and there is no such thing as a normal or average breast, though we are fed images of perfect breasts – models' breasts, film stars' breasts – and consequently we are sometimes made to feel inadequate. Breasts are as much a part of you as your hair color, eye shape and the rest of your body contours, and their size is largely determined by genetic factors and the amount of fatty tissue. It is quite normal for one breast to be slightly larger than the other.

Although your breasts can't be altered except through surgery, they do change throughout your life. They start out as a nipple, projecting from a surrounding ring of pigmented skin called the areola. Then, about two or three years before the onset of menstruation, the fat cells specific to the breast tissue enlarge in response to the sex hormones released during adolescence. During pregnancy, your breasts increase in size as the milk glands prepare for feeding; breastfeeding itself does not bring about these changes. Finally, with age, the supporting ligaments, skin and breast tissue thin and become inelastic and the withdrawal of the female hormones after menopause makes the breasts lose their fat and their uplift.

Breasts also change monthly in response to the menstrual cycle and the action of the female hormones, estrogen and progesterone. Prior to your period, they may have the consistency of orange pips, feeling rather lumpy and solid.

Support

The breasts have only one support. They are slung in a ligament which goes around the breast, both ends being attached to the chest wall. The two muscles that cover the front of the chest and support the loop of ligament are the pectoral muscles, major and minor. If your breasts grow

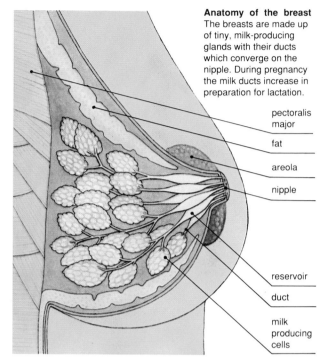

Anatomy of the breast
The breasts are made up of tiny, milk-producing glands with their ducts which converge on the nipple. During pregnancy the milk ducts increase in preparation for lactation.

- pectoralis major
- fat
- areola
- nipple
- reservoir
- duct
- milk producing cells

very large during adolescence or pregnancy, the ligament may be irreparably stretched and the breasts will sag. You can go some way to prevent this by wearing a proper fitting bra while your breasts are growing, and one with support during pregnancy and lactation. In fact, the fashion of going bra-less is deleterious to the shape of any breast except the smallest and lightest, and the best way of looking after your breasts is to wear a good bra. Breasts cannot be made larger by exercise, and your pectorals can't help them to stand up higher on your chest.

The benefits of breastfeeding

All breasts have the capacity to feed a baby, even those with flat and retracted nipples. Anatomically speaking, a breast is simply an overgrown sebaceous gland secreting milk and not sebum. The amount of milk you produce is a response to the amount of milk your baby takes, and therefore the amount he or she needs.

Mother's milk is the perfect food for human babies – it meets all the nutritional requirements for the first four to six months of life. In addition, it contains antibodies and other substances that can protect the infant against harmful viruses and bacteria. Breastfeeding is good for women too. Many women are put off breastfeeding because they think it will spoil their figures - in fact, the changes in the breast happen during pregnancy, not while feeding. The woman who breastfeeds will probably lose more weight and return to her pre-pregnant figure faster than the one who bottle feeds because breastfeeding uses up more than 1000 calories a day and stimulates the hormones that contract your internal organs back into shape. Breastfeeding is also ideal for promoting bonding, that close attachment between mother and child.

Breast milk can be your baby's only nourishment until he or she is four to six months old. After this time, mixed foods are essential for continued healthy growth and development. Even when you are weaning your baby, however, you can mix the food with expressed breast milk.

How to breastfeed
Successful breastfeeding depends on you feeling comfortable in yourself and your surroundings. There is no point in feeding your baby if you hate every minute of it, or are only doing it because you feel you should. To care for your breasts, wash them in water only several times a day. Moisturize them with baby lotion or put a dab of lotion, olive or peanut oil on your breast pad to keep your skin

supple. This will act as an emollient. Surround yourself with everything you need and support yourself or the baby with pillows so there is no strain on your shoulders or back.

SEE ALSO

BENIGN BREAST DISEASE
BREAST CANCER
BREASTFEEDING PROBLEMS

BREAST OPERATIONS
BREAST SELF-EXAMINATION
NIPPLE PROBLEMS

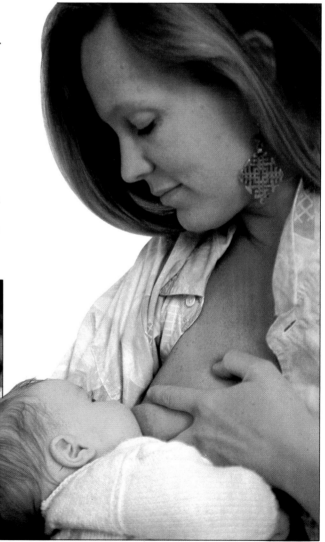

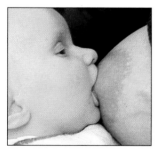

Successful breastfeeding
The baby is only feeding properly if the whole of the nipple is in her mouth and her tongue is underneath the nipple. When the feed is finished, don't pull your nipple away; break the suction with your finger to ease the baby off.

NUTRITION

There is no question that we are what we eat. Good nutrition is the key to general fitness and health. What constitutes a healthy and protective diet? Primarily, cutting down on saturated fats. Fat gives us concentrated energy and any we don't use gets stored in our bodies, making us overweight. Fat is linked to heart disease because it raises levels of cholesterol in the blood, clogging the arteries, leading to heart attacks.

Sugar and salt are the other two problems. Sugar provides only empty calories which give energy but nothing else. It also promotes tooth decay. As sugar provides no nutrients, it should be easy to cut it out, but many of us are hooked on the stuff because we have developed a sweet tooth, either in childhood or from eating commercial junk foods which have sugar in them to make them more appealing. Fructose, glucose and dextrose are all forms of sugar and are not necessary to our diets.

Salt is added to most commercial foods and most cooks add it in varying amounts when cooking. We do need salt to help maintain fluid levels in our bodies but nothing like the amount we consume. Some people will suffer high blood pressure because they eat too much salt but there is no way of knowing which people, so it's best to be spare with salt when cooking, and to avoid putting mountains of it on your plate while eating. Sea salt crystals have some minerals which iodized salt doesn't have, but it is still salt.

Even armed with basic information, many women find it difficult to change their eating habits, because it means a change of lifestyle. But poor diet affects women more than men because of changes in hormone levels throughout life. For example, extra calcium is needed to prepare for the post-menopause years when the reduction of estrogen weakens bones.

Nutrition plan

The way to start is to familiarize yourself with the right foods and choose a program you can cope with. Like dieting, if the plan is unrealistic from the start, willpower may not be enough. Accept your personality; some people love food and eating, others can't be bothered, but they are expected to prepare food daily and enjoy the accla-

mation when family or friends comment on it. You don't have to do everything at once; choose one or two points and start with them so that you ease yourself into the new program.

Don't
◆ eat lots of meat
◆ use salty commercially processed food
◆ add salt when you're cooking
◆ buy sugar and sugar-laden foods
◆ fry your food
◆ use cream

Do
◆ start to read the labels on prepared foods
◆ look out for additives such as salt, sugar, etc.
◆ choose and prepare wholewheat products - bread, pasta, cakes
◆ eat potatoes in their skins
◆ cook with brown rice
◆ learn to cook with legumes and whole grains
◆ make sure your diet contains a lot of fresh food that requires no cooking or preparation

Snacks

Many of us don't eat three square meals a day any longer and snack instead. Look at your snacks, are they cookies and processed food? If they are, substitute with fresh fruit and vegetables, dried fruit, broiled food, salads, low fat cheese, yogurt, and wholemeal bread without butter.

Additives

These are put into food to increase its attractiveness, taste and shelf life. Don't get obsessive about additives; there is no evidence to suggest that you should eat none at all.

Nutrients may be added to food. For example, margarine has added Vitamin A and D. This is good news since Vitamin D helps in the absorption of calcium. Added calcium to milk and the availability of milk with lower fat content means that there is now no reason for calcium deficiency.

Main constituents of our diet

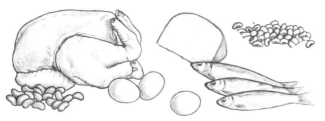

Proteins are the structural material of our bodies. We need protein throughout our lives; children need protein for growth and adults need it for repair and replacement. Few people in the western world eat too little protein, and as any excess is used as energy or converted into fat, this can lead to an increase in weight.

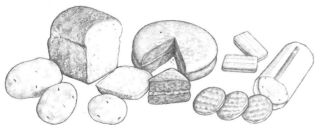

Carbohydrates are divided into two groups; the sugars and the starches. Foods containing unrefined carbohydrate, such as potatoes and wholewheat products, are rich in essential nutrients, including fiber, and give us energy at the same time. Sugars and refined carbohydrate, such as cakes, give us only energy, so overeating these and a sedentary lifestyle will cause obesity.

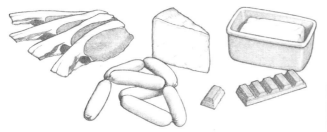

Fats are essential to a healthy body as fuel and for building body components but again we eat too much. They are divided into two groups. Saturated fats are the ones we need to cut down on. These are contained in animal fat – meat, cream, butter and cheese – and in some vegetable products such as coconut oil and, of course, any dishes made with these ingredients. Saturated fats tend to increase the level of cholesterol in our blood and this is a factor in heart disease. The other group is the polyunsaturated fats which are necessary for the repair of body cells. This group reduces cholesterol levels slightly. These are contained in vegetable oils, nuts and oily fish. A good way of differentiating is to avoid those fats that turn solid when cold and oils from tropical countries (i.e. palm, coconut).

Vitamins are chemicals that help to regulate our body's internal chemical system. Most of us obtain sufficient amounts in our daily diet. Deficiencies tend to occur only during times of ill health or changes in our metabolism, such as during pregnancy. Claims are made about using vitamins for treatment, such as reducing the severity of the symptoms of premenstrual syndrome and the common cold. Although none of these has received wholehearted backing from the medical profession, folic acid, one of the complex B vitamins, has been given in higher doses to women who have previously had a baby with brain or neural tube defects such as spina bifida.

Minerals are essential to our metabolism in quite small amounts. Most of us get quite enough from a balanced diet. Any deficiencies are usually only a problem if, because of some intestinal disorder, we fail to absorb the mineral properly.

Many women are unaware of the basics of good nutrition, or they may follow the correct road with their children, but ignore guidelines themselves, making them vulnerable to illnesses such as diverticular disease (caused by lack of fiber), and anemia (caused by lack of iron).

SEE ALSO:

ACNE
ANEMIA
DENTAL PROBLEMS
DIGESTIVE
 PROBLEMS
HEART DISEASE
HYPERTENSION

OBESITY
PREGNANCY
 PROBLEMS
PREMENSTRUAL
 SYNDROME

DIET

So much has been spoken and written about good eating and a balanced diet that many people are turned off because they feel it is too mammoth a task to change their lifestyles and what they eat. Others feel you have to be really radical, but this is simply not true. All you need to do is to make small changes to your diet to achieve substantial changes to your health. None of the changes is very difficult, and you don't have to be obsessive about it. It is better if you don't eat a lot of saturated fats – butter and cream – or sugar or salt. But you don't have to exclude these foods all of the time. My own working rule is that if you do the right thing 80% of the time, the other 20% won't matter too much.

Vegetarianism

Many people are turning to vegetarian diets; some exclude all animal products, even dairy products and eggs. A vegetarian diet of any kind is a healthy option but requires eating a wide variety of foods. The vital factor is to combine the vegetables with grains so that the complete protein is made up. (Animal protein contains the correct number of essential amino acids to make a complete protein; vegetable protein does not.)

Milk is a major source of vitamins and minerals so everyone on a vegetarian diet should include skimmed milk (all the goodness with none of the fat) and a great variety of plant foods – nuts, lentils, legumes, grains. If you are a vegan and therefore taking in no animal products at all, you should supplement your diet with Vitamin B_{12} which is not found in great quantity in vegetable products. Also calcium, iron and Vitamin C might be in short supply. One good sensible rule is that there is no such thing as an essential food – there is always an alternative.

Supplements

Do we need to take minerals or vitamins in a supplement or tablet form? In the western world, it is generally supposed that no one eating a balanced diet should be short of minerals and vitamins. The problem, however, is that there are certain sections of the population who are not eating a balanced diet. The main groups of women who may find they need supplementation are teenage girls who eat irregularly and the wrong foods, any woman on a diet not prescribed by a doctor and any woman who is post-menopausal or pregnant.

Times for careful eating

These are times in a woman's life when she needs to take care of her diet. During adolescence the rate of growth in a girl is second only to that in infancy. Her growth spurt usually begins and ends earlier than in boys, but it is not possible to predict when it will happen.

The greatest influence on a teenager's diet is her peer group. It is more difficult to have control over an adolescent's choice of foods the way parents can when children are younger. Eating also becomes part of a social activity and family meals assume less importance. Most teenage girls are very concerned about their shape and weight and as many as one girl in ten may try to control her weight by some means. This usually involves excluding nutritious foods such as bread, cereal and protein and filling up on empty calories – junk food in the form of snacks and soft drinks.

In pregnancy, your body is providing nutrition for both you and your baby. There are foodstuffs that you may not be able to tolerate, particularly during the first four months. This is an important time for the baby and you need to eat well when you feel like it. The best idea is to snack often with healthy foods. That way you won't feel uncomfortable and you'll be well fed. Your medical advisers will suggest supplements with folic acid, iron and calcium if this is necessary. Don't take supplements unless your doctor advises.

One of the major problems for post-menopausal women is osteoporosis which is the loss of protein from bones. Research has shown that osteoporosis can be halted (not cured) by having hormone therapy. This doesn't mean that every woman needs hormone therapy, but if you get aches and pains in your bones and muscles, backache and pins and needles in your hands and feet, go to your doctor to ask for a diagnosis. If your bones are beginning to look thin on X-ray, your doctor should consider hormone therapy.

A balanced diet

So what is this balanced diet? It is taking food from

GETTING FIBER INTO YOUR DIET

Progress in food technology in the past has tended towards refining foods to take out the roughage. We now know that this is not the correct approach. You should make a conscious effort to include unrefined products, and fruit and vegetables in your diet so that you digest your food properly and your body eliminates waste efficiently.

Casseroles and stews
Red meat can be replaced by vegetables in sauce.

Pasta
Commercial brands now include wholewheat pastas in all shapes.

Salads
Fresh raw vegetables and fruits should be the major source of fiber in your diet.

Brown rice
The fibrous outer coating is not removed and so supplies plenty of fiber and flavor.

Potatoes
Cooked in their skins, these versatile vegetables provide a nutritious package.

Bread
Wholewheat flour combined with other grains make this a tasty dietary staple.

Pastry
Wholewheat pastries and cakes are a nutritious treat, especially if the sugar content is reduced by the substitution of dried fruits.

as many different sources as possible and eating food in its natural state – that is fresh, unprocessed and, where possible, raw. The problems in our Western diet center on our concentration on foods which narrow down the spectrum of our diet and contain many foods that are unhealthy. Too many processed foods – prepacked, precooked, junk food, fast food – contain too much animal fat, salt, additives and too little fiber. The food companies are now coming under pressure to reduce the salt, sugar and additives in their products. This is easier to monitor with improvements in labelling.

Our methods of cooking are also hazardous to health. Frying is a common method of preparing food, adding butter to vegetables is almost a ritual, sauces are progressively richer and creamier. So changing to broiling food instead of frying, limiting butter on vegetables and reducing sauces instead of thickening them with butter, cream or flour would lead immediately to healthier eating.

If you feel that you need the discipline of a diet program, look at it carefully: Is it too expensive?

Will it fit in with your family meals? There is no point in preparing two meals and watching the others eat your favorite foods. Is the diet balanced nutritionally? Stay clear of diets that confine you to one or two foods. Nobody is meant to survive on a limited number of foodstuffs and it could throw your metabolism awry. Do you like the foods that are permitted in the diet? Are there any indulgences? You know yourself. Do you want to stretch your willpower to the limit or adopt a more flexible attitude? Your responses to these questions should help you organize a plan for reducing your weight by yourself.

SEE ALSO:

ANOREXIA NERVOSA
BULIMIA
HORMONE
  REPLACEMENT
  THERAPY
PREGNANCY
  PROBLEMS
OBESITY
OSTEOPOROSIS

NUTRIENT	SOURCES	WHY IT IS NEEDED
Protein	Red and white meat, dairy products, legumes and lentils, seeds and nuts.	Maintains and supports all body growth.
Iron	Red meat, liver, egg yolk, dried fruits such as apricots, raisins, dried legumes and spinach.	With protein, it forms hemoglobin to carry oxygen through the body. Vitamin C taken simultaneously helps absorption; tannin and antacid medication limit absorption. Deficiency causes anemia resulting in fatigue.
Calcium	Dairy products, whole fish (sardines), sunflower and sesame seeds.	With other minerals, and Vitamin D, helps strengthen teeth and bones.
Vitamin A (retinol)	Carrots, margarine, fortified dairy products, liver, green vegetables.	Important to health of mucous membranes and resistance to infection.
Vitamin B1 (thiamine)	Wheat germ, liver, whole grains, nuts.	Aids digestion and utilization of energy.
Vitamin B2 (riboflavin)	Milk, yogurt, cottage cheese, liver, whole grains, green vegetables.	Promotes health of skin and eyes.
Vitamin B3 (niacin)	Oily fish, whole grains, liver, fortified breakfast cereals, peanuts.	Aids digestion and normal appetite needs.
Vitamin B6 (pyridoxine)	Meat, bananas, dried vegetables, molasses, brewer's yeast, whole grains.	Helps to regulate your body's use of fatty acids to fight infection.
Vitamin B12 (cyanocobalamin)	Milk, eggs, meat, dairy foods.	Essential for maintenance of red blood cells and nervous system. No vegetable source sufficient for daily needs. Vegans should see their doctor about synthetic forms.
Folic acid (folacin)	Green leafy vegetables, nuts, dried vegetables, whole grains.	Essential for blood formation. Vital during pregnancy as lack leads to higher incidence of neural tube defects in babies.
Vitamin C (ascorbic acid)	Broccoli, oranges and most citrus fruits, red, green and yellow vegetables.	Increases resistance to infection, blood coagulation and iron absorption. More required during illness.
Vitamin D	Fortified milk, oily fish, liver, sunshine on your skin, eggs, butter.	Helps in absorption of calcium and builds calcium and phosphorus into bones and strengthens them.
Vitamin E	Vegetable oil, green leafy vegetables, wheat germ, egg yolk, whole grains.	Protects fatty acids from destruction.
Phosphorus	Milk products, meat, fish, whole grains, beans.	Combines with calcium to strengthen bones and teeth.
Iodine	Seafoods, fortified salt.	Regulates energy use in body.
Zinc	Lean meat, seafood, whole grains and dried beans.	Makes up some enzymes and releases Vitamin A from liver.

EXERCISE

To be healthy and fit you need to exercise as well as eat the right foods. Exercise keeps you supple and strong, helps to improve the efficiency of your heart, lungs and other vital organs. It helps to counteract fatigue and stress and will help you to sleep. Exercise builds stamina, so the more you do, the more you are able to do.

In the past, women were normally discouraged from exercising too much. These days, some form of exercise is a regular part of most women's lives. Enthusiasts rhapsodize about exercise and if you've never tried, you may be irritated and bored by this. Even if you know why you should exercise, you may still be reluctant to do so. The important thing therefore is to find some exercise that suits you. Don't underestimate the amount of exercise you, as a woman, already take running up and down stairs, cleaning the house, rushing to work and around the supermarket. As long as you're not lazy, you probably are getting quite a bit of exercise. Although exercise in the form of a sport or leisure activity should be part of your life and that of your children from the earliest age, it is never too late to start.

Benefits of exercise
Different types of exercise affect the body in different ways: some improve muscular strength; some improve physical endurance; some improve flexibility; and some improve the efficiency of your respiratory and cardiovascular systems.

After energetic exercise, the blood sugar is high and appetite is depressed, so you won't feel hungry. If you exercise vigorously for more than 30 minutes, your body begins to produce its own morphine-like substances, endorphins, and this makes you experience a "high." You will feel tranquil, satisfied with yourself and pleasantly happy. The calming after-effects can last for several hours, and that's better than taking Valium! Regular exercise usually leads to a reduction in blood pressure. It also is thought to help protect against atherosclerosis and heart attacks.

Exercising muscles and skeleton
Muscles help us to maintain posture and give us a range of movements encompassing voluntary actions as well as instinctive reflexes. They should be exercised to keep up our strength, stamina and fitness. The muscular system in the body requires the most fuel to keep it going which is why a manual laborer needs twice as many calories a day as an office worker. For women, certain areas of our bodies require more attention. These are the muscles affected by childbirth – the pelvic floor muscles and the abdominal muscles – and those areas that we feel uncomfortable about because our body shape isn't what we want it to be, such as the upper arms, thighs and pectorals. However, vigorous work with a muscle or group of muscles, even for a short time, leads to an increase in its size and strength, and improves your shape. As well as the muscle strengthening, the effort uses up calories which, accompanied by a sensible diet, will help you to lose weight.

Starting an exercise program
Most of us start an exercise program because we take up a new sport or we feel unhealthy or overweight. Unfortunately fat is difficult to take off selectively, because it tends to be taken off the last place it was deposited.

When you start to exercise, be careful. If you lead a sedentary lifestyle, don't start off suddenly on a strenuous exercise program. Our lifestyle almost ensures we won't get enough exercise to be healthy – cars, television and automation in the home and at work. Consult your doctor to see how fit you are. If you're overweight, or have recently had surgery or been ill, you'll need to start gently and carefully. A history of asthma, bronchitis, back pain, arthritis, high blood pressure or heart disease means that medical advice should be taken before you start.

Good exercise is not painful. Muscles do need to be stretched and conditioned and they should never be made to burn or ache. To prevent injury, warm up before you start and cool down afterwards. Stop exercising immediately if you feel breathless, dizzy or in any kind of pain. Using stairs instead of elevators and taking a brisk walk every day is a good way to begin. If you want to take up a sport, do you want a solitary activity such as jogging, or a sociable sport such as golf or tennis? Make sure you have the right shoes whatever you decide to do. A slow game of tennis can be just as enjoyable before your fitness improves because of the social aspect. Swimming is probably the best all-round exercise for women. It exercises all the muscles in the body, is good for joints and can be done at your own pace. Because you are supported in the water and are working against water resistance instead of gravity, you appear to take less effort and there is little risk of injury.

However, as a general rule for women after the age of 35, the best sports are those taken upright, such as cycling, horseback riding and tennis, although jogging, for example, is not a very good activity, especially after the menopause when there may be some thinning of the bones. The hammering of your feet on the ground can cause joint problems in the legs and spine. If you decide to join an exercise class or something similar, make sure the instructor is qualified to teach, and not just an enthusiastic amateur.

Now that exercise and fitness have a higher priority in our lives, you may come across technical terms or approaches that tend to make your jogging or sit-ups program sound like a scientific experiment. Here are some definitions of the theory and practice of certain types of exercise.

Aerobic Exercise

These exercises raise your heart rate significantly, thereby increasing the demands of your body for oxygen. Regular exercise of this sort improves your heart muscle and your respiratory system, increasing their efficiency. The type of exercises in this category are jogging, walking briskly, cycling or dancing. To help realize how your heart is coping, you need to be able to take your pulse before, during and after the exercises. These exercises aren't the sort you would do to get rid of a tummy bulge or fat on your thighs, although obviously calories are used up and therefore your weight stays under control, depending on the sort of food you eat.

Isometric exercise

This is a still form of exercise in which one group of muscles acts against another group or a fixed object, usually weights. This increases the strength and improves the tone of your muscles.

HOW FIT AND FLEXIBLE ARE YOU?

Many women think that because they are naturally slim, they are fit. This is not the same thing at all. Specific types of exercise, such as those to improve suppleness or stamina, may be what you really need. To give yourself some indication of whether you need to take a more positive view about an exercise program, ask yourself these questions. If the answers are mostly in the affirmative, then you need to do something soon to improve your stamina and flexibility.

▲ Are you out of breath after walking up three flights of stairs, or up a steep hill, or after running for the bus?
▲ Do your legs ache after climbing three flights of stairs?
▲ Do you have to haul yourself out of the bath?
▲ Do you find it difficult bending down to pick something up or to secure your shoelaces?

The exertion, however, needs to be great which means this form of exercise raises blood pressure abruptly.

Isotonic exercise

This is exercise with movement and includes weight training and calisthenics. It is a more fluid method of exercising combining the rhythmic, reptitious movements of calisthenics and the body working against its own weight or external weights – a simple exercise is clenching your hands to exercise the pectoral muscles. This system increases muscle strength, size and endurance and is good for women whose muscle tone is poor, particularly around the stomach and back.

Isokinetic exercise

This is a mixture of isotonic and isometric exercise and is the sort of exercises you do in a specially equipped Nautilus gym. You should combine this with aerobic exercises to warm you up and cool you down.

SEE ALSO:

BACKACHE   HEART DISEASE
FITNESS TESTING   SPORT INJURIES

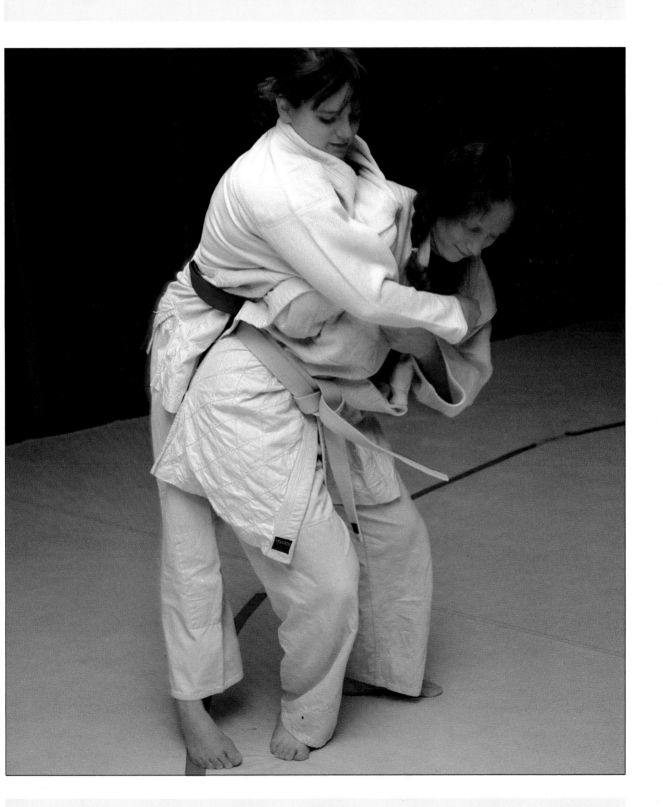

SLEEPING

When you are asleep, your heart rate slows down, your temperature drops and your digestive functions almost stop. However, your muscles keep contracting every now and then and you may move about more than you think. Babies need at least 16 hours of sleep a day on average but by the time we are into childhood, seven or eight hours a night is enough. It isn't really for our bodies that we sleep; it is the brain that needs recharging. The adrenal gland secretes a hormone, cortisol, and the levels of this hormone in the blood relate to periods of wakefulness and sleep.

Dreaming is an essential part of sleep; dreams manufacture chemicals needed for intellectual functioning. Dreaming takes place at least four times a night during quite light sleep. This coincides with REM - rapid eye movement. However, if you take barbiturates, you are less likely to dream and may awake exhausted even though you have slept for eight hours.

Insomnia

Women seem to suffer from insomnia more than men. Maybe this is because most women find that their agenda of life, children, work, housekeeping, continues on into the night after they have gone to bed. They cannot stop their minds working, remembering things that they ought to have done, things that they have forgotten and that they have to do tomorrow.

At particular points in a woman's life, insomnia is quite a common feature. For instance, one of the first effects of becoming pregnant is fatigue and, paradoxically, the inability to sleep when you lie down at night. Waking in the early hours of the morning is also common in pregnant women, and towards the end of pregnancy you may become an insomniac because you simply cannot find a comfortable position to lie in. In the first two thirds of pregnancy, the reason for insomnia is that the baby's metabolism does not shut down at night but yours does. The baby continues to grow, develop and feed all the 24 hours.

Certain emotions will certainly preclude sleep. The worst is resentment. If you reverberate about an incident that occurred during the day in which you felt you were treated unfairly, or make a choice of words which you wish you had said at the time, then there is no chance of sleeping. Resentment raises the blood pressure and the pulse rate and this is exactly the opposite of what has to happen before you can go to sleep. It follows from this that there are certain parts of your body on which you should concentrate in order to get to sleep. Sleep will come more easily if your pulse rate is slow and your blood pressure is down. This can be helped by lying fairly still and controlling your movements by taking deep slow breaths and concentrating on the process of breathing. The slower you can make your breathing, the nearer you are to sleep and the slower your pulse rate will be. To help you to do this, you can concentrate on relaxing various parts of your body.

Start with your forehead and relax a frown, relax the muscles of the jaw, chin and neck. Make your arms feel limp. Become aware of the pressure of your torso lying on the bed and then gradually down your legs until they are completely relaxed, including your toes. Many people find this process so soporific that they are asleep before they get to their feet.

Another trick is to empty your mind and think about a favorite thing. Mine is black velvet. Every time another thought creeps in, concentrate on the favorite thing again. This is an almost infallible cure for going without sleep.

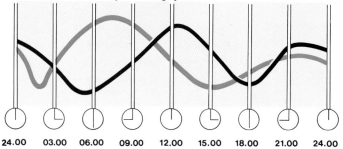

Cortisol levels
These are usually lowest at around 2am. Different peaks and troughs account for "morning" or "evening" people. The colored band represents a woman with high levels in the morning. The black band represents the other woman who finds it hard to wake up but is alert in the evening.

24.00 03.00 06.00 09.00 12.00 15.00 18.00 21.00 24.00

SEE ALSO:

DRUG DEPENDENCY
FATIGUE
INSOMNIA
PREGNANCY
 PROBLEMS

GETTING ON IN A "MAN'S" WORLD

Besides the emotional crises of youth with the problems of school exams and coping with your sexual experiences, and the emotional upheavals in later life of possibly divorce and, more certainly, bereavement and the empty nest syndrome, there are added stresses for women today. Very often we find ourselves in an unequal position with men in a society that is itself unequal. This can be extremely difficult and frustrating to live with, especially when obvious inequalities persist in our society.

The feminist movement has achieved much in raising consciousness about the inequality between men and women. However, sexism is still everywhere – in advertisements, the media and at work. The latter is one of the most difficult to deal with as men are often given preference for promotion. Sexism at work is, however, breaking down, with the laws allowing maternity leave and the continuing battle for equal pay for equal work. More women are becoming managers and supervisors. If a woman wants to succeed and is prepared to meet the challenge, then she can surely achieve her ambitions; the basis for all the arguments should be that you are treated fairly as a person and not because of your gender.

Some women feel hopeless and helpless at having to make their way in a man's world. This system is not going to go away overnight but it is changing slowly. What women are uniquely gifted and empowered to do is to manage the system to suit them. Workplace day-care facilities and flexible hours or work-sharing are slowly being established in the business world.

How to set realistic goals
Whether you are determined to succeed because of a personal life plan or you are like the majority of us, working to support yourself and your family, it is important that you realize that perhaps it is not possible for you to control your world completely. One of the greatest causes of unhappiness and mental ill health is the disparity between expectation and achievement, between make believe and reality, between hope and the actual result. Setting realistic goals lessens stress. You will only find real happiness and satisfaction in your work if you come to terms with reality.

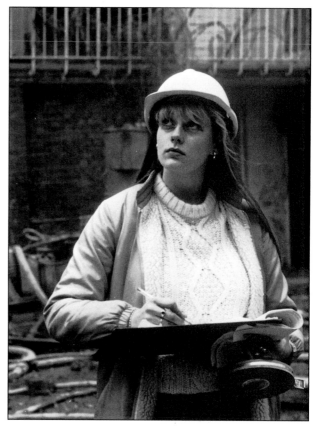

Other women can be very supportive, particularly those women who have experienced what you are going through. You may find support from groups in your area such as working mothers groups and projects for establishing professional standards in day-care. Many problems result from mismanagement of time such as getting behind in your work, or things that need doing for the family or the house. Give all your tasks priorities and do the important ones first. Write down all your activities, their relevance and how they can help to sort out your problem. It will be quite a lesson to realize just how much time you have wasted and how much you have put to a useful purpose.

SEE ALSO:	
ANXIETY	FATIGUE
DEPRESSION	MOOD CHANGES

MENTAL FITNESS

The greatest obstacle to mental fitness is stress. Today women are suffering from stress more than ever before. Stress is not all bad of course. Up to a point it increases our productivity and efficiency. Beyond a certain point, these advantages are outweighed and can lead to insomnia, illness, neuroses and an inability to cope. One of the sad things about our lives is that the inability to cope is seen as a failure; a disease that has been medicalized, hence the millions of prescriptions every year for minor tranquilizers.

Avoiding or managing stress is not easy. Although diet and exercise are rightly at the top of our health priorities, mental health is not grouped in with these and ways of improving it and increasing mental fitness are not openly discussed. Women can be subjected much more to mental pressures than men. We are more prone to psychological disturbances because of the activity of our hormones and also because we live longer and consequently suffer more bereavement and loneliness. Also, women sometimes do not have as much choice as men so they find themselves frustrated by marriage, or career, or financial insecurity and are unable to do anything about it. Even if you manage to escape this trap, you may suffer from guilt because you're trying to bring up children while keeping your career alive.

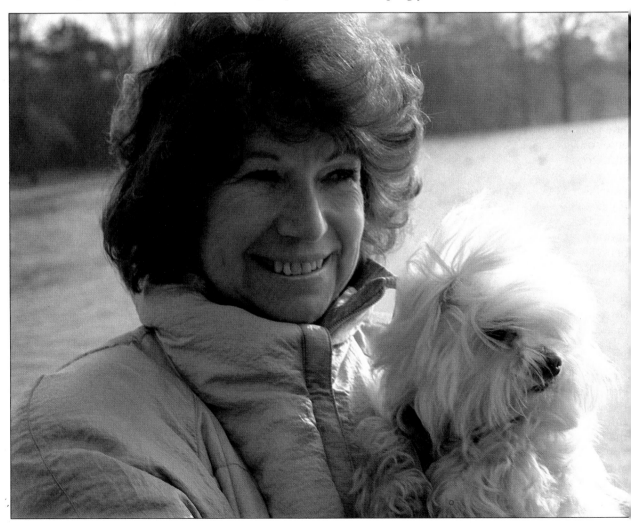

To keep ourselves mentally fit requires realism. While maintaining emotional growth, we still need to see that conflict is normal and certain conditions will always increase problems. Poverty, divorce, bereavement, ill health – all these things will obviously cause mental strain. Coming to terms with the conditions that affect our mental well-being is part of the way to ensure we are mentally fit. This doesn't mean you shrug everything off; that would be foolish. It does mean coming to terms with things. Look at yourself and accept yourself for what you are; if you set your standards too high, for example, you are bound to be disappointed at some time. Even the unpredictable catastrophes can be dealt with if you accept help and know where to find it.

What is good mental fitness?

You need not resort to Valium or any other medication if you learn to manage your personality. It can be done, though you have to be determined and make some effort. You may even need help. You will need to be realistic and keep a correct emotional balance so that you don't overreact to situations or circumstances. Nothing is hopeless and if you have good friendships and support in your family, any problem can be solved – in time. If you can't decide whether you have a sensible attitude to life and its vagaries, talk to someone about your responses. Do you always put the blame elsewhere? Do you feel self-pity when there is no occasion to?

One technique you might try to achieve mental fitness is, in calmer moments, to write down the sorts of things that make you feel stressed or insecure and then consider ways to prepare yourself for them or to manage them. If the time when you all get home at night is chaos, organize the routine carefully so everyone knows what is expected of them and your responsibilities are reduced. Even simple breathing exercises are calming. Ten deep, slow breaths help me reduce the feelings of panic. An extension of this would be yoga which gives an overall calming effect that aids tranquillity. Meditation can have the same effect. You should go to a qualified teacher in either of these disciplines to get the best results. They can take a year or more to study and perfect.

Relaxation

Psychological fitness is only possible if you can relax. After exercising, you'll probably feel tranquil and calm; so physical exercise is an important step towards achieving mental relaxation.

Irritation and aggression will be dissipated if you can achieve some measure of relaxation. The simplest is to lie down and rest your body. In this position, you then rest your mind by clearing it of worries and stressful thoughts. Complete relaxation is only possible when you are freed of your thoughts – as with meditation techniques.

RELAXATION TECHNIQUES

1. Let the thoughts flow freely through your head.
2. If a thought recurs, stop it by saying "no" under your breath.
3. Imagine a calm scene. Blue is a relaxing color, so try a clear blue sky and calm sea.
4. Become aware of your breathing and that it is slow and natural. Follow each breath as you inhale and exhale.
5. You may find it helpful to repeat a soothing word such as "love," "peace" or "breath." Think of this word or sound silently in your mind.
6. Remind yourself to keep the muscles of your face, eyes and forehead cool and relaxed.

Biofeedback is a more mechanical means of inducing relaxation. By use of a machine you read various physiological signs such as pulse rate, finger temperature or muscle tightness. Such readings help you learn to reverse these messages of stress – which you can combat by making a drink, or calling a friend, or writing down possible solutions to the problem. When the crisis is over, think about what happened and what it felt like to bring the crisis down. Very soon you may be able to calm yourself without going through the whole procedure; you just have to remember that you have calmed yourself once before and you can do it again. This is a means of imposing your mind over your body.

SEE ALSO:

ANXIETY	INSOMNIA
DEPRESSION	MOOD CHANGES
FATIGUE	

FACING CRISES

Many domestic crises have very serious effects on women. Bereavement, especially of a partner or child, is one of the greatest stresses for either sex to suffer. Divorce also means a tremendous upheaval. Children leaving home and becoming independent can leave a woman feeling isolated and unneeded.

Divorce

Since 1940, when one in five marriages ended in divorce, the divorce rate has soared. According to the U.S. Census Bureau, one out of every two couples married in the 1970's ends up divorcing. While divorce is always traumatic, many women are now taking the view that it makes a change in lifestyle possible. This feeling perhaps emanates from the reconsideration of marriage by many women, who expect a lot more of marriage than they used to, and rightly so. Modern marriages fraught with modern stresses can require a great deal of work and compromise.

One of the major aspects of marriage break-up is that middle and old age are longer than they used to be. For some couples the post-parenthood phase, if it hasn't been anticipated and planned for, can be traumatic, especially if the couple feel their interests are diverging. If you are to spend 20 years as a couple after the children have gone, you need to explore new areas to extend yourselves and fulfill the promises of your early life together without getting on one another's nerves.

Emotional upsets are unavoidable after divorce but several things may help you back to normality. Try to resume a social life as soon as you can. Join clubs, participate in outings and, if friends polarize with the split up, be understanding and accept that you won't be seeing some people much.

Remember you are not unique; there are lots of people who have gone through a similar experience. Life must go on and it could get a lot better. Don't start searching for a lost youth and allow your fantasies to supplant reality. Be astute and calm about assessing your future life and seek guidance, or talk to someone, rather than do all this on your own. Remember you can probably live quite happily with a few friends helping you.

Ensure the happiness and security of the children before that of yourself or your partner. Don't let yourself or your children become the victim of divorce. Rather think of yourself as a survivor. If you look at the divorce through your children's eyes, you may be better able to help them cope with their own problems like facing friends and trying to understand your emotional conflicts. Your children may be suffering pangs of guilt and believe it to be their fault that the marriage broke up. Reassure them that this is not so. It is comforting to know that most children feel that it is better for warring parents to split up than for them to stay together for the sake of the children. Explain to them that, while it may feel like the end of the world, it will be very much better in the long term.

Widowhood

More than half of the women in the U.S. population over the age of 65 have been widowed. You will find it very difficult in the early stages to come to terms with widowhood, so deep is your grief, but understanding the stages you are likely to go through may help.

You will certainly feel numb for the first terrible days. This is helpful because it enables you to get through the funeral and the family gathering and deal with the financial matters. Sometime later you may become depressed as you perceive the emptiness in your life. If anxiety about the future accompanies your depression, you may experience the physical symptoms of colitis, gastric problems and mental upset. These physical symptoms of bereavement may then lead you to take more alcohol or seek tranquilizers and drugs to combat the insomnia, agitation and tearfulness. This state of depression may last six to nine months. It does go, so it is important that you try to battle with it. The next phase is the acceptance when you start making positive plans for the future. Be assured that you will triumph over despair.

There are ways you can help yourself after bereavement. You may find out more about yourself and your reactions, and about the important question of how strong you are without your partner.

Expect to be confused and to experience emotions such as shock, disbelief, denial, rage – these are all normal and healthy. Don't put mourning aside. It lasts for different times for different people but you must go through it – indeed we all go through it at some time. In addition you must

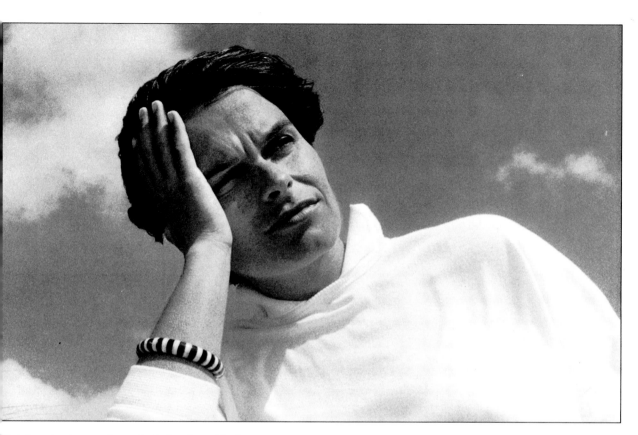

finish grieving and not indulge in self-pity so you can get on with life.

Set a time limit on how long you are going to allow your initial grieving period to continue. A minimum of 6 to 12 weeks seems realistic but you should try not to go beyond that. Welcome friends and relatives who are keen to help and support you. Accept invitations to visit but don't stay too long. Be prepared to push yourself to go out and meet new people to avoid loneliness.

If you become severely depressed, seek medical help. Your doctor will supervise the anti-depressant therapy and should you contemplate suicide, contact someone immediately.

Empty nest syndrome

When the children grow up and leave home, you are bound to feel the silence even if you are involved in a full working life of your own. The house is empty, and it feels like nobody needs you anymore. The best way to protect yourself from feelings of loneliness and isolation is to plan ahead. You can work out a loose timetable that allows you to fill any spare time. It is not fair to allow this syndrome to creep up on you without doing anything about it. If you don't work, you could retrain or go back to your old career. Take up new hobbies or travel or even move to a smaller house for your retirement.

This syndrome normally occurs about the time of menopause and may be accompanied by feelings of insecurity and inadequacy. Planning for the rest of your life with your partner will help you to overcome any symptoms.

SEE ALSO:

ALCOHOLISM	INSOMNIA
DEPRESSION	MENOPAUSAL
DRUG DEPENDENCY	PROBLEMS
DIGESTIVE	MOOD CHANGES
PROBLEMS	

AGING

We all begin to age from about the age of 24 so it is odd that we make such a fuss about aging in our middle years. The signs do become more obvious then but if we take care of our bodies through exercise and good diet, we can learn to adjust to aging and see each stage of our lives as being different and bringing new joys and excitements. So while at 50 you may not be able to play tennis at the same pace as when you were 25, the game played leisurely can be just as enjoyable as the competitive games of your youth.

The most obvious signs of aging are on the face and hands. Wrinkles and crows feet should be seen as character lines of life rather than signs that the best is over. It is sad to see older people searching for the elixir of life, wearing clothes suited to a younger generation, taking hormones and remedies whose effect is imaginary rather than real.

Those who complain hardest have usually done nothing to try to stay youthful. I can never understand why everyone doesn't take up some form of exercise from 35 onwards. One of the most attractive images of youth is a supple body – mobile and agile despite creaking joints and weakening muscles. A continued program of exercise can give you this image. Another characteristic associated with youth is a slender physique. We can all be our natural shape without rolls of fat if we eat sensibly. Careful eating and a program of exercise can do a great deal to keep us youthful and good looking. However, few people are prepared to make the effort, although women are generally more aware of health and fitness, they may not do anything about it.

Menopause
This is the most dramatic event for women because it signals the end of our reproductive life. Even if you have had your family or made the decision not to have any children, this is a very clear sign that you are no longer fertile. This may be difficult to accept. The physical changes, caused by waning female hormones, include weight gain, depression, irritability, tearfulness, night sweats and aching joints and muscles. Not all women have an uncomfortable menopause; at least half will have no symptoms at all. For those who do, hormone therapy has proved a boon.

There are physical changes of menopause that affect the genital tract, including thinning of the lining of the vagina and cervix. Secretions become scantier and so lubrication can be difficult. But even on the sexual side the news is good. Most women do become lubricated well enough to make entry comfortable – it just takes longer. If you ask your partner to be more understanding about foreplay, you should have no difficulty. Contrary to popular belief, there is no waning of interest in sex. The level of desire and enjoyment is hardly different, though sexual relations may be of a different nature.

There is a widely held belief that sex must inevitably decline with age. Because the older generation spoke so little about sex to their children, the myths about the old having no interest in sex were born. However, studies show that where frequency often reduces, the only obstacle for 70 and 80 year old women is finding available men. This is a heartening prospect.

Emotional changes
Some women feel anger at the prospect of getting older and the fact that they can't do the things they used to do. This is a wasted emotion to my mind. There is no point in trying to change the unchangeable. You should only worry about things that you can control and not those you cannot. There are so many ways you can enjoy yourself; if you are better off now than before, treat yourself. While you can't control aging, you can control the way you age. Clothes, hair, make up – they all help. Think of each year at a time and explore new activities and new things to try – travel, study, hobbies. Though you may not have the physical strength, you have the wisdom and experience which will make many tasks achievable.

Physical changes
You will notice your body changing in many ways. In general, "the machinery" turns over more slowly and the joints and muscles begin to lose their power. Your hair grows thinner and may become white. Your teeth change too. There is nothing more aging than cracked, yellow teeth with receding gums but they can be preserved with good preventative dentistry.

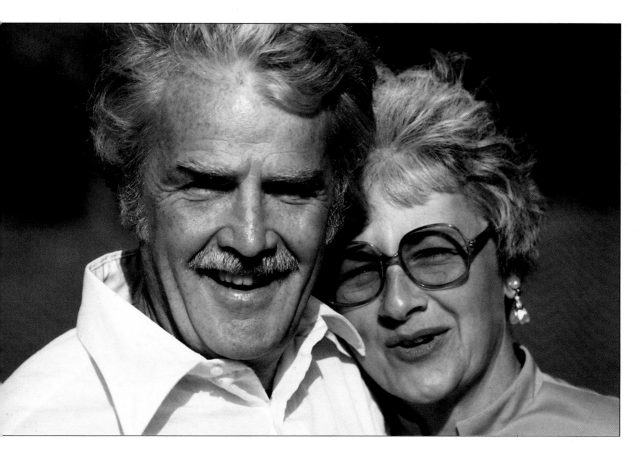

In general the skin all over your body becomes drier, so rub body lotions and moisturizers all over yourself whenever you can remember, especially on your face and hands. Use a bath oil so that a fine protective layer of grease is left on your skin; this will also suppress the itchiness that you may experience as you get older. Your circulation will become more sluggish, and you will feel the cold more quickly after 70. Keep your hands and feet warm; chilblains are a nuisance so make sure the lower part of your legs are kept warm in cold weather with well-insulated boots. Your feet are of paramount importance. Any small injury can take a long time to heal and walking can be uncomfortable due to corns, calluses and thick toenails.

Your senses will start to diminish; sight fails, hearing becomes less acute and your senses of smell and taste may change. The likelihood of illness is greater as you get older and depending on your condition, the symptoms can be difficult to cope with.

As women tend to outlive men, there are more of us over the age of 70. Maintain links in your community and keep yourself alert and interested in what is going on around you. A good doctor is a real bonus in old age. If your doctor is sympathetic and interested in your aches and pains and worries, and you have support from your family and friends, old age can be the time you catch up on those things you always meant to do, but never found the time.

SEE ALSO

DENTAL PROBLEMS
FACE LIFT
FOOT PROBLEMS
HORMONE
  REPLACEMENT
  THERAPY

MENOPAUSAL
  PROBLEMS
OBESITY
WRINKLES

Human beings are a drug-taking species and many drugs are part of our everyday lives. Stimulants such as caffeine, alcohol and cigarettes are freely available and advertised everywhere. Marijuana, cocaine and even hard drugs like heroin may be encountered at parties or on the streets.

Alcohol

The escalation from social drinking to a dependency on alcohol can creep up on women without their being aware of it. Some people are more at risk from becoming alcoholics than others. The pressures of some stress-laden professions can contribute greatly toward the development of alcoholism, particularly in those people who are predisposed.

Not all drinking is bad. Indeed the occasional drink can have a beneficial effect in that it tranquilizes and this brings positive effects to the heart, circulation and blood pressure. There are rough guides to safe measures. About 45ml (1fl oz) of alcohol a day is the level you should keep to. This is the equivalent of half a bottle of wine or one liter (2 pints) of beer or three measures of diluted spirits. By quoting these figures, I'm not encouraging drinking. You should try to keep below these levels. You should never lose sight of the fact that alcohol is an addictive drug and the addiction could harm you physically and socially, ruining your job prospects, your life within your family and your health.

How does it affect you?

Alcohol makes you feel bright and interesting. In small quantities it is not a stimulant; it relaxes you and helps you to shelve any inhibitions you may have. This is a particularly desired effect in a social situation where you may feel shy and insignificant. After a few more drinks, you will feel warm because alcohol is a vasodilator which causes the veins to dilate and increase blood flow to the skin.

Some time later, however, the pleasant effects wear off, and you could feel weak and dizzy as the levels of sugar in your blood fall. The effects of a heavy drinking session are known as a hangover and these vary from person to person. The major effect is a headache and dehydration; alcohol is a diuretic and so your body will lose a lot of fluid even though you've taken a lot in. You therefore should drink plenty of water so that the alcohol is diluted in your body and the loss through the diuretic effect is compensated for.

Certain drinks have a greater potential to produce a hangover. The worst offenders are the brown and red drinks such as brandy, rum, whisky and red wine. Gin, vodka and white wine contain fewer of the substances that help to produce a hangover.

SENSIBLE DRINKING

Here are some tips to help you drink sensibly if you think you might be drinking too much:
◆ Never drink alone.
◆ Don't drink on an empty stomach. Try to eat something at the same time as you drink – cut out the aperitifs.
◆ Don't gulp your drink; sip it and make it last. Always try to dilute the drink by having water or juice between drinks.
◆ Try to pace yourself through an evening so you don't take in too much early on.
◆ If you don't feel like a drink, have water and lemon or a soft drink.
◆ Never drink and drive.
◆ Don't be bullied into having a drink with every round. Put your hand across the top of the glass if your host is being too swift topping you up.

Smoking

Tobacco smoke contains three substances which are dangerous both to people who smoke and to those who just breathe in air which contains other people's smoke. The three are tar, nicotine and carbon monoxide. In addition to the hazards to health associated with lung damage from inhaling smoke containing tar and carbon monoxide (a poisonous gas), nicotine is an addictive substance which is absorbed from the lungs and acts on the central nervous system.

Except for women and teenage girls who still find the image glamorous and grown-up, smoking is declining in all other sections of the population. Nicotine addiction is not easy to control. Once cigarette smoking begins, the likelihood of being able to give smoking up recedes as the occasional cigarette becomes more frequent, and then turns into a daily habit.

The rise in smoking among women is alarming and, as you would expect, there is a parallel rise in lung cancer. The rate of lung cancer in women who smoke is now higher than that in men. We have overtaken them in this nearly always fatal disease because of the change in our smoking habits.

Smoking on its own is bad enough, but this habit also has an effect on those who don't smoke. It is known that there is a 30% higher risk of a non-smoker who lives or works with a smoker getting cancer of the lung than a non-smoker who lives in a tobacco-free environment. The worst effect of smoking is on children. Children who live with smokers have more chest infections, more respiratory ailments and they have a greater chance of growing up into smokers than the children of non-smokers. There is no question that smoking is extremely harmful to your health. Ignoring this fact puts you, and those close to you, in peril.

SMOKING DURING PREGNANCY

If a woman can't give up smoking during pregnancy, then she should think about her unborn child. The effects of smoking will affect practically the whole of the baby's development. The babies of smokers tend to have a low birth weight. This means that their resistance to disease, their ability to breathe normally, even the way they feed can be detrimentally affected if their mothers smoke. Every puff of smoke sends nicotine, tar and carbon monoxide across the maternal placental barrier to your baby.

Probably the worst effect of smoking during pregnancy is the fact that the carbon monoxide present in the mother's bloodstream prevents hemoglobin from taking up oxygen. Instead, the hemoglobin is converted to carboxihemoglobin which is resistant to oxygen. This means that the baby is being deprived of the most important substance supplied by the mother, oxygen.

EFFECTS OF SMOKING ON YOUR BODY

The average smoker smokes 15–20 cigarettes a day. The effect on your pocket alone can be as much as a month's salary in one year – money literally going up in smoke. The cigarette smoke lingers in clothes and hair and is an unpleasant odor for those around you. The physical effects touch most parts of your body but almost all the health risks will diminish as soon as you give up, so it's worth doing so.

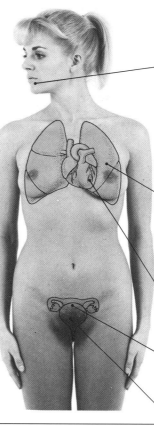

Cancer of the mouth and throat is more common; as smokers swallow some smoke, the esophagus may also be at risk.

Most smokers experience morning cough because they produce more phlegm. The destruction of the tiny hairs (cilia) in the lungs leads to this build-up of phlegm and lung infections such as bronchitis. This usually weakens the chest and can cause chronic emphysema. Chemicals in the smoke cause lung cancer.

Nicotine causes blood vessels to constrict and this raises the blood pressure, making all kinds of heart disease more common. If crucial blood vessels supplying the heart constrict, this, and other factors, can bring on heart attack.

Smokers are more likely to miscarry, and babies born to smokers have lower birth weights and more respiratory problems.

Because of the presence of certain chemicals in the urine, cancer of the bladder is more common.

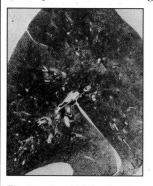 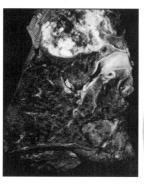

The tiny cilia, which in a healthy lung (left) filter out any inhaled particles, can be damaged by smoking and the destruction exposes the lung to infection and the build-up of phlegm. In a cancerous lung (right), the cells lining the bronchi are damaged by tobacco smoke, leading to the development of a tumor. This spreads to the lungs and the cancer cells are carried in the bloodstream to other parts of the body, such as the brain, liver and skin.

Giving up

Millions of people all over the world have stopped smoking and testify to the fact that it is possible to stop. If schools have campaigns against smoking, I think the message does get through. In one school I know in England, only two out of nearly 100 sixth-year pupils smoke and they are looked down upon by the others. More and more politicians and public authorities have taken up the case for abolishing smoking from public places and making the habit prohibitive through taxes and ostracization of smokers. The lobby of the large tobacco companies is still strong, however, and their advertising campaigns particularly encourage young people to take up the habit.

Three quarters of those who stop say that it wasn't as difficult as they thought. I am not saying it is easy, but as someone who has experienced the problems, it is possible. You need to prepare yourself and be ready for various side effects, such as weight gain because you're eating more. This isn't necessarily going to happen and it can be brought under control again after the initial withdrawal period. You must convince yourself that the habit is worth giving up before you start or you'll only go back on your promise to yourself and make excuses.

Social drugs

Nowadays, drugs that used to be considered too strong, too easy to abuse and habit-forming, are passed around at some social gatherings even though their use is illegal. You no longer have to search hard to find viciously addictive drugs such as heroin. Caffeine, on the other hand, is a drug that most of us take in some form every day in tea, coffee or cola drinks. Although the stimulating effect of caffeine varies widely from person to person, if taken in large enough quantities it can cause palpitations and anxiety. Most of us, however, use this effect to wake us up in the morning or keep ourselves alert during an evening and the thought of excess and abuse is far from our minds.

Contrary to popular belief, smoking marijuana does not automatically lead to an addiction to harder drugs. There is a whole group of people who smoke marijuana, and never wish to proceed any further. In terms of the effect it produces and the way it is perceived by people who use it, smoking marijuana is regarded by some as akin to drinking alcohol, which is used as a stimulant by those in positions of the most influence in our society. The difficulty is that often young people see marijuana as an escape or an excitement. This can lead to a tendency to seek greater escapes and greater adventures, and to experimentation with stronger and more addictive substances. It is these illegal drugs with their fearsome side effects and addictive qualities that pose the greatest threat to people's health.

Heroin

This drug is very addictive. In recent years the street price of heroin has dropped and consequently it has claimed many more addicts. There are now even "heroin babies" whose mothers were addicts when they were born so the babies inherit the addiction. The first weeks of their lives are usually agonising. Unless the mother confesses to her habit, it will not be known what the baby is addicted to. This can lead to a dangerous situation when sudden withdrawal can actually kill the baby. Even if death doesn't occur, there may be convulsions and coma. The baby will be extremely irritable and impossible to pacify. These babies need constant supervision in special units to ensure their comfort and return to good health. There is now an added danger for heroin users in that the needles they share to inject themselves can carry the AIDS virus if they are contaminated with infected blood. This is one of the fastest means by which the virus is passed through a community.

Cocaine

The effects of cocaine on the brain have led to its abuse. It produces feelings of euphoria and increased energy and has become fashionable in certain professions where it is used to improve performance. However, regular inhaling of the drug can damage the lining of the nose and lead to psychological dependence. Psychosis may even develop if high doses are taken and overdoses can cause seizures and cardiac arrest. Crack, a purified form of cocaine, produces a more rapid and intense reaction that wears off very quickly. It has been responsible for many deaths.

TAKING PRESCRIBED DRUGS DURING PREGNANCY

During pregnancy, drugs should be treated very warily; certainly you should never treat yourself. After the experience of using hormones to treat pregnant women in the 1950s and 60s and the resulting tragedies of thalidomide and DES, no drugs should be taken during pregnancy unless absolutely necessary. Many well-known drugs can interfere with a pregnant woman's proper physiological functioning and thus indirectly affect her fetus. The fetus itself may be directly susceptible to drugs crossing the placenta, as with tobacco smoking and heroin addiction. The following drugs definitely have been associated with fetal defects:

Tetracycline antibiotics	Depress bone growth and cause tooth staining.
Synthetic progesterone	Hormones used in pregnancy testing can masculinize the female fetus.
Tranquilizers	Taken in high doses can cause retinal damage and impairment of intellectual development in the fetus.
Iodine and antithyroid drugs	Can cause hypothyroidism and goiter.
Antihypertensive agents	Can result in problems of breathing and heart beat for the baby.

Other drugs are also under suspicion for ill-effects and these include:

Analgesics	Can be bought easily over the counter but don't take them without your doctor's advice. Those that contain opiates or salicylate should definitely not be taken. This includes aspirin which, if taken in large amounts towards the end of your pregnancy, can cause a prolonged labor and excessive bleeding during childbirth.
Anticonvulsants	Prescribed for epileptic sufferers, can result in fetal abnormalities. These are twice as common in children of epileptic mothers.
Oral anticoagulants	Are associated with internal bleeding.

As so many commercially available drugs contain alcohol and other unfamiliar drugs, treat even cough medicines and hayfever preparations with caution.

Prescribed drugs

I feel the medical profession must take some blame for the increase in dependency, particularly of tranquilizers. With the increase in stress-related disorders in women, more doctors are prescribing tranquilizers instead of helping their patients sort out the underlying problems which cause stress in the first place. Unfortunately this takes time, and many doctors are too busy to stop and listen.

If you visit your doctor because you feel depressed, and are prescribed a minor tranquilizer, this may worsen your symptoms if they in fact result from anxiety rather than a depressive illness. A correct diagnosis needs to be made. This may take some probing by your doctor. Sleeping pills or barbiturates are a daily item on the menu too. Those with a sleeping problem may be prescribed these instead of being advised on how to overcome sleeplessness and the basic difficulties that cause it. Doctors are becoming aware of this problem but

you have a responsibility to yourself and to your family to avoid dependence on habit-forming drugs given to you on prescription. You need to question yourself about whether you are heading for addiction. Tranquilizers are extremely habit-forming and may be difficult to stop. Expert advice is available and self-help groups will support you.

SEE ALSO:

AIDS	HYPERTENSION
ALCOHOLISM	INSOMNIA
ANXIETY	MISCARRIAGE
BODY ODOR	NAUSEA AND
CANCER	VOMITING
DEPRESSION	PALPITATIONS
DES	PREGNANCY
DIGESTIVE PROBLEMS	PROBLEMS
DRUG DEPENDENCY	
HEADACHE	
HEART DISEASE	

DANGER SIGNS

There are certain symptoms or danger signs which you should take notice of because, to a doctor, they are very important indeed. They may be a sign of cancer or some other life-threatening disease and a doctor should investigate them. In many cases, there may be no cause for alarm, but if you experience any of these symptoms, contact your doctor to rule out any problems.

DANGER SIGNS	WHAT SHOULD I DO?	WHAT WILL THE DOCTOR DO?
Blood in sputum with sore throat, persistent cough, or chest infection — it could be a burst blood vessel caused by the coughing.	If there is a lot of blood, go to an emergency room; otherwise, keep the sputum and show your doctor.	You may be referred for a chest X-ray and/or throat swab.
Blood in vomit after taking drugs such as aspirin, eating something unusual, drinking a lot of alcohol, or a bout of indigestion. You may have a duodenal ulcer.	If you feel faint or if there is a lot of blood go to the emergency room; otherwise, make an appointment to see your doctor. Keep a specimen of vomit to show your doctor.	Question you about food, your stomach and digestion. Examine your abdomen, look at your vomit and your stools. Possibly order an Upper GI series.
Blood in stools commonly because of hemorrhoids or severe diarrhea. It may occur with diverticulitis. Black, tarry stools occur when a duodenal ulcer bursts.	If you feel faint or if there is a lot of blood, go to the emergency room; otherwise, make an appointment to see your doctor. Keep a specimen of stools to show your doctor.	Question you about your stomach and intestines. Examine your abdomen and rectum (internally). Examine your stools. Possibly order a barium enema.
Blood in urine with kidney or back pain or a recent urinary infection such as cystitis.	If there is a lot of blood, go to the emergency room; otherwise, make an appointment to see your doctor. Keep a specimen of urine to show your doctor.	Question you about your bladder, urine and kidneys. Examine your urine and arrange an intravenous pyelogram(IVP).
Bleeding after intercourse usually dark brown, may be accompanied by an unpleasant, itchy vaginal discharge, could be an erosion of the cervix (see Cervix problems).	Question your partner in case it is from him. See your doctor immediately.	Question you about any blood or discharge, and about your periods. Examine your abdomen and breasts and give you an internal examination and Pap smear.
Inter-menstrual bleeding could be a minor menstrual irregularity or benign growths of the cervix or vagina.	See your doctor immediately.	Question you about any blood or discharge, and about your periods and your form of contraception. Examine your abdomen and breasts and give you an internal examination.
Sudden heavy periods out of the blue the commonest cause is probably a miscarriage. If habitual, it is probably fibroids.	If it doesn't stop, call an ambulance immediately; otherwise, see your doctor.	Question you about your periods, your method of contraception and whether you could be pregnant. Examine your abdomen and breasts and give you an internal examination.

DANGER SIGNS	WHAT SHOULD I DO?	WHAT WILL THE DOCTOR DO?
Lump in breast The commonest cause is a benign cyst of the breast, or premenstrual syndrome symptoms.	See your doctor as soon as possible, immediately if there is discharge from the nipple.	Question you about the lump. Examine both breasts and armpits and possibly suggest a mammogram.
Discharge from nipple The commonest cause is lactation or a benign cyst of the breast, or of the nipple ducts. This may happen when using the pill because of a change in hormone balance.	Take your temperature if you feel hot or your breast is tender. See your doctor as soon as possible.	Question you about the discharge. Examine both breasts, nipples and armpits. You may be referred for a mammogram.
Sudden onset of indigestion The commonest causes are starting to take medication for the first time, or eating strange foods.	If it persists for more than 3 days, see your doctor.	Question you about food and digestion. Ask for a stool specimen for analysis. Try a course of treatment, order a barium meal. Look for signs of gallbladder disease.
Onset of persistent headaches The commonest causes are migraine, tension headache, post-herpetic neuralgia (related to shingles) and dental problems.	Take over-the-counter analgesics. Any related signs, e.g. pins and needles in the skin, flashing lights, nausea, see your doctor. If the headaches persist or wake you up from sleep, consult your doctor.	Question you generally. Give you a physical examination. Take your blood pressure. Examine your eyes or perhaps refer you to a dentist or neurologist.
Sudden pain or tenderness of calf or swelling of one ankle The commonest cause is deep-vein thrombosis; especially if you have varicose veins, recently had a baby or surgery or take oral contraceptives.	Rest and put your leg up on a stool. Call your doctor.	Question you. Examine your leg, give you a bandage; give you a course of treatment, if necessary. May advise you to stop taking the contraceptive pill.
Loss of consciousness The commonest cause is a vasovagal reaction, a slowing of the pulse and a decrease in blood pressure caused by your autonomic nervous system. Not all loss of consciousness is fainting, however. Seizures and heart rhythm disturbances can also cause you to lose consciousness.	If you feel faint, lie down and elevate your legs. Don't drive a car or climb ladders. Make an appointment to see your doctor.	Question you and give you a full physical examination.

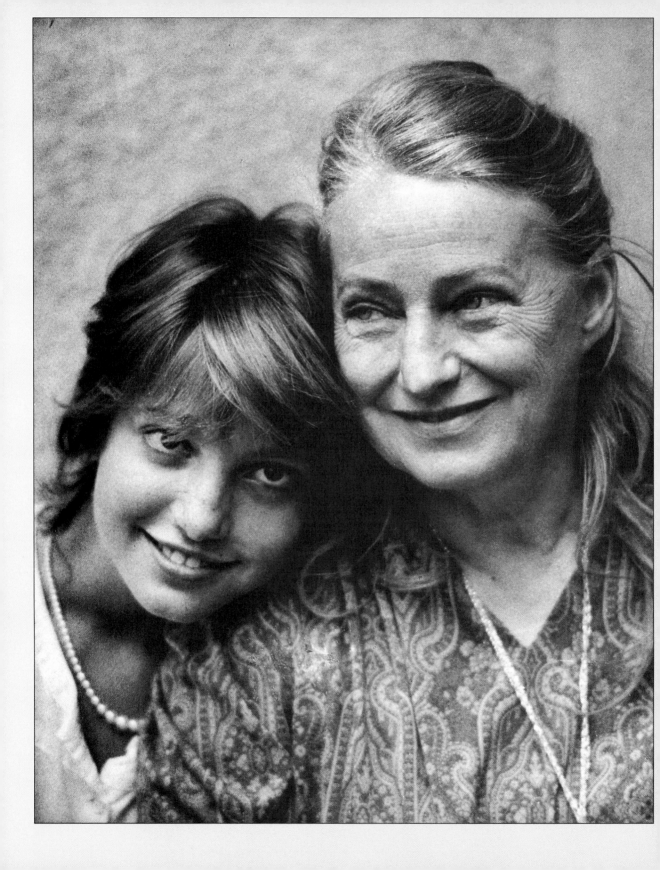

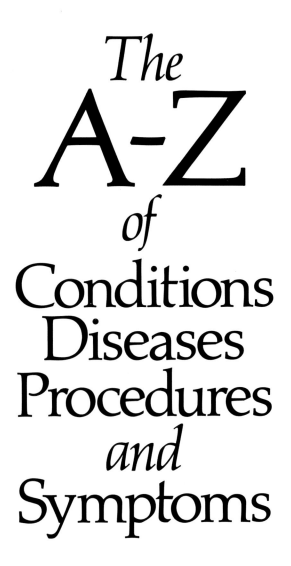

The
A-Z
of
Conditions
Diseases
Procedures
and
Symptoms

ABDOMINAL PAIN AND CRAMPS

Abdominal pain or cramps, which can occur anywhere between the rib cage and the groin, signals disorders of the digestive or urinary tract or the reproductive system. In the majority of cases, the pain will probably be due to menstrual problems or eating something that disagrees with you.

Recurrent abdominal pain is most likely to be caused by a digestive upset. The most severe abdominal pain of all is that associated with stones in the gallbladder or kidneys.

Women suffer pain in their pelvic region with menstruation but the site of undiagnosed pelvic pain can be difficult to identify. If there are no other symptoms, such as vaginal bleeding or discharge or frequency and pain during urination, the task of diagnosis is more difficult. A pelvic examination will help. Ovarian and fallopian tube disorders, for example, are localized. Sometimes ovarian pain radiates to the inner thigh. If the pain was preceded by intercourse, for example, this can give a clue.

Cases of chronic pelvic pain may indicate a psychosomatic disorder relating to sexual problems.

Abdominal pain in pregnancy may be alarming but it is rarely serious unless you are suffering a miscarriage in which case there will be bleeding from the vagina. Pain near to term could be the onset of labor.

There are so many abdominal organs that it can be very difficult to work out exactly the cause and site of the pain. You can help your doctor if you can describe the pain. For example, colicky pain, like sharp waves, can indicate that an organ has been distended and the pain comes from the contractions of that organ. Cramping pain on the other hand is closely associated with menstruation. Also note whether the pain began gradually or started suddenly and without warning. This may indicate that something has ruptured. To help with the diagnosis, note any other symptoms.

SITE AND NATURE OF THE PAIN	PROBABLE CAUSE
The pain is below the waist and urination is painful and frequent	This could be *cystitis*.
Your normal period pains become worse and increase in severity during the period	This could be *endometriosis*.
Your skin burns and feels tender	This could be shingles, a viral infection like chickenpox. Apply soothing calamine lotion and consult your doctor.
You suddenly have cramping pain and diarrhea	You may have eaten something within the last 2-4 hours to inflame your digestive tract. This is gastroenteritis (see *Digestive problems*). Pain with *diarrhea* may have been caused by a parasite, when it is known as dysentery, but this is rare unless you have recently been travelling in the tropics. If you have influenza, this can affect your bowel and cause mild diarrhea with cramping pains. Consult your doctor if the symptoms persist for more than 24 hours.
You haven't moved your bowels for some time	The pain could be caused by *constipation*. Change your diet for 24 hours, drink lots of fluids and see if this improves the problem.
You can put your finger on the ache in the middle of your ribs	This is probably indigestion if you've recently eaten. If it doesn't go away, it could be an ulcer, or if it gets worse when you stoop, a hiatus hernia (see *Digestive problems).* If the dull cramping pain extends up your chest or down your arm, this may be heart pain. Consult your doctor.
The pain is severe and centered around the lower right side (or has moved from your navel to the right side) which is very tender and swollen, and when you touch it, it springs back	This could be appendicitis. Consult your doctor immediately.
Abdominal pain is accompanied by bleeding from the vagina	If you are pregnant, this may be a miscarriage. Go straight to bed after calling your doctor. Keep your legs raised. If you pass any clots or membranes keep them for the doctor to help discover the cause of the miscarriage. Don't take any medication.

SITE AND NATURE OF THE PAIN	PROBABLE CAUSE
The pain is severe and you have a fever, with or without a vaginal discharge	This could be a pelvic infection (see *Pelvic inflammatory disease*). If you might be pregnant, this could be an *ectopic pregnancy*, or a *miscarriage* if there is bloody discharge from your vagina. See your doctor immediately.
The pain runs around from your back down to your groin, with or without fever	This could be a kidney infection or stones in your kidney. Consult your doctor.
The pain is high up under your ribs on the right side, and you are vomiting and the pain spreads around to your back	This could be acute cholecystitis, the result of *gallbladder disease*. Consult your doctor immediately.
In the second trimester of your pregnancy, you may experience pain on one side. It feels like a length of elastic is about to snap	This is round ligament pain (see *Pregnancy problems*). Consult your doctor.
During pregnancy, your abdomen may tense and feel hard for a couple of seconds	Your uterus will be practising for childbirth with periodic mini contractions, known as Braxton Hicks contractions. There is no cause for alarm but do check with your doctor if they are prolonged or become intense. Try to lie on your side to relieve them.
You are intermittently constipated and have bouts of diarrhea, causing cramps in the lower abdomen	This could be diverticular disease or a stress related condition, known as irritable or spastic colon (see *Digestive problems*).

If you suffer abdominal pain for at least four hours without respite, and the pain is accompanied by vomiting, dizziness or diarrhea, get urgent medical attention, lie down while you wait and don't eat or drink anything in case surgery is necessary. Never take aspirin because this may inflame your stomach lining further. A hotwater bottle or heating pad can help relieve the pain.

Treatment for abdominal pain, where surgery isn't immediately necessary, is usually given after a pelvic examination, laparoscopy or dilatation and curettage for pelvic problems; and biopsy, or blood, urine and stool tests for other problems. You may have X-rays and ultrasound if a digestive disorder is suspected.

If you are unable to make a diagnosis from this information, consult your doctor.

ABORTION

To doctors, abortion and *miscarriage* are synonymous. Very few lay people see abortion and miscarriage as the same thing. This is because for decades the word abortion was only used with the prefix "illegal" or "procured" which had damning connotations; miscarriage was seen as a natural event which was uncontrollable. When you hear a doctor using these words, remember that they mean the same thing. The term for a legal abortion is *termination of pregnancy*.

Legal versus illegal abortions relate to the length of time that the pregnancy has been in existence. In the U.S., the Supreme Court has ruled that during the first trimester (up to the 12th week of pregnancy), the federal and state governments cannot place legal restrictions on a woman's choice to have an abortion. Only a woman and her doctor have the legal right to make a decision about an abortion. However, during the second trimester (between the 12th and 24th weeks), individual states may impose certain restrictions on where and how abortions are performed – to protect a woman's health. Beyond the 24th week, a state may prohibit abortion, except when necessary to preserve a woman's life. (To determine the laws which apply to your individual state, you can contact Planned Parenthood or your state attorney general's office.)

Threatened, repeated, and incomplete abortions are medical terms used to describe certain situations when a miscarriage occurs. Abortion occurs quite naturally in one third of all first pregnancies; it is "Nature's way" of preventing malformed fetuses from being born. It also gives the uterus a trial run in preparation for a full pregnancy.

By far the best way of dealing with an unplanned or unwanted pregnancy is with prevention in the form of sound *contraception*. Abortion should not be seen as a method of contraception; it carries its own risks. The womb may become infected and vigorous therapy with antibiotics will be needed. Repeated abortion carries with it the greatest risk of all – *pelvic inflammatory disease* and the possibility of *infertility*.

ACNE

Our skin is covered with sebaceous glands which secrete sebum to keep it supple and moist. If the exits from these glands become blocked, sebum is released into the deeper layers of the skin. This causes inflammation which can become infected. The result of this is pustules and the characteristic pimples of acne. As the pimples heal, scar tissue and pitting of the skin may result.

What causes it?

The cause of the overgrowth of the cells of the sebaceous duct is usually a response to the male hormones, androgens, which circulate in the blood and are highest at puberty when they outnumber estrogens. Sometimes, acne persists well into the teens and rarely into the twenties and thirties. This is a more difficult time for treatment and is often the reason for scarring and discoloration.

Acne in a milder form may occur prior to menstruation and during treatment with certain drugs, particularly cortisone.

Acne isn't caused by eating rich or fatty foods, or not washing thoroughly or by drinking too much or leading a slovenly life. There does seem to be a tendency for acne to run in families.

Should I consult the doctor?

Acne is graded in stages of severity:
stage 1 - an oily skin with blackheads
stage 2 - pustules
stage 3 - deep, tender, hard purplish spots
stage 4 - pitted and scarred skin.

If you feel that self-help treatment isn't working, see your doctor if the acne is severe or you are upset and you feel self conscious about it. Acne invariably causes stress and worry because of its unsightliness. This emotional reaction increases the production of androgens by the ovaries and makes the acne worse.

What will the doctor do?

The basis of treatment is to reduce bacteria in the glands, stop the multiplication of cells in the ducts which result in the blockages and eliminate the spots and whiteheads. A small daily dose of the antibiotic tetracycline has been found to improve acne considerably. This reduces the bacteria. This is a treatment if there are a lot of pustules. The antibiotic needs to be taken for some time to be effective. There are usually no side effects and the dose is reduced according to the progress of the treatment.

In women and girls who have stopped growing, the oral contraceptive pill may be prescribed. This can often settle the acne down because the estrogen in the pill reduces the rate of production of sebum. This treatment takes a few months to work. The doctor is unlikely to prescribe the pill before the age of 17 as acne does not justify the giving of hormones before growth is completed. It will not be prescribed if there are contra-indications or if this is not a method of birth control favored by the acne sufferer. Medications for moderately severe acne applied directly to the skin include benzyl peroxide. This is a cream, lotion or jelly with an antibiotic that also peels the skin. As there are side effects, this treatment must be supervised and you should avoid extremes of temperature on your skin because your skin will be more sensitive.

Another treatment is based on retinoic acid (Retin-A), a derivative of Vitamin A. This increases the speed with which the cells are shed and therefore the side effects include cracked lips and extensive drying and peeling skin. (Eating foods rich in Vitamin A is not the same thing and won't treat your acne.)

Carefully measured doses of ultraviolet radiation cause the skin to peel gently, unblocking the glands. In severe cases with deep pitting, there may be blue-purple lesions which are deep in the skin. Injections of special steroids directly into these lesions may ameliorate this condition. This is only done in a specialist clinic.

For scarring and pitting, techniques such as dermabrasion and chemical skin peel may be recommended.

What can I do to help?

◆ Never squeeze anything but a blackhead.
◆ Try to keep your fingers away from the acne as this simply spreads the germs into the surrounding skin.
◆ Don't use proprietary acne cleansers as these abrade the skin and break down the pustules spreading germs all over the skin, thereby encouraging acne lesions.
◆ Moderate exposure to sunlight is helpful as it dries your skin out.
◆ Cleanse the affected area of your skin meticulously. Use soap, brought to a lather and massage it into your skin for at least two minutes. The aim of this is to de-fat the skin. Wash this way at least three times a day.
◆ While your treatment is in progress, wear a heavy textured makeup to cover the acne. Many people mistakenly feel that this will block the glands further. Makeup will not make acne worse and it does improve morale.
◆ Don't let the acne affect your diet. Research has shown that foods such as chocolate don't have the slightest effect on acne. However, if you are run down or anemic, this could have an effect. So eat a good balanced diet to improve your general health.

SEE ALSO:

ANEMIA
DERMABRASION
FACIAL TREATMENTS

AIDS

AIDS stands for acquired immune deficiency syndrome and it is caused by the human immunodeficiency virus or HIV. While HIV is infectious, meaning that it can be passed on from one person to another, it is not as contagious as some other viruses we know, such as the common cold or influenza. It can't be caught simply by social contact; it's not spread by coughs and sneezes. Indeed it is quite difficult to catch and can only be transmitted by the mixing of body fluids – mainly restricted to blood and semen. So while the virus has been found in saliva and tears, it is in far too low concentrations to be infectious.

AIDs affects us so dramatically because it weakens the body's natural defences, the immune system, to such an extent that we are unable to fight off any infections or cancerous growths. AIDS sufferers contract deadly diseases that the general population rarely do.

The body's response to infection with HIV is to produce antibodies and, at this point, if a person is AIDS tested, the antibody test will be positive. These people are called HIV-positive. Contrary to public belief, they do not have the AIDS disease. They are, however, carriers of the disease and may spread it to others.

The virus has the capability of lying dormant in the body for quite a long time, some researchers say up to 10 years, so unless tested, carriers may spread the disease to sexual partners without being aware of it. This is what happened within the gay community.

Where did it come from?
There are many theories about how the virus first entered the gay community and how it spread. The route accepted by most authorities is originally from West Africa, thence to Haiti and to San Francisco. Haiti at the time was a favorite holiday resort for American homosexuals from the West coast.

It did not take long for this pool of infection to rise to alarming proportions. In 1980, around 1% of San Franciscan gay men had been infected by HIV. In 1987 it is estimated that half of the 80,000 homosexuals there now carry the virus.

How does it spread?
The main route of infection of the virus is sexual contact because the virus is present in very large numbers in semen. It can be passed, therefore, through sexual intercourse, vaginally or anally to women, and anally to men. Women can also infect a man sexually. It can also be passed on by sharing hypodermic needles, a practice very common among drug addicts. It has also been transferred to hemophiliacs by previously contaminated blood transfusions, and an HIV positive mother can infect her baby in the womb or at the time of birth.

In theory, the transmission of the AIDS virus from one person to another during intercourse could be blocked by any barrier which prevents mixing of blood, seminal fluid and female genital secretions. Until recently this has been no more than theory but evidence is gathering that the condom provides a way of having "safer sex." Research has shown that the AIDS virus is unable to permeate

WOMEN AND AIDS

Dr Helen Kaplan, a leading sex therapist from America, believes that women should be assertive in protecting themselves from AIDS. She urges women and their partners to take an AIDS antibody test before engaging in what she calls "wet sex"– any practice that involves the exchange of body fluids.

Because the skin covering the nipples is also a mucous membrane, she says they shouldn't come into contact with a man's saliva or semen. Most researchers think it is extremely unlikely that AIDS could ever be transmitted this way. Similarly, any open sore including a hang-nail could be a port of entry for the virus.

Since it takes up to six months after exposure to AIDS for the body to develop the antibodies detected by the test, couples are advised to abstain from wet sex during this "window of infection" and get tested a second time. During this period Kaplan recommends a variety of sexual activities including mutual masturbation, sensous massage, vibrators, erotic films and fantasies and rubbing rhythmically against each others bodies while fully clothed. Many women actually enjoy such techniques of extended foreplay as much as they do full intercourse.

Women should be prepared for the man who will want to proceed to penetration. Simply to ask him to wear a condom at this point is not being assertive enough; Kaplan sees it as being compliant. Women should be wary of any man who is guarded about his sexual past or who is reluctant to submit to an AIDS test. If a man makes you feel bad for bringing up the subject, you should avoid him, she advises.

Many men are probably as worried as women about AIDS and are grateful if you raise the subject of testing as long as it is done tactfully and not accusingly.

Kaplan describes the current status of the AIDS epidemic as two islands: one consisting of homosexual and bisexual men and the other of intravenous drug users. The islands are surrounded by women who provide the potential route for the virus to escape into the heterosexual population on a massive scale. We should not hesitate therefore to protect our bodies and ourselves.

any of the commercially available brands of condoms; spermicides help too. Something as simple as the wearing of condoms and the use of spermicides could be a way of helping to control AIDS.

Theoretically only one sexual contact is enough to contract AIDS and this has resulted in many tragic cases among women. A woman may have sexual contact with a man without knowing that he is a drug addict sharing equipment with others. Similarly, a married woman may be infected by her husband who has had homosexual affairs. Any pregnant woman carrying AIDS, in theory, can infect her unborn baby. The numbers of HIV-positive babies is still quite small – but these infants will certainly die, probably before the age of four. As many AIDS mothers are also intraveneous users of heroin, a baby can be born with AIDS and addicted to heroin.

What is the treatment?
Most people with full-blown AIDS die within two years of the disease developing. However, no one actually dies of AIDS; death is nearly always from an unusual form of pneumonia which hardly ever effects the general population – Pneumocystis carinii – or a skin cancer called Kaposi's sarcoma, or other opportunistic infections which under normal circumstances the body would be strong enough to fight off with ease. Most recently it's been found that the virus can affect the brain directly, thereby destroying the body's ability to function properly.

The possibility of finding a cure for those who are already infected by AIDS and of finding a vaccine to prevent anyone else from becoming infected is only conjecture at present. Most authorities, however, believe that neither of these things will come in the next five years. Producing an AIDS vaccine is infinitely more difficult than with other viruses because AIDS destroys the immune system which produces the anti-

A NEW DISEASE
Compared with the slow evolution of humans, viruses can evolve into new viruses and produce new diseases amazingly quickly. The AIDS virus is an example of a new disease that is still evolving.

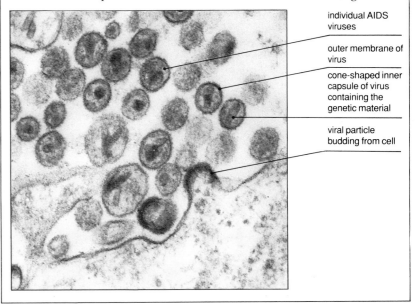

individual AIDS viruses

outer membrane of virus

cone-shaped inner capsule of virus containing the genetic material

viral particle budding from cell

bodies that are stimulated by the vaccine. Also, different forms of the virus seem to be appearing. At the present moment there is no known cure for any disease caused by a virus, whether it's 'flu, the common cold or AIDS. There are early signs that Zidovudine (AZT) and drugs like it may have a restraining effect on HIV and therefore prolong the lives of AIDS sufferers, without curing the disease completely.

At present the screening test is applied to all blood in blood banks as this is a route by which hemophiliacs have been tragically infected. The question of who should be tested is at the center of controversy and no doubt this will continue. A positive result only indicates past exposure to the virus and does not show whether the disease has been contracted or indeed ever will be.

What can I do?
If you feel that you have been exposed to the virus, you can request a blood test, although it is wise to obtain counseling first on the advisability of the test, and the implications of the result. If you have been infected, you must alter your sexual life-style to avoid transmitting the virus.

To avoid becoming infected adopt "safe" sex procedures; reduce the number of sexual partners, and ideally limit them to those whose sexual histories are known; avoid unprotected anal and vaginal intercourse – always use a condom, and spermicide as a lubricant; avoid ejaculation into the mouth.

SEE ALSO:
SEXUALLY TRANSMITTED DISEASES

ALCOHOLISM

Alcoholism and alcohol-related problems continue to be a serious issue among women. With emancipation from traditional roles of a home-centered life, many more women now find themselves in stressful positions of responsibility in their work and in high-risk professions. Where a woman is also a single parent and the sole breadwinner, she can expect more stress.

The stresses for many women are therefore greater than ever before and many seek relief in alcohol. Even those who have maintained a relatively home-centered life are at risk. Women sometimes turn to alcohol when their children leave home and they come to believe that their lives are empty and lonely.

What is it?
Alcoholism is an abnormal dependence on alcohol and varies from a mild degree such as social drinking whenever possible, to a very advanced state where alcohol is necessary to start the day. Drinking is a pleasurable and acceptable custom but such social drinking may lead to dependence, though this can take from 10 to 15 years to occur.

Treatment for alcoholism is often complicated by the double standards that exist in society. While social drinking is acceptable, heavy drinking, especially when it affects work, is not, and this encourages people to become secret, furtive drinkers. Many alcoholics therefore tend to drink alone frequently during the day, but nearly always deny doing so, making detection and treatment difficult to start up. Eventually, the social drinker who is at risk comes to rely on alcohol to allay tension and to feel good. Alcohol taken regularly or in large quantities has terrible effects on the body – it damages the liver irreparably, causing cirrhosis, and it affects the nervous system.

Why are women at risk?
Physically women are less tolerant of

· S y m p t o m s ·

▲ Heavy drinking, either constantly at all times of the day or in two or three day binges
▲ Blackouts or loss of memory while drinking
▲ Drinking alone
▲ Needing a drink to face the slightest stress
▲ Irritability
▲ Aggressive behavior
▲ Secretiveness about drinking
▲ Flushed, blotchy face
▲ The veins in the nose are purple and pronounced
▲ Trembling
▲ Slurred speech

---

alcohol than men. Our bodies contain less water so that our blood absorbs the same amount of alcohol much more quickly. At certain times of the month, some women respond differently to alcohol; for example, premenstrually, women complain of a reduced tolerance to alcohol.

Alcohol is much easier to come by now too. Some supermarket shelves groan with wine and spirits and social pressures have been removed. Once women were discouraged from drinking in public, now we drink openly in bars.

Could I be an alcoholic?
If you answer yes to one of these questions, alcohol is affecting your life in a major way and you should seek help.
1. When faced with a problem, do you turn to alcohol for relief?
2. Are you sometimes unable to meet home or work responsibilities because of your drinking?
3. Has someone close to you expressed concern about your drinking?
4. Have you ever needed medical attention as a result of drinking?
5. Have you ever experienced distressing physical or psychological reactions when you stopped drinking?
6. Have you ever had a blackout or total loss of memory while awake when drinking?
7. Have you ever failed to keep promises to yourself about controlling or stopping drinking?

Should I see the doctor?
Despite the dereliction of the body that results from heavy drinking, there is no one who can make you give up alcohol other than yourself but all alcoholics need help to do it. If you answer yes to one of the questions opposite, see your doctor as soon as possible. It is usually difficult for alcholics to admit their problem, but admission is the first

---

ALCOHOL IN PREGNANCY

Drinking alcohol in pregnancy can harm your growing baby and leave it with physical and mental defects for life, such as cleft palate, hare lip, abnormal limb development and heart defects as well as lower than average intelligence. This condition is called fetal alcohol syndrome (FAS) and is characterized by distinguishing features in the newborn baby. The eyes have a fold at the top giving the baby a mongoloid appearance, the chin recedes and the bridge of the nose is flat and low. This syndrome results from excessive drinking whether in binges or constantly throughout pregnancy, although like all toxins the major effect is probably felt in the first 8 weeks when the fetus is developing and is most at risk. Some part of every drink reaches the baby through the mother's bloodstream, so beware of alcohol during pregnancy and if you must drink, limit yourself to two glasses of wine or one can of beer in one day.

major step. If you are seriously dependent, the problems are increased when you have to abstain from alcohol; for example, withdrawal often leads to intense anxiety.

What will the doctor do?
Depending on the severity of your problem and of your symptoms, your doctor will advise on the best course. Voluntary organizations such as Alcoholics Anonymous exist to help all people who want to give up drinking. All members have been alcoholics and they share their experiences in order to help others with a drinking problem stay sober and rebuild their lives.

For alcoholics with a serious problem, hospitalization and drying out is the first step. Detoxification is for the most seriously affected alcoholics who need to recover from the acute effects of drinking. They need to dry out before any withdrawal is possible. Sedatives and other drugs help to overcome the cravings and hallucinations that patients suffer while the body is being detoxified of alcohol. After this initial drying out, the next step is counseling. Therapy helps drinkers to answer the important question as to why they were drinking. The final step is to try to avoid the stresses that caused the problem in the first place.

What can I do?
You have real difficulties if you develop an increasing tolerance for alcohol – when you need more and more to achieve the desired effect. Surreptitious drinking means that dependence has developed to an unacceptable degree and marks the beginning of a critical phase when it becomes increasingly more difficult to stop drinking. One result of this is neglect of your social responsibilities and your diet.

If you want to give up alcohol, you can do it with the help of doctors, counselors and ex-alcoholics, but you have to really want to. The stresses or difficult situations that caused you to find solace in alcohol will need to be faced or avoided. Perhaps changing your job or reorganizing your life will be the only way.

EFFECTS OF LONGTERM ALCOHOLISM

The head
Headache caused by the dilation of the blood vessels in the brain may be an immediate after effect but this usually goes after a good sleep. There is an increased risk of cancer of the mouth, pharynx, larynx and esophagus; if you smoke as well, this greatly increases the risk. You may develop ulcers in your digestive system.

The brain
Alcohol impairs various sensory, perceptual, mental and motor functions so that thought and bodily coordination become disorganized. Thus, drinking and then driving is extremely dangerous. Chronic alcohol ingestion can cause a variety of psychotic states and neurological disorders including Korsakoff's psychosis, hallucinations, polyneuritis, and Wernicke's encephalopathy.

The liver
Cirrhosis of the liver results from longterm, heavy alcohol intake. This impairs the liver functions which process the nutrients from your food intake. Hepatitis, fatty liver and cancer of the liver are other possible disorders. Pain and tenderness in your liver leads to loss of appetite.

The skin
The skin becomes warm and sweaty. The veins in your face and nose are blotchy and purple. In later stages of liver failure, the palms of your hands are permanently red.

The heart
A heavy drinker tends not to eat a balanced diet and as alcohol contains only calories, you will eventually become vitamin deficient, particularly in thiamine (Vitamin B1). This will affect the heart's muscular tissue which will be damaged as a result of this lack of essential nutrients.

The stomach
A lot of alcohol in one bout can make you vomit or feel nauseous with gastritis when the mucous membrane that lines the stomach becomes inflamed. This can become a chronic condition with a constant high intake of alcohol.

SEE ALSO:

ANXIETY
DEPRESSION
DRUG DEPENDENCY
HEART DISEASE
PREGNANCY PROBLEMS
PREMENSTRUAL SYNDROME

AMENORRHEA

This means a lack of menstrual periods. The condition is known as primary if the periods have never started at all, or secondary, when normal menstruation is interrupted for four months or more. Primary amenorrhea is usually due to the late onset of puberty but less commonly it may be caused by a disorder in the reproductive or hormonal system.

Reasons for amenorrhea

The commonest reason for secondary amenorrhea is pregnancy. However, if the hormonal balance is interrupted for any other reason, this can also cause periods to be absent. For example, the suppression of hormonal production in the brain by suddenly stopping the birth control pill can lead to amenorrhea for up to a year. Many women who breastfeed have no periods until they wean their babies.

More seriously, amenorrhea can be a side effect of being grossly underweight, such as with anorexia nervosa. (Abnormal weight control will be suspected if your weight is as much as 25lbs below average body weight for your height and frame). Stress, certain chronic diseases such as thyroid disease or anemia, and long-term medication with drugs such as tranquilizers and antidepressants can be other causes of amenorrhea.

Amenorrhea may also result from excessive physical activity – some highly trained athletes experience this condition.

Amenorrhea is a permanent condition after the menopause or if you have your uterus removed in a hysterectomy.

· Symptoms ·

▲ Failure of the onset of menstruation and pubertal development – no development of sexual characteristics such as body hair, breasts and pelvic broadening
▲ Periods stop quite suddenly or gradually cease with each successive month until the flow literally dries up

Is it serious?

Even though amenorrhea does not necessarily mean you are ill, it does usually mean that you are not producing eggs and so cannot conceive.

Should I see the doctor?

The tendency to start menstruation late may be inherited, so if your mother started her periods late, don't worry if you aren't developing at the same rate as your friends. However, if you are 18 and have not menstruated, you should be seen by a doctor to check that there is no abnormality. If periods suddenly stop, pregnancy could be the cause, so see your doctor or do a pregnancy test first. In any case, see your doctor if your periods have been absent for four months.

What will the doctor do?

If you have never had a period, your doctor will probably give you a physical examination and take a sample of blood to measure the level of pituitary hormones.

With secondary amenorrhea, once pregnancy is excluded, a full medical examination should be undertaken by a specialist and if you are taking any long-term medications, these should be checked and stopped if necessary. Your doctor may arrange for you to have an X-ray to see if the gland that controls the secretion of hormones, the pituitary gland, is healthy.

Ultrasound scanning or laparoscopy may be undertaken to check your ovaries and pelvis. Hormonal therapy will determine if you are ovulating or not. Your doctor will probably only give you treatment if you want to become pregnant. This is most likely to be with fertility drugs or pituitary hormones.

What can I do?

The lack of menstrual periods is not dangerous to your health and in most cases of amenorrhea, there is no cause for alarm; just be patient and your periods will start up naturally. You may need to change your lifestyle to correct any dietary or physical problems if this was found to be the cause. Remember that after childbirth and during breastfeeding, cessation of periods does not necessarily mean you cannot become pregnant, so you should take precautions if you don't want another pregnancy right away.

OLIGOMENORRHEA

This is a condition when periods are regular but infrequent, that is not approximately every 28 days. There is usually no problem if these periods are preceded by ovulation. Oligomenorrhea is commonly experienced as women approach the menopause.

SEE ALSO:

ANOREXIA NERVOSA
BREASTFEEDING
HYSTERECTOMY
INFERTILITY
LAPAROSCOPY
MENOPAUSAL PROBLEMS
OVARIAN PROBLEMS
ULTRASOUND

AMNIOCENTESIS

This is a procedure in which a small amount of amniotic fluid is drawn off from the amniotic sac in the uterus, without harming the fetus. The fluid is then chemically tested to check on the health of your unborn baby.

Because the amniotic fluid is swallowed by the fetus and passes out through its mouth and bladder, it contains cells of the baby's skin and other organs, which when analyzed under a microscope can give clues to the baby's condition and its sex.

The chromosomes in the cells can be analyzed to give information about 75 different genetic disorders. Not all the tests are done routinely, so it is important for your doctor to authorize all the tests that could apply to you because of your medical and family history. There is a new technique called chorion villus sampling which also diagnoses genetic disorders, but it is still in the experimental stage.

Why is it done?

The major reason for doing this test is to check for chromosomal abnormalities. These are more likely to occur if:

◆ The mother-to-be is over 35. Such women are more at risk of delivering a Down's syndrome baby and may be offered this test routinely at between 16 and 18 weeks of pregnancy. Maternal age is an important factor in Down's syndrome; the incidence rises sharply after 35.

◆ Either parent has a known chromosomal abnormality. For example, if a woman is a carrier of a genetic disorder such as hemophilia, her sons will have a 50% chance of being affected. Amniocentesis reveals the sex of the baby, so if she is carrying a boy, she will need to make the decision whether to terminate her pregnancy.

◆ A chromosomally abnormal child or one with another birth defect

HOW IS IT DONE?

Amniocentesis needs to be done 14 weeks after your last menstrual period because until then there is not enough amniotic fluid or cells to analyze. Before the fluid is removed you will have an ultrasound scan to determine the position of the fetus and placenta. Some women feel no pain, just the sensation of pushing and pulling; others find it more painful. Some report cramps afterwards.

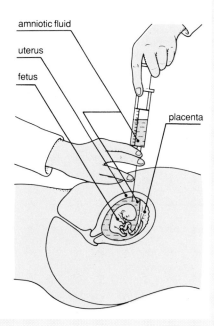
amniotic fluid
uterus
fetus
placenta

Extracting the fluid
After the possible application of a local anesthetic to your stomach, a hollow needle will be inserted through your abdominal wall into the uterus. About 14g (½ oz) will be removed in the syringe. This will be spun in a centrifuge to separate the cells which are then cultured from 2½ to 5 weeks.

has been born previously.

◆ Certain diseases which run in either parent's family including muscular dystrophy and certain errors of metabolism such as phenylketonuria.

◆ The mother has suffered three or more miscarriages.

◆ The baby is to be induced prematurely or delivered early by Caesarean section. The test is done late in pregnancy to determine lung maturity. Premature babies are prone to respiratory distress syndrome.

◆ Neural tube defects such as ancephaly are suspected. It can check also for spina bifida if alpha fetoprotein levels are raised.

◆ There is a Rhesus incompatibility. The test will indicate whether the baby needs an intrauterine blood transfusion or careful attention after birth.

What are the risks?

The risk of fetal injury is practically nil and those of spontaneous miscarriage are slim – approxi-

mately one out of 200 – with trained staff and an ultrasound scan. Other complications such as infection and bleeding are also rare. Some fetal blood cells may leak into the maternal circulation, possibly resulting in complications for Rhesus negative women. The test is about 99% reliable.

The procedure, however, should not be undertaken lightly. You must weigh the reasons for having it and whether you are prepared to have your pregnancy terminated if the tests give you cause for concern. Waiting for the results can be agonizing because your pregnancy is well established and termination will be the same as an induced labor.

SEE ALSO:

DOWN'S SYNDROME
CHORION BIOPSY
GENETIC COUNSELING
PRENATAL CARE
RHESUS INCOMPATIBILITY
ULTRASOUND

ANEMIA

A precise definition of anemia is a lack of hemoglobin in the blood. Hemoglobin is the red pigment which carries oxygen around the body and makes the red blood cells look red. Anemia may be due to a reduced number of circulating red cells, or to a fall in the hemoglobin content of the red cells, or to a combination of both. Therefore anemia must be caused by a deficiency of certain factors which are necessary for the formation of red blood cells, such as iron, folic acid, Vitamin B12, or to a diminished production of red cells. The latter group includes conditions such as leukemia, bone cancer and malignancy of the blood-forming material.

What causes it?
There isn't space here to go into all the causes of anemia, so I am only

discussing the iron and vitamin deficiency anemias to which women are particularly prone. All of us lose some blood and therefore hemoglobin each month with menstruation. During pregnancy there are changes in the way our bodies use folic acid, which is one of the B vitamins. Both folic acid and iron are needed to help the baby's development. If your body has too little folic acid, folic-acid deficiency anemia will result and this is why folic acid and iron are routinely given to pregnant women. We only need small amounts, but we need them daily, the best source being green leafy vegetables. The latest research indicates that all women may not need these supplements when pregnant, but deficiency is so serious that all women have their blood tested rigorously throughout pregnancy.

Vitamin B12 anemia, also known as pernicious anemia, is usually the result of some abnormality in the way our bodies absorb Vitamin B12. Most of us get enough Vitamin B12 from our diets, but if there is a lack of a certain substance in our

WOMEN AT RISK

Poor eaters
Most healthy women eat a balanced diet to provide enough iron, folic acid and Vitamin B12. However, some women who eat junk food or are on a poor diet because of economic circumstances or old age, or those who adopt extreme measures to combat their compulsive eating (bulimia) may become anemic. All deficiency anemias are most common among the elderly and poor.

Menstruating women
If your periods are excessively heavy (menorrhagia), you may lose more hemoglobin than you can make up in the following three weeks and over a period of time this may lead to iron-deficiency anemia. Therefore, if you have heavy periods or frequent periods, make a special effort to include a foodstuff rich in iron in your diet.

Pregnant women
Pregnancy is a time of regular blood tests to check for deficiency anemias. The increase in the volume of blood (a pregnant woman has about $1^1/2$ liters (3 pints) more blood) means that more iron is needed to supply the red blood cells. Folic acid is needed for the development of the baby and iron is laid down in the fetus' liver as a store for the first six months of life because breast milk contains only traces of iron. If you have a multiple pregnancy, make sure you take the folic acid supplements and eat foods rich in the vitamin; mild folic acid deficiency is 3 times as common among women with multiple pregnancies.

New mothers
After the birth of your baby the tiredness and lethargy that often occurs may mask a mild

case of anemia. You will need to build up your strength again, so continue to keep an eye on your diet and make sure it is full of iron-rich foods.

Heavy aspirin users
Aspirin taken in large amounts can lead to irritation of the stomach lining. If this causes internal hemorrhaging which goes unnoticed, anemia may be the first symptom of this form of drug abuse which is common among women.

With affected relatives
The tendency to have insufficient quantities of intrinsic factor is inherited so if a close relative suffers from this type of anemia you may be at risk.

Post-surgical
Pernicious anemia may be the result of surgery on the intestine.

stomachs, known as intrinsic factor, Vitamin B12 won't be absorbed. Pernicious anemia not only affects the production of the red blood cells, but it is vital to the central nervous system.

Should I see the doctor?

If you are pale and tired, especially if you are not eating a well-balanced diet for any reason, see your doctor to check for anemia.

What will the doctor do?

You will be referred for a blood test to find out what the specific deficiency is. Normal hemoglobin levels are about 14g of hemoglobin per 100ml of your blood. If your reading is below 11g/100ml, your doctor may treat you for anemia, although you may need further tests to determine the precise reason for your condition. As most deficiency anemias can be cleared up by dietary means, your doctor will probably give you supplements in the form of pills or injections, depending on the severity. Severe cases may require a blood transfusion. If it is discovered that you have a Vitamin B12 deficiency because of an absorption problem, you will require further tests to confirm this and you will need Vitamin B12 supplements for life.

What can I do?

The best form of treatment for any iron and folic acid deficiency anemia is prevention. All menstruating women should eat a diet rich in iron – green leafy vegetables, fish, red meat, liver, watercress, dried fruits. The B vitamins are plentiful in brewer's yeast, wheatgerm products and in whole grains. If you are a strict vegetarian, you may need to supplement with synthetic Vitamin B12 as the best sources are found in animal products such as fish, white meats, milk, cheese and eggs.

Iron is quite difficult for the body to absorb efficiently and taking Vitamin C at the same time increases absorption. Antacid medications, on the other hand, limit the absorption of iron. You can greatly increase the content of iron in your food by cooking in iron pots.

SEE ALSO:

BULIMIA
MENORRHAGIA
PREGNANCY
PRENATAL CARE

ANOREXIA NERVOSA

This is an extreme example of using food as a weapon to cope with seemingly insoluble problems. It can be interpreted as a weapon to use against family, teachers and oneself. Anorexia may start at different ages, but usually it is at a time when the issues of autonomy, independence and self esteem come to a head. Many anorexics feel they are involved in a struggle for autonomy they can't win. That would explain why anorexia arises frequently with the onset of puberty. The pressure of coming to terms with the physical and mental changes of adolescence may be very hard for an anorexic girl to take, as she feels forced into maturity before she thinks she can cope with it. She may fear growing up because she feels she is not ready to approach the pressures this brings. She feels that if she is not developing and retains a child-like form, she won't have to shoulder adult responsibilities. As a result, these girls often find lectures on sex and puberty the opposite of reassuring; they interpret them as threatening.

What causes it?
However, all anorexics are different and anorexia arises differently in each sufferer. The term anorexia nervosa literally means loss of appetite due to nervous causes. An insecure girl may feel that in a culture that regards the thinner figure as attractive and desirable, it is tempting to go on a strict diet in order to maintain a slim shape. If this gets out of control it results in emaciation and other physical side effects such as the suppression of menstruation (amenorrhea) and the growth of soft downy hair. Vitamin and mineral deficiencies occur because too little essential nutrients are eaten. At this point all the body tissues begin to waste away, particularly those with protein. This is why anorexics appear to have no muscles whatso-

ever. Eventually, the persistent anorexic will starve herself to death.

Anorexia must be thought of as a state of mind and not a physical illness that can be cured like a cold. Many anorexics feel that they'd rather be dead than fat and go to extraordinary lengths to avoid putting on weight. They starve themselves – often secretly so their families and friends may not realize the true extent of the problem – and exercise frantically but they still don't see the bones sticking through their skin as grotesque. In a mirror they see themselves as fat, so they're constantly on a treadmill not to gain weight.

· S y m p t o m s ·

- ▲ Extreme thinness – emaciation
- ▲ Cessation of menstruation
- ▲ Growth of soft downy hair
- ▲ Regression to pre-adolescent physical state
- ▲ Inability to eat to the point of starvation
- ▲ Secretive eating habits to mask the true food intake

Should I consult the doctor?
As anorexics tend not to recognize they are ill and need help, you as parent, relative or friend may have to make the first move. You should first talk the problem over with your family doctor. Even more helpful may be one of the voluntary organizations who are sympathetic to anorexics. They will advise you on the best approach. In many cases, the anorexic may be so devious that setting up treatment becomes very difficult.

What will the doctor do?
Counseling is the basis of treatment. It is very important for anorexics to get the kind of help they need and initially they must be encouraged to recognize that something is wrong. Self help groups have excellent results. This involves

working together with other women where common problems can be shared, discussed and worked on.

In severe cases, medical treatment may be necessary; the anorexic may need hospitalization for controlled feeding and psychotherapy. Force feeding may save a life in extreme examples, but it will not exact a cure, so time and patience is important, especially with very young sufferers. Systems of reward and encouragement are important for young patients. However, if there is mental illness, drugs may be administered to promote weight gain. One such drug is chlorpromazine.

What can I do?
You must try to build up the anorexic's confidence and help her to be kinder to herself and not to set such high standards. It's very good for an anorexic to hear over and over again that she is quite good enough the way she is. To prevent a relapse, she may need psycho-therapy for years.

Watch the way you treat your young children at mealtimes. Children learn to use food as a manipulative tool early in their lives. Parents who show a fussy concern at mealtimes and use bribery to achieve the object of a clean plate will set problems for themselves later. As long as a child has a healthy selection of foodstuffs, and some freedom of choice, there should be no reason for her to use food as a weapon against a parent.

SEE ALSO:

Amenorrhea
Bulimia
Depression
Eating problems

ANXIETY

We all feel anxious at some time in our lives – whether about nuclear war, our financial or sexual affairs, or on behalf of others – but real anxiety with symptoms of panic and excessive uneasiness can put these worries out of all proportion to reality. The true definition of anxiety is a fear reaction. The whole body is in a state of tension – jumpy, nervous and agitated. The brain is confused and unable to sort things out quickly and clearly. In the short term, in the case of an accident for example, the anxiety reaction increases our efficiency and is a protective mechanism. However, if we experience anxiety as a reaction to emotional stress, there can be a deleterious effect on the body.

What causes it?

Long-term stress usually results because of certain events that occur or recur in our lives and over which we have little control. This could be difficult working conditions, marital problems, illness, separation, bereavement and financial problems. In fact, any difficult situation can give rise to varying degrees of stress. You may not even be aware of the effect the stressful situation is having upon your physical well being and after trying to cope, you might suffer a nervous collapse.

If stressful situations prevail and anxiety becomes long term, chronic anxiety may manifest itself with many physical symptoms such as headaches, stomach pains, sweaty palms and compulsive eating. The symptoms are mainly due to the hormones from the adrenal glands. The brain sends messages to the two adrenal glands and it is the physical effects of adrenalin in the system which give rise to anxiety symptoms.

Real anxiety is normal in daily life but neurotic anxieties, such as obsessional behavior about cleanliness, are reactions out of all proportion to the actual problem.

Certain professions are more stressful than others – journalism for example – but one of the most stressed people in our frenetic modern life is the working mother. However, anyone can be subjected to stress leading to intense anxiety; there appears to be no specific causative effect.

· S y m p t o m s ·

- ▲ High blood pressure
- ▲ Increase in menstrual disorders
- ▲ Panic attacks involving the physical symptoms of fear – fight or flight reflex
- ▲ Heart rate increases as blood flow increases
- ▲ Breathing rate increases for oxygen to help muscular activity
- ▲ Blood pressure increases so blood supply to organs increases
- ▲ Pupils enlarge so we can see better
- ▲ Blood sugar level rises for maximum energy
- ▲ Skin pale and clammy due to sweating
- ▲ Shivering, shaking, clattering of teeth as adrenalin levels tail off; normally this passes, within about half an hour. However, in some people even slight stress can cause these symptoms and panic attacks.

Should I see the doctor?

If you suffer frequent anxiety attacks, you may be convinced that you are suffering from real physical ailments such as a heart condition. If you are aware that you are often anxious, see your doctor soon.

What will the doctor do?

Your doctor will question you about your symptoms and possibly give a complete physical examination to rule out any underlying physical basis for the anxiety. He or she may prescribe anti-depressive drugs or tranquilizers, but these will not be much use in preventing further

attacks. Successful treatment needs to address itself to the root cause of the anxiety. Relaxation techniques in the event of an attack can help but essentially you need to come to terms with the cause of the stress. Your doctor may recommend a therapist to help you deal with your worries and the stress in your life.

What can I do?

While doctors and counselors can help treat anxiety, success relies eventually on the sufferer.

- ◆ Try to control stressful situations and desensitize yourself to stress.
- ◆ Keep yourself in good physical health with a proper diet and regular exercise.
- ◆ Observe how your body works during panic attacks – only so much adrenalin is liberated at any one time and the worst panic fears subside in a few minutes. Once you realize this, try to be still and wait.

How can I cope with a panic attack?

During a panic attack, help yourself by concentrating on something other than yourself and your problem. Look around you and concentrate on a picture or pattern of shapes as hard as you can. You'll find that in a short time, your feelings may start to come back to normal. Stay calm. Try to continue what you are doing slowly. Don't rush at it. Take your time and work towards it. Once you've reached your target, set a new one. Always make the targets achievable and make sure they happen quickly. With the reaching of each goal, reward yourself – success brings success. Once you've learned to control your feelings with these techniques you'll find that you react to situations with less anxiety.

Self knowledge is very liberating and worth working towards because it means that you are well on your way to being able to deal with life's

ANXIETY

LEARNING HOW TO RELAX

Relaxing tense muscles can counteract the effects of stress. The simplest way to relax, without using any special equipment except for a cushion or two, is to lie on your back on the floor, with your legs hip-width apart, in a quiet, comfortable place. Loosen any tight clothing and remove your shoes. Breathe in and tense each part of the body as described below and count to ten. Breathe out as you relax.

Face
Close eyes, slightly open mouth, smooth your forehead upwards

Head and neck
Lower your chin to lengthen the back of your neck

Shoulders
Pull your shoulder blades together and down, and then flatten and spread them into floor

Abdomen
Tense your stomach

Buttocks
Push hard against the floor

Toes
Curl them downwards or towards yourself

Calves
Point toes to face

stresses. Also remember that your feelings can't harm you. You are not in danger. Say this to yourself over and over again. You may have to control these anxiety reactions all your life if you find that you can't prevent them.

STRESS

There is no medical treatment for stress – it would be wrong if there were. Too much in our lives is medicalized. We need to learn to avoid unnecessary stress and cope with any we run up against.

Certain factors in all our lives at some time lead to stress in healthy individuals. Because of a woman's traditional role within the family, her central involvement in some of these may lead to a high degree of stress with a higher chance of stress-related illness. Some of the more stressful occurrences are death of a spouse or family member, pregnancy, sexual difficulties, marriage and children leaving home.

Coping with stress

React only to stress that is unavoidable. Ignore the rest. Try to discriminate and save your energy for combatting the unavoidable situations. Try to put the problems out of your head and relax. Get another opinion on the problem.

You may be mismanaging your time, so look at the way you apportion your energy and time. Examine your limitations and scale down your expectations to realistic levels. Stress will eventually weaken your performance anyway. Realistic expectations will make you more efficient and more satisfied with your performance.

Any kind of physical activity is a tranquilizer and helps deal with stress, so try to incorporate some into your life every day.

Take action. Analyze the problem on paper. Write down a list of the possible causes of your stress. This should scale down the problem, and help suggest solutions and pinpoint what is causing the stress or the

component in your life that gives you most anxiety. The problem once defined, may no longer seem insurmountable. Try to work through optional solutions. Select the most realistic and opt for the one you think most likely to succeed. Give yourself a timetable for each part of the action plan.

What can stress lead to?

If stress builds up, this can lead to serious symptoms such as migraine headaches, skin conditions such as dermatitis, functional disorders such as duodenal ulcers, spastic colon and dyspepsia, asthma and diabetes. People under stress are more susceptible to viral illnesses.

SEE ALSO:

ALCOHOLISM
DIGESTIVE PROBLEMS
DRUG DEPENDENCY
HEADACHES

ARTHRITIS

Arthritis means inflammation of the joint. The different types of arthritis all affect women more commonly than men. *Rheumatoid arthritis* is the form most common in young adult women. It is one of the *autoimmune diseases* caused by an allergic reaction in the body, mainly affecting the joints and especially those of the hands, feet, wrists and ankles.

Osteoarthritis is quite different from rheumatoid arthritis; there is, in fact, no inflammation. It usually begins in late middle age. It is said to be the natural aging process of joints, which in some people occurs earlier in life than it should.

Degenerative Joint Disease
A particular form of arthritis occurs in post-menopausal women, and mainly affects the terminal joints of the fingers. As with osteoarthritis, this type is characterized by bony out-growths. Small, pea-sized lumps may occur on either side of the joint – Heberden's nodes – and this is a classical sign of the condition. As this is not a destructive joint disease, it is treated symptomatically with analgesics.

Infectious arthritis
Whenever you have an infectious disease such as influenza, there may be arthritic pain in the joints. These pains disappear with the infection and leave no permanent effect. True infectious, or septic, arthritis occurs when there is a bacterial infection in the joint. This only occurs with one joint. Antibiotic treatment is essential or the joint will be permanently damaged. This infectious arthritis may result from bacterial infection with an *STD* such as *gonorrhea*.

Spondylitis
The spine takes a great deal of strain during one's lifetime. When its joints are affected by arthritis, they may put pressure on the nerves and give rise to pain down the arms with numbness and tingling in the fingers, and in the lumbar region, to sciatic pain spreading through the buttocks to the back of the legs. This is known as spondylitis.

Sufferers of the skin condition psoriasis sometimes develop swollen, painful joints.

ARTIFICIAL INSEMINATION

This is a relatively simple method of trying to achieve a pregnancy in couples who have failed to conceive. There are two types: AIH – artificial insemination using your husband or partner's sperm, and AID – artificial insemination using an anonymous donor's sperm.

Why is it done?

AIH is the option for men whose sperm count is normal, but there is a problem with intercourse either because of psychosexual difficulties, physical injury or handicap. Sometimes the semen may have been stored by a man who has to undergo treatment that leaves him sterile, such as chemotherapy. It is also used to ensure the sperm reaches the cervix when the sperm count is low, or there is a low volume of ejaculate or the woman's vaginal acid is too hostile.

If a woman's partner has too few sperm, or too many abnormal sperm, or he is the carrier of a genetically transmitted disease, or if she simply wants a baby but has no male partner, the sperm of a donor is used.

Donor selection is not yet standardized. Donors tend to be students or people from a group known to the doctors. They are screened for as many physical and mental disorders as possible, including the AIDS virus. Some centers try to match physical characteristics such as hair color and stature. These checks are as yet only guidelines. Although legal, some doctors regard AID as being ethically questionable and some refuse to co-operate.

How is it done?

Artificial insemination is done in special centers on the day before ovulation, and sometimes again in the next two days after that. Ovulation is deduced from temperature and menstrual charts and from measuring hormone levels daily in the urine. Just before ovulation

DEPOSITING THE SPERM

Fresh sperm collected from one's partner, or frozen donor sperm can be used.

With a speculum holding the vaginal walls apart, the semen is injected into the cervix with a small syringe. Sometimes semen is sprayed around the vagina. Afterwards the woman lies with her buttocks slightly raised for 30 minutes or a cervical cap is fitted.

speculum

pool of sperm

there is a marked increase in certain hormones in the urine. Depending on her situation, the woman may have been given fertility drugs to ensure ovulation occurs.

The semen is collected fresh, usually via masturbation, from the male partner, and frozen in the case of donor sperm. A speculum holds the vaginal walls apart while the semen is injected into the cervix with a small syringe. Some doctors spray semen around the vagina too. The woman will need to lie down with her buttocks slightly raised for about 30 minutes. Sometimes a cap is fitted over the cervix so she can get up right away.

If pregnancy doesn't occur, the routine is repeated for up to five more cycles. However, provided tests have been done and the woman is healthy and there are no impediments to conception, with fresh semen the success rate in bringing about a pregnancy within six months is 60-70%; with frozen sperm, it is 55%.

What are the complications?

Whether AIH or AID is sought, the couple should be given counseling routinely. Some couples view AID as a kind of adoption, but with the

feeling of having a closer relationship with the child. With fewer children for adoption, AID is now one of the only alternatives. Divorce rates in couples who conceived with AID are very low, so it would appear that the children are brought up in stable homes.

AID is not straightforward, however. There is the legal aspect of the legitimacy of a child born with AID. Though this is not as much of a stigma or problem as before, there is still the question of the status of the child, and the legal position of the wife if she uses AID without her husband's consent.

SEE ALSO:

INFERTILITY

AUTOIMMUNE DISEASE

Autoimmune disease results when the body becomes allergic to its own tissue and attacks it as though it was foreign. Symptoms depend on whichever tissue is most dramatically involved in the specific disease. The commonest of all the autoimmune diseases is *rheumatoid arthritis* where pain, stiffness, immobility and destruction of joints are the most obvious signs. In another condition, polyarteritis nodosa, it is the arteries that become most inflamed; in dermato-myositis it is the skin; and in polymyositis, the muscles where the allergic reaction takes place. Nevertheless, the joints and other organs are involved. The autoimmune diseases are a "family" of diseases, all of which share the same symptoms to a greater or lesser degree. This is because the allergic reaction takes place within the connective tissue that forms the architecture of most organs. The basic component of connective tissue is collagen. These diseases are sometimes called collagen vascular diseases.

The natural history of autoimmune diseases is that they go through periods of waxing and waning. Each relapse has to be treated on its own merits but can vary from mild to very severe. Some of the autoimmune diseases such as rheumatoid arthritis burn out after several years and become inactive, but usually only after a fair degree of joint and organ destruction. Others may go on chronically for many years.

Other autoimmune diseases include *systemic lupus erythematosus*, 90% of whose sufferers are women, mainly in their early childbearing years. Still's disease is a juvenile rheumatoid arthritis that affects girls between the ages of two and five. Attacks last a few weeks and the disease usually runs its course by the time the child reaches puberty. Scleroderma is a rare condition that affects the skin making it shiny, tight and thickened.

Hashimoto's disease is a form of hypothyroidism (see *Hyperthyroidism*) in which the body's antibodies attack the thyroid gland.

BACKACHE

Your spine is made up of about 30 vertebrae. Between each pair of vertebrae is a disc and the disc and vertebrae are held together with ligaments. Mild backache is usually caused because some part of this mechanism is twisted or stretched. Severe backache, however, is more usually the result of pressure on the nerves because of a malalignment of one of these bones or discs. This type of back pain can be disabling because the nerves are affected, making movement excruciatingly painful. Other back pain results from bad posture or a sagging mattress.

Pain in the low part of your back is the most common back pain in women because it usually has a gynecological cause. The most common is with menstruation. Throughout pregnancy, and in labor, particularly if your baby is lying in the posterior position with its head pressing against your sacrum, you will experience some backache. A labor position on all fours is recommended for a backache labor.

If you are unable to make a diagnosis from this information, consult your doctor.

SITE AND NATURE OF PAIN	PROBABLE CAUSE
The pain goes round and down the sides of your abdomen, and you have a fever and/or notice a burning sensation when you pass urine	This may be a kidney infection. Consult your doctor.
You have recently had a fall or an accident, and you notice other symptoms such as tingling down your legs, difficulty moving a limb and loss of bowel or bladder control	You may have damaged your spinal cord. See your doctor immediately.
You have been doing strenuous exercise or spring cleaning, gardening or decorating, and the pain prevents you moving and shoots down one leg	You probably have sciatica which can be caused by a prolapsed disc. Consult your doctor. It could just be a muscle strain in which case rest, painkillers and hot water bottles or heating pads will help.
The pain is in your joints and you are over 45	This could be the beginning of *osteoarthritis* or the symptoms of *osteoporosis* if you are post menopausal.
You are into the second trimester of your pregnancy	Backache is quite common in middle to late pregnancy. If your baby is due, this may be the first sign of *labor*.
You are overweight	*Obesity* can lead to backstrain.
You are menstruating and the back pain gets worse towards the end of the cycle	This could be *endometriosis* which causes severe pain before and during your period.
You suffer from low back pain nearly all the time	This could be a pelvic disorder such as *ovarian cysts*, *fibroids* or a fallopian tube infection.

BATTERED WOMEN

We tend to think that wife battering is a recent phenomenon. It was first reported in the 1870s but not until the 1970s did the general public begin to recognize this hidden violence as a common problem. Since 1972, many communities throughout the United States have developed crisis intervention, emergency assistance, emergency shelters, peer counseling and other services for battered women. A major breakthrough occured across the country when states passed legislation that made spouse abuse a criminal offense and gave abused wives access to the criminal court system.

Media attention focused on the issue has forced society to question some men's behavior within marriage and now the law is beginning to recognize rape within marriage. Battering is often linked to sexual violence. Wives describe other forms of brutality such as punching, kicking, the use of weapons, boiling water and even attempted strangulation. Battering is rarely only physical; it can involve humiliation and mental torture as well.

Who does the battering?

In the United States, researchers estimate that some 1.8 million American wives are beaten by their husbands each year, and that 16 out of every 100 couples are involved in marital violence. According to some researchers, incidents of violence perpetrated against women by the men they love and live with, whether married or not married, reaches well into the millions. There's also an association between spouse abuse and child abuse, in investigations of child abuse; a great number of the cases involve cruelty to the mother.

Who is battered?

Certain erroneous views have built up about wife battering.

- Few, if any, battered women are masochistic and enjoy or invite being beaten.
- It is not only the lower classes but middle and upper class women who are beaten.
- Women of every religious and ethnic background and at every educational level are beaten.
- The majority of wife beaters are professionally successful. They are often charming and loving and do not exhibit necessarily psychopathic personalities.
- Battering is not always lessened during the lifetime of a marriage or after marriage if it was present earlier in a de facto relationship.

Why does it happen?

When looking for a cause, we find that men who beat their women have several qualities in common. They may have "learned" domestic violence from their own parent's behavior. An immature personality and low self-esteem is common, leading to the acquisition of macho attitudes from their peer groups. Very often they are traditionalists with a strong belief in family unity and their wife's subordinate role. They may blame others for their actions, be pathologically jealous, exhibit severe stress reactions and an aggressive use of sex. Other related factors include a history of childhood violence and ambivalent relationships with their mothers. Aggravating factors can also include alcoholism, drug abuse, stress and obsession with their wife's sexual fidelity.

Why do women stay?

Generally a woman who has suffered battering feels that she must be in some part to blame and that her behavior warranted physical violence from her partner. Many people ask why a woman does not leave her man but, in fact, very few battered women are in a position to do so mainly due to economic, social and psychological pressures. Others are fearful that they will be stigmatized if they tell family or friends, or even the authorities about the abuse. Many women have an unswerving love for their partners and are unwilling to break up their families. Isolation and depression may result in apathy which prevents them from taking any steps to rectify a deteriorating situation.

A woman with small children is often totally dependent on her partner for money. In many countries, the home is the property of the husband alone, meaning the woman will find difficulty securing alternative accommodation should she leave home.

A woman who leaves home with small children and is then considered homeless, runs the risk of having her children taken into care by the local authorities. A woman with children may despair of her ability to raise them alone.

What can you do?

Despite the difficulties, a woman must be helped to leave a physically abusive partner and she should ruthlessly enlist the aid of friends and relatives to do this. Many cities offer hotlines for battered women. Once out of physical danger, she will need help and counseling to develop feelings of self-esteem and competence. More than that, she will need services including refuges where she can be helped to reorganize her life with her children. More effective means of enforcing financial payments would provide maltreated women with financial resources.

Legal protection is available to women through restraining orders handed down by the court, banning a husband from approaching his wife. Medical treatment as an out-patient in hospital emergency rooms is always available but women should be admitted to hospital to have their injuries treated and as a refuge, and to get witnesses to their conditions.

By far the most important and useful change that is necessary to lower the prevalence of wife battering is the rejection of the macho view of male aggression, particularly in the husband's role.

BENIGN BREAST DISEASE

Fibrocystic disease and other non-malignant lumps in the breast are often referred to as benign breast disease to differentiate them from malignant cancer. Some of these conditions are normally found in many women with no ill effects.

The most serious disorder of the breast is breast cancer but even this can be detected early at a treatable stage by regular self-examination.

What causes it?
Cysts or benign tumors found in the breast are uncomfortable rather than painful and in many cases they can be effectively treated. If one of the milk-producing ducts or sebaceous glands around the areola becomes blocked, a fluid-filled cyst may develop.

A fibroadenoma is another non-malignant condition which occurs when the milk-producing glands thicken, causing firm, painless lumps that seem to move about within the breast. These are harmless and don't usually require treatment. This is usually found in young women.

Fibrocystic disease, also known as cystic mastitis, chronic cystic mastitis, or cystic disease of the breast, is present in about 30% of all women. This is usually found during the years when women are producing estrogen – the childbearing years.

Nearly all women can detect some mild fibrocystic disease in the breast prior to menstruation. The breast feels as though it is filled with nodules about the size of orange pips. This is because the breast is primed by estrogen, then stimulated by progesterone, prior to menstruation, as it prepares itself for pregnancy by growing tissue in the milk-producing glands. These are swollen just before menstruation but the swelling subsides and the breast is back to normal by the time menstruation has ceased. The swelling makes the breasts heavy, tender and tingling. Sometimes they may be so sore they cannot be touched. These symptoms are reported as part of premenstrual syndrome.

Very rarely fibrocystic disease becomes chronic and takes the form of more solid masses and it is largely this more solid type that runs the risk of developing into breast cancer. Therefore, women with this disease should examine their breasts carefully every month and if they are over 35 or in a high risk group, they should ask their doctors for a baseline mammogram and direction on how frequently they should follow up with additional mammograms. Many doctors recommend that starting at age 40, women with fibrocystic disease have annual mammograms.

· S y m p t o m s ·

▲ Lump or lumps in the breast – some as small as orange pips, others up to 2cm (1in) across
▲ Heaviness and tenderness of the breasts
▲ Solid masses in the breast – this is a chronic condition

Should I see the doctor?
See your doctor if self-examination reveals anything different in the character and shape of your breasts.

What will the doctor do?
Your doctor will examine you and arrange for you to have a mammogram. You will then be treated according to the nature of the lump. Only about one in ten lumps is cancerous.

Treatment for a cyst is usually under a local anesthetic when a long needle draws off the fluid, or by surgical removal of the cyst and, if there is infection, with a course of antibiotics. The fluid will always be tested for malignant cells.

If fibroadenomas cause pain, your doctor may prescribe hormone therapy to get rid of them.

The treatment for fibrocystic disease is not always satisfactory, but depending on the most uncomfortable symptoms, relief can be gained.

Water retention can contribute to discomfort prior to menstruation and many patients respond to diuretic drugs which do reduce heaviness and tenderness in the breasts. These drugs can flush valuable minerals out of the system, so watch your diet.

Some women get relief by taking a low dose oral contraceptive pill or drugs containing sex hormones which prevent the secretion of estrogen and progesterone by acting on the pituitary gland.

Your doctor will usually surgically remove a benign tumor and give you regular check-ups in case of malignancy.

In cases where cysts and tumors recur and with them the obvious anxiety about possible malignancy, the specialist may do a sub-cutaneous mastectomy and reconstruct them with silicone implants.

What can I do?
If your breasts are heavy and tender, wear a firm supporting bra. Examine your breasts routinely, once a month, to check for any changes.

SEE ALSO:

BREAST CANCER
BREAST SELF-EXAMINATION
BREASTFEEDING PROBLEMS
HORMONE REPLACEMENT
  THERAPY
MAMMOGRAPHY
MASTECTOMY
PREMENSTRUAL SYNDROME

BIOPSY

A biopsy is a minor operation most often performed under local anesthetic either superficially (on the skin) or deep (in the bone marrow for example), to extract a small piece of body tissue and examine it under a microscope for the presence of disease or abnormality.

Why is it done?

Biopsy is most often performed to detect malignant change. An excision biopsy would be performed on a pigmented mole where there were signs that it might be undergoing malignant change. With a suspicious breast lump, a needle might be passed into the center of the lump and a few cells drawn off into a syringe to see whether it was benign or malignant.

In someone who is a chronic drinker where cirrhosis of the liver is suspected, a needle biopsy would be performed to take a specimen of liver cells. This would be done under a local anesthetic. The operation is simple and quick, taking about 10 to 15 minutes with the cells examined under the microscope the same day to give a rapid result.

The liver is rarely treated surgically so it is sometimes necessary to do a biopsy to check on the efficacy of treatment.

One of the investigations performed on a patient with anemia might be a bone marrow biopsy, quite often taken with a wide-bore needle inserted into the middle of the breastbone or hip to remove a specimen of liquid bone marrow. Pathologists would be on the look out for an arrest of red and white cell development.

A biopsy may be done when there is a lump, a tumor, a cyst or a swelling of unknown character and doctors feel that they can only reach an accurate diagnosis by taking a bit of that lump and looking at the cells directly. Only then is it possible to decide what is going on, what treatment should be recommended, and with what vigor a cure should be pursued.

HOW A BIOPSY IS PERFORMED

A biopsy can be done in a variety of ways depending on whether the area to be tested for abnormal growth is on the skin or within the body. Most biopsies are performed under a local anesthetic, either:

◆ by means of a scrape which simply removes a thin film of surface cells, such as during a Pap smear or a D & C, to assess if underlying malignant change is causing symptoms.

◆ by surgery to take a specimen of skin or remove a gland or excise a melanoma. During major surgery a small piece of suspicious tissue could be removed or examined microscopically for cancerous change.

◆ with a needle to remove a sample of fluid in the breast; this investigates cysts or other lumps detected in the breast.

◆ with a hollow needle passed into the liver via an incision made over the right lower ribs and a slim needle inserted through it to remove a sample of tissue.

◆ by means of a fiberoptic excision, when a fine tube with a lens and a light is passed into the body so the inside can be visualized. A small specimen is removed with a tiny knife in the head of the instrument. This is done for ovarian cysts, to prove a gastric ulcer is malignant or to confirm the tumor type of a growth in the colon or rectum.

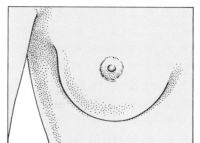

A breast biopsy is an alternative to mammography. A small piece of tissue is removed for analysis; the incision quickly repaired.

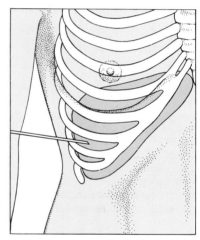

In a liver biopsy the patient holds his or her breath while the needle is inserted between the ribs or through the abdomen.

When is a biopsy done?

A biopsy is taken so that treatment and follow-up can be properly planned. The inevitable consequence of a biopsy is a decision that the lesion is benign and no further action is necessary, or that it is malignant and anti-cancer treatment should start. Follow-up treatment with chemotherapy, or deep X-ray therapy may be advised. In this sense, a biopsy is only a means to an end.

An open biopsy is done as part of an operation under general anesthetic when an endoscopic investigation is impossible. In this case, prompt analysis is vital in case the surgeon needs to remove the diseased area immediately, thus avoiding another general anesthetic and surgery later.

In order to get a quick result, for breast cancer for example, the sample of tissue is prepared for

BIOPSY

BREAST LUMPS AND BIOPSIES

The biopsy of breast lumps and cysts is worth a special mention. In the past, far too often the possibility of a mastectomy was never discussed with patients prior to investigative surgery. Quite often the first a woman knew about the possibility that she had breast cancer was when she woke up after the operation to find that one of her breasts had gone. This is brutal and intolerable and no woman should allow herself to be put in this position.

If you have any kind of a lump or cyst in the breast, demand that you have a prior breast biopsy so that

you can be told of the diagnosis and participate in the decision as to what kind of surgery will be performed. It's your breast and it's only just and fair that you should be involved. It will also give you some time to make the psychological and emotional adjustments to losing a breast. Request that you see a counselor who has experience in helping women in the same position as you. You will also have the opportunity of discussing what kind of breast reconstruction or prosthesis you would want to wear.

analysis by freezing it in liquid nitrogen and cutting it in a section or smearing it on a slide to study its cytological features. A method that is more time consuming is when the sample is embedded in wax for firm consistency so that after about 24 hours it can be cut into fine slices and placed on a slide.

How a result is obtained

To obtain a result, the slide is viewed under a microscope by a pathologist who notes any distortion or alteration of the tissue structure. If the biopsy was taken to check for an infection, such as after a throat or vaginal swab, the sample will be tested with specific antibodies or a specific tissue culture may be required, as happens with the fluid aspirated during an amniocentesis test in pregnancy.

An electron microscope is used to distinguish the cell origin of certain tumors and with tissue taken from the kidneys. Special enzymes and antibodies are used to stain samples in other cases. These procedures take longer but give a more accurate diagnosis and provide more information about the future activity of the tumor or disease.

BIRTHMARKS

These are discolored patches or lumps in the skin varying in size and color. The thing they have in common is that they are present at or shortly after birth.

What are they caused by?

Birthmarks or nevi are usually either a collection of pigmented cells or a lump of tiny capillary blood vessels in the skin. The pigmented nevi are brown in color and may contain hairs, when they are called moles. The capillary or vascular nevi are pink, red or bluish-purple in color.

Many tiny birthmarks, such as a stork's bite at the nape of the neck, are so common they are accepted as almost normal. They often disappear within the first year. Many larger capillary nevi also disappear, particularly those in the upper layers of skin. They may wither, shrink and become so pale that they are hardly visible.

Whether pigmented or vascular, nevi can vary in size, shape and texture from something small, flat and pale to an extensive dark, colored lump. The less noticeable the birthmark, the less interference the better. Even the most disfiguring vascular marks may fade and whiten with time.

The only birthmark that tends not to fade spontaneously is the port wine stain. If this is large and diffused and on exposed parts of the body, it can be very disfiguring. The color can be intensified by crying, exertion and exposure to heat and cold. Thickening of the skin with age and tanning may obscure the stain.

Should I see the doctor?

Consult your doctor if the birthmark worries you or makes you feel self-conscious and if it cannot be disguised with makeup. If there is any change in a birthmark, consult your doctor.

What will the doctor do?

If you have a pigmented birthmark, any change in the appearance of the mark will be treated with caution by your doctor. Without fail your doctor will recommend a biopsy to check that the true nature of the nevus can be interpreted and any malignant changes identified.

If you have a strawberry nevus, the doctor may advise you to wait and see.

What is the medical treatment?

If there is no cause for concern, and you want the birthmark removed, moles and pigmented birthmarks can be excised. This is usually done under a general anesthetic.

If you have a vascular nevus, a wide variety of treatments are available depending on the depth of the network of blood vessels. A shallow vascular nevus can be burnt off with laser treatment, or cautery, when an electric current burns away the tissue.

Small birthmarks can be frozen with carbon dioxide. There may be some white scarring, but with a trained technician this is a simple, well-tried method.

Sclerosing agents, which cause the skin to harden, can be injected into the nevus, causing it to wither and shrink.

Very deep marks can only be helped with excision and a skin graft.

What can I do?

As most birthmarks are small and flat, they can be disguised by camouflage. There are several ranges of excellent, well-pigmented camouflaging creams on the market in a range of colors. Go to your pharmacist and find one to suit your skin type. With a little practice, the majority of birthmarks can be hidden completely.

BLEEDING (VAGINAL)

As all women bleed from the vagina during menstruation for part of their lives, this is not usually a cause for concern. However, any change in your normal cycle or bleeding between periods should be treated with suspicion.

If you notice any bloody discharge during pregnancy, call your doctor and lie down and wait (see *Pregnancy problems*). The cause of the bleeding will depend on whether you are in early or late pregnancy.

If you are post-menopausal, remember that irregular vaginal bleeding is not normal.

If you are unable to make a diagnosis from this information, consult your doctor.

NATURE OF THE BLEEDING	PROBABLE CAUSE
You are younger than 15 and older than 45	Irregular bleeding can be the result of hormonal changes. An occasional irregularity may not be cause for concern, but after two months, see your doctor if the cycle hasn't settled down.
Bleeding follows intercourse	This could be cervical erosion (see *Cervical problems*). Go to your doctor for a *Pap smear*.
Your periods become unusually heavy	This is known as *menorrhagia*. You may suffer from *anemia* if you lose a lot of blood every month. See your doctor.
You are or could be pregnant	This might be a spontaneous *miscarriage*, or if there is severe abdominal pain, an *ectopic pregnancy*. See your doctor immediately.
Bleeding is only spotting, and you're on the pill	This may be breakthrough bleeding. If it is bothersome, see your doctor, you may want to change your method of *contraception*.
You are going through menopause	During the menopause, your periods may change in character, but if they are heavy, see your doctor immediately. Irregular heavy bleeding is not a symptom of menopause (see *Menopausal problems*).
You feel heavy or swollen in the lower abdomen, suffer backache and your cycle changes	This could be some disease of the pelvic organs, such as *ovarian cysts* or *fibroids*. See your doctor immediately.
You have an IUD fitted	This can cause the bleeding. See your doctor or go to the family planning clinic (see *Contraception*).

BODY ODORS

To a degree, all body odors, whether they come from the mouth, armpits, genital area – including the vagina and rectum – or the feet, are normal. A basic level of body odor is unavoidable because bacteria inhabit these areas, and in the course of their metabolism, break down normal body substances – sweat, secretions and fluids – into chemicals which smell. Whether you appreciate and enjoy these smells is largely due to per- sonal preference and conditioning. However, they do have a clear biological function.

Body odor from the armpits and genital area, for instance, is due to chemical attractants which both males and females find arousing. This is obvious in the behavior of animals. Female pigs will only allow males to mount them if the male is giving off a strong body odor called "boar taint." Furthermore, in early experiments with oral contraceptives, it was found that male primates (chimpanzee) would not mount the female because the pill had eradicated her natural, female odors. Even in insects, the chemical attractants, pheromones, play an important part in reproduction: some are so strong that a female butterfly can attract a male over a distance of 200 miles.

What are they caused by?

There are specialized sweat glands, the apocrine glands, in the armpits and genital regions of humans, which are found nowhere else in the body. These glands are activated by normal activity and by emotion – excitement, fear and sexual arousal.

To most noses, the accumulation of body odor in a strong concentration is unpleasant, particularly in hot, sweaty conditions, where odiferous breakdown products are released in large quantities.

However, these smells are natural and an obsession with hygiene and the use of artifical, perfumed chemicals to disguise the natural can lead to irritation and possibly

HALITOSIS

This is bad odor from the mouth. It is a mysterious condition and has been attributed to mouth ulcers, bad teeth, infected gums, a coated tongue and a variety of stomach problems. A thorough investigation rarely reveals a specific cause, though in most people lack of food and drink will increase mouth odor. This is because drinking, chewing and swallowing process the saliva in your mouth. Without this the saliva stagnates. This degree of halitosis can be overcome simply by eating or drinking something – a sort of self cleansing.

infection. Vaginal deodorants are a case in point.

Foot odor varies from person to person. The manmade fibers used in shoe production don't allow the feet to breathe naturally. Nylon panty hose and panties also increase accumulation of sweat in the groin, increasing the risk of infection.

Should I consult the doctor?

If the body odor is unusual for you and unpleasant, this could be a symptom of an infection. For example, a vaginal discharge and smelly fishlike odor could be trichomoniasis. Consult your doctor if you notice a different or unpleasant smell.

What can I do?

Almost all body odors are perfectly normal, and basic hygiene takes care of most excesses. This means you should:
- brush and floss your teeth regularly
- bathe your armpits and genital area at least once a day – in exceptionally hot weather, when sweating is profuse, it may be necessary to wash more frequently
- wash sweaty feet daily in the evening
- wear cotton socks which are absorbent or open shoes or sandals which allow air to get to your feet
- wash all socks and stockings after one wearing

I am very much against the use of chemical cleansers and deodorants inside any of the body's orifices because they can upset the delicate chemical balance of bacteria and yeasts which normally live there. If the balance is disturbed, inflammation and allergy may result. I therefore do not recommend you use vaginal deodorants, mouthwashes, chemical douches or sprays. Don't put antiseptics in the bath water as this can act as an irritant.

Anti-perspirants and deodorants can be used according to personal taste under your armpits and eau de cologne or perfume provides an astringent for your face and neck to cool you down and freshen you. Special foot deodorants and anti-perspirant foot powders may be helpful.

SEE ALSO:

DENTAL PROBLEMS
FOOT PROBLEMS
GENITAL PROBLEMS
MOUTH PROBLEMS
TRICHOMONIASIS

BODY SCAN

Scanning machines, whether they are used for the body or the head, combine computers and X-rays. Unlike the first generation of X-ray machines which don't show clear images of soft tissue in the body and whose X-rays come from a single source and direction only, modern scanners take pictures of soft tissue, such as a tumor, and send X-rays from all sides – from a circumference of 360° – with no greater amount of radiation than regular X-rays. The computer then builds these cross-sectional images up into a two-dimensional slice. This means that a total body picture can be received.

Old machines were only able to take an X-ray picture at one particular point on the body. Scanners, particularly those used in computerized tomography, although originally developed to look at the brain, because of improved technology can take pictures at every point through the body, fractions of millimeters apart – almost in fine slices. This means that extremely precise

pictures of the body can be taken. For example, a tumor can be measured in fractions of a millimeter.

It is clear that scanners with image intensification present a leap forward in terms of the amount of information they yield and the accuracy of that information. This allows doctors to make a more accurate and precise diagnosis, guides the technician during a biopsy, improves surgery and helps with prognosis.

Why is it done?

By far the greatest application of body scanners is with malignant disease to assess the size and spread of tumors, particularly in the brain. It is used after a stroke if there is no clear indication of what part of the brain is affected. It can also be used for certain serious abdominal diseases such as liver tumors. One of the ways the body scanners have revolutionized medicine is that they allow doctors to see where they have never been able to look before

without the intervention of surgery or fiberoptics.

Scanning machines are enormously expensive to buy and to run. Several skilled operators are needed and the computer terminals and the expensive scanning equipment are costed by the minute. There is always great pressure on a scanner from the many departments in a large hospital as well as from smaller hospitals which require its use too. A scanner cannot therefore be used for routine investigations where lesser machines will do a good job.

How is it done?

The procedure is painless. Sometimes a substance may be injected into a vein to make certain vessels and organs more visible. If the abdomen is being scanned, a drink of a dye will be given to make the bowel show up more clearly.

You lie on a moveable bed which lies inside a circular apparatus. If your brain is being scanned, your head will be the part covered by the machine. You will be strapped to the table as any movement will blur the pictures. The machine rotates around you.

Examinations can be taken in a multitude of positions with X-ray sources coming from various directions. The images show up on a television screen.

Body scans don't take long to complete but they are somewhat longer than standard X-rays. A recent development, a scanner known as Cine-CAT, takes only milliseconds to achieve an image. This is useful for moving parts in your body, such as the flow of blood through an artery, greatly increasing the diagnosis and treatment of heart disease, for example.

CAT SCANS

In computerized axial tomography, hundreds of X-ray pictures are taken as the machine revolves around the head. The pictures are

then fed into a computer which shows how they relate to the skull, building up a picture of sections of the brain.

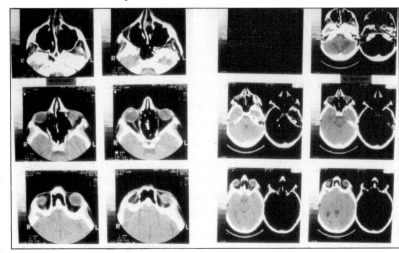

OTHER SCANNING SYSTEMS:

Magnetic Resonance Imaging (MRI)

This is quite often used to view soft tissues such as the brain. MRI machines do not use X-rays to penetrate the body but instead employ a combination of radio-waves and a strong magnetic field.

MRI is particularly useful as it ignores bones and shows up soft tissue which is the opposite of our standard X-ray pictures. It actually reflects the presence of water in cells because it focuses on the behavior of hydrogen atoms in water molecules. This allows MRI to do certain things better than CAT scanners, such as distinguishing between the brain's white matter and the much more water-rich grey matter. Teeth and bones, which contain little water, do not appear at all in MRI enabling doctors to see tissue surrounded by bone such as the spinal cord. MRI has also been used to spot the tiny lesions of multiple sclerosis on brain and spinal tissue.

Digital Subtraction Angiography (DSA)

This is an X-ray picture often used to show up blood vessels, such as those of the heart which would pin-point a blockage that had caused a heart attack. The computer can measure the degree of constriction by converting the image into a digital code and comparing it to others made from different angles.

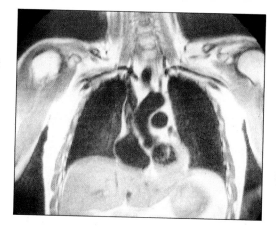

Magnetic resonance imaging is particularly useful for viewing soft tissue. In this scan of a normal healthy person, the heart and circulation are clearly imaged. The blood-filled ventricles are seen pumping blood to the lungs and around the general circulation. The blood vessels supplying the head and arms (the carotid and subclavian arteries) are also visible. The heart is at the center right of the picture with the lungs behind.

It can also measure the rate at which blood diffuses into the heart muscle, giving doctors a good indication of whether or not a heart attack is likely to occur.

Sonography

Ultrasonic scans make pictures with ultrasound and the first snap-shot in the family album may be an ultrasound scan taken at the sixth month of pregnancy which can show the baby's face, organs and limbs clearly. Intra-uterine sono-graphy gives us this sneak preview of what the baby will be like at birth. A computer translates the sound echoes that bounce back into an image of the fetus.

Sonography is the only body scanning technique recommended for pregnant women; it's also well suited for examination of the breasts, heart, liver and gall bladder.

Radioisotope Imaging

This system does not use X-rays but an image is made by a Single Photon Emission Computed Tomography. This shows blood flow by displaying trace amounts of radioisotopes in the blood. So, for instance, in a brain scan, a decrease in blood flow would show up quite clearly as a dark bluish-black patch against a healthy orangey-red background.

Positron Emission Tomography (PET)

This is a refined, versatile technique, which can measure metabolism revealing how well the body is working. Radioactive tracer substances are used in this scanning technique which can study epilepsy, schizophrenia, Parkinson's disease and cerebro-vascular disorders.

SEE ALSO:

CANCER
HEART DISEASE
ULTRASOUND

BREAST CANCER

This is a malignant growth of the tissues of the breast. There are varying malignancies according to the type of cell they grow from; the commonest kind of tumor grows from the milk-producing glands. Some cancers grow very rapidly and others more slowly, depending on the rate of cell division and this factor determines the treatment which will vary according to how aggressive the cancer is. The American Cancer Society projects that one out of every 10 white women born in 1985 will develop breast cancer during her lifetime, and one out of 28 will die from it. They also project that one out of 14 black women, who have a lower overall percentage of breast cancer, born in the same year, will develop breast cancer and that one out of 34 will die from it. Despite these sobering statistics, this is a curable disease. The tumors can be detected in the early stages by regular breast self- examination and by modern screening techniques such as mammography. As the breast is a detachable organ, it can be surgically removed along with any tumours before cancer cells invade other organs via the

bloodstream. However, this depends on early detection because except for the painless lump, there are usually no other symptoms.

Should I see the doctor?
If your monthly self examination or regular check-up detects a lump in your breast, consult your doctor immediately.

What will the doctor do?
If your doctor dismisses a lump and tells you not to worry, get another opinion or visit a family planning or health clinic. If manual examination detects a lump, your doctor

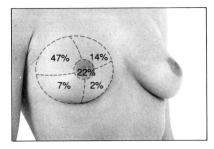

Distribution of cancers
For the purposes of diagnosis, the breast is divided into 4 quadrants – the upper, outer one contains the most tumors.

should refer you for a mammogram. This is a technique that uses X-rays to examine the breast and show up variations in consistency. A tumor will appear as a white patch, denser than the rest of the breast and therefore impenetrable to certain X-rays. However, the only means of determining for certain that a lump is cancerous is through biopsy, in which a small portion of tissue is removed for microscopic examination. If the lump is found to be a fibroadenoma or a benign tumor, you will need to have the lump surgically removed. At this time, you may have another type of biopsy to check further for cancerous cells. If these are found you will need to discuss with your surgeon *before the operation* the

action to be taken while you are under the anesthetic. In the past, too many surgeons removed the breast immediately if the biopsy showed cancer.

What is the treatment?
Once there is a positive diagnosis, you should have further tests to ascertain the extent of the cancer. These include more X-rays, checking the lymph nodes for possible spread of the cancer, blood tests and scans. You should be involved in discussions about the course of your treatment, and the doctors should try to determine where the cancer might have spread in the rest of your body.

The surgical treatment for breast cancer will either be a lumpectomy when the lump is surgically removed on its own, leaving the rest of the breast intact, or a mastectomy, when part or all of the breast and surrounding nodes and muscles are surgically removed. These may be followed by radiation therapy treatment which kills cancer cells by radiation. This will be started when the skin has healed after breast surgery. The frequency of treatment varies, but is usually for a six week period, two or three times a week. You will be required to attend regularly at a radiation therapy clinic at your hospital for this treatment.

Drugs may also be given to interfere with the multiplying cells themselves. These are known as cytotoxic drugs. They have unpleasant side effects because they interefere with other cells as well. However, a specialist will be able to offer different combinations and different drugs to combat your cancer and reduce side effects.

Some cancer cells are responsive to your hormones and during the childbearing years, a plentiful supply of female hormones will encourage the growth of the cancer. Until recently, the removal of those glands that produced hormones –

ovaries, adrenals and pituitary – was the treatment. Now there are chemical means of suppressing the production of the hormones and avoiding surgery.

For a relatively trauma-free and effective treatment of breast cancer, a combination of careful timing, a wide variety of treatment, and specialist medical teams is necessary.

What can I do?

Breast cancer is a chronic illness and you must follow up your treatment with a regular timetable of screening visits to check that the disease has not started up again. A recurrence is known as metastasis, and even if your breast has been removed, there is always the danger of cancer developing in your other breast or secondary cancer in another part of the body.

You should also watch for any minor but lingering symptoms which could indicate problems elsewhere, such as changes in your menstrual cycle or the condition of your lungs.

Contact a self-help group if you feel you need support for yourself and your family. You may be able to help others with your experience. If you feel nervous and lack confidence in the medical staff, take someone with you to help you state your case and support you when you express your feelings to your doctor.

If you fall into a high-risk group, be meticulous about self examin-

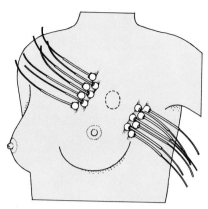

Iridium implants
For a relatively small tumor, one new treatment is to surgically remove the cancerous lump then insert radioactive wires in the breast which kill any stray cancer cells. These wires are later removed. Conventional radiation therapy is also required.

ation. Go to see your doctor for an annual check-up and ask if you can have mammography more regularly. Ask that the lowest dose of X-rays possible is used.

If you discover you have breast cancer, try not to panic. Take time to adjust to your condition and the treatment. Seek psychological help as well as medical treatment. Studies have shown that women who have a chance to discuss the implications and results of their condition are better able to face up to it with their doctors.

SEE ALSO:

BENIGN BREAST DISEASES
BREAST OPERATIONS
BREAST SELF-EXAMINATION
COSMETIC SURGERY
MAMMOGRAPHY
MASTECTOMY
NIPPLE PROBLEMS
RADIATION THERAPY

WOMEN AT RISK

There are certain factors which make you a more likely candidate to develop breast cancer.

 Previous breast disease
a past history of benign breast lumps seems to increase the chances.

 Race
white women are more at risk than other races.

 Heredity
breast cancer tends to run in families.

 Fertility
women who are childless are at greatest risk.

 Age
increased risk after the age of 40.

 Bottlefeeding
only nursing your children at the breast appears to have protective effect.

Diet and environment
the high-protein, high-fat, low-carbohydrate and low-fiber diet favored in developed countries predisposes to breast cancer.

BREAST OPERATIONS

There are four main forms of cosmetic surgery to the breasts, all generally referred to as mammoplasty. Breast reduction makes large, pendulous breasts smaller; breast uplift raises droopy breasts; breast augmentation increases the size of small breasts; and breast reconstruction builds new breasts after mastectomy. The major factor in the success of these operations is the skill of the surgeon and how familiar the operation is to him or her so that the physical and emotional repercussions can be minimized. Another major factor is patient expectation.

BREAST REDUCTION

Reduction mammoplasty is usually done for medical reasons. The breasts may be so large that their size and weight causes pain in the shoulders or back, their size may cause chaffing and skin rashes and make any athletic activity difficult or impossible. Breastfeeding may be impossible with very large breasts. Large breasts may be unfashionable and out of proportion to the woman's height and weight or very embarrassing to a young girl. In some cases one breast is considerably larger than the other.

The size of your breasts may be related to your weight. If you are obese, reducing your overall weight will reduce the size of your breasts.

You should discuss the size and shape of your new breasts with the plastic surgeon and he or she will prepare you for any scarring and the fact that your nipples may lose their sensations. If you want to breastfeed, let the surgeon know. Operations involving the free grafting of the nipple make breast-feeding impossible.

What happens?
You will be in hospital for about five days. The operation takes about three hours under a general

BREAST REDUCTION

This corrects large, pendulous breasts that alter posture, or produce shoulder pain.

Before surgery, an outline of the incisions and future nipple site are drawn by the surgeon.

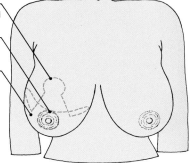

keyhole pattern incision

incision around areola

area to be removed

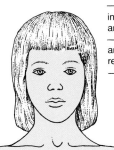

transplanted nipple and areola

incision pattern brought together

Skin, fat, excess breast tissue, and part of the oversized areola are removed. The remaining tissue and fat is secured within the skin covering and the nipple is located higher up.

anesthetic. There are a number of different methods but generally the incisions are made around the nipple and areola and the under-lying fat and breast tissue removed. The nipple is then relocated to a more natural position.

The nipple may be completely numb and there will be soreness and tingling. The stitches will be removed after about six days and you won't be able to play active sports, for example, for about a month. The scars will be red for six months or so, but they eventually fade. Most women who have this operation are delighted with the results. The only problem that may arise is the healing of the scar tissue.

BREAST UPLIFT

Sagging breasts aren't fat, they only need to have excess skin removed and the breast contoured with the nipple relocated to a more natural position. This is called mastopexy. The incisions and surgical procedure is similar to reduction mammoplasty, but simpler and quicker. You will be hospitalized and the operation is done under general anesthetic with the same restrictions on your activity afterwards as with breast reduction. There is little scarring and the results are excellent. The sensations in the nipple won't be lost and you should be able to breastfeed.

BREAST AUGMENTATION

Known as augmentation mammo-plasty, this is the most common cosmetic breast operation. It has few medical implications, as small breasts are just as efficient at breastfeeding as larger ones. Women may have both breasts enlarged or if they have one breast smaller than the other, may have the smaller breast augmented to match the larger. Breast size cannot be increased by any other means such as exercising, although some women on the contraceptive pill experience an increase in size.

What happens?

The operation involves the implantation of silicone gel behind the breast. There have been few recorded instances of allergic reactions to silicone, although sometimes the body may react to it and form a fibrous shield around the implant. If this becomes too hard it can distort the breast shape, but further surgery will correct this.

Before the operation you should talk to the surgeon and discuss the shape and size of your new breasts. Pre-operative mammograms are normally taken to ascertain that no unsuspected malignancy is present.

BREAST AUGMENTATION

The prosthesis' size and shape depends on the chest capacity, the skin available to cover it and the size of the "pocket".

The incision may be below the breast, at the armpit, or at the junction of the areola with the skin.

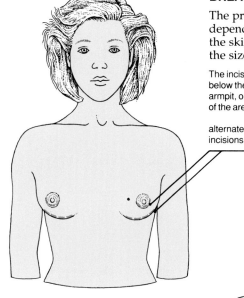

alternate incisions

implant

The implant, a silicone bag containing silicone gel, may be surrounded by an additional bag containing fluid. The breast and overlying tissue are separated and the implant inserted between two inner layers or two muscular layers.

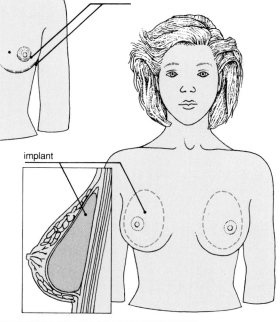

The surgery is usually performed under a general anesthetic though some centers do it with local anesthesia only. You will have discussed where you want the scar which can be made on the curve below the breast or around the areola. A pocket is formed to take the implant and the jelly-filled silicone sac of the agreed size is inserted in place and the incision stitched.

You will experience tingling around the nipple with bruising and soreness for a few days. Active exercise or stretching should be avoided for a month. The scars soon fade and results are very good with the most up-to-date methods. Breastfeeding should still be possible.

More modern advances include a tissue expander which is an inflatable device placed in the breast with a tube to the outside through which a saline solution is gradually introduced to make space for the silicone implant. Other expanders can be left in place and the exterior tube opening closed off when the desired size is reached.

BREAST RECONSTRUCTION

Many women who have had a mastectomy are constantly reminded of it whenever they bathe or undress. Therefore, breast reconstruction, if it is available, is an ideal solution. The first factor to be considered, however, is the timing of the reconstructive surgery. Some surgeons perform the reconstruction at the same time as the mastectomy. This is still a matter of controversy because other medical specialists believe that spotting recurrence of the cancer is difficult with implants. You need to be reassured that no cancer has spread before the operation is undertaken, otherwise you will only be disappointed.

BREAST OPERATIONS

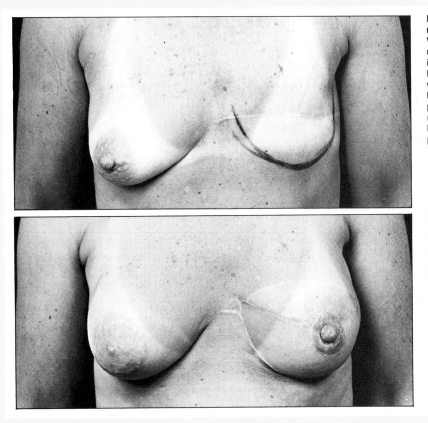

Before breast reconstruction
When a breast is removed, one technique is to allow the incision to heal before proceeding with an implant. Shortly before beginning the procedure the surgeon marks where the new breast is to be positioned.

Post surgery
The implant is covered by skin grafted from elsewhere on the body. A nipple has been created and the scars are practically healed.

What happens?

If you had a subcutaneous or partial mastectomy, then some skin, the nipple and areola will be left in place to cover the implant. If not, skin grafts or flaps of skin will be taken from other parts of your body. Another method is the tissue expander (see previous page) which slowly stretches the skin and tissue so that a silicone implant can eventually be put in its place.

There are many methods of reconstructing a breast after mastectomy and the results are not always as good as new. Some surgeons take fat from the buttocks or abdomen and fashion a nipple from similar skin elsewhere on the body, such as the genitals. This would appear extreme as there are then problems post-operatively with other parts of the body and so

techniques such as tattooing are used to give good results.

This is a more radical operation than the other breast procedures and it will take you about three months to full recovery - you must undertake no active sports or stretching for the first month. There may be some swelling, discoloration and possibly infection after the operation. Scars will occasionally be visible but as the major reason for women having reconstruction has been shown to be for their own peace of mind, this small matter will probably not be an overwhelming problem.

SEE ALSO:

BREAST CANCER
COSMETIC SURGERY
MASTECTOMY

BREAST SELF-EXAMINATION

In the U.S. every year, breast cancer is diagnosed in approximately 135,000 women. There are nearly 42,000 deaths from breast cancer annually. For many of these women, regular breast self-examination would have revealed changes in tissue caused by an early stage of cancer when the disease is most easily treated without further serious consequences.

Why is it done?

By examining your breasts regularly, you can detect lumps and changes in shape or discharge from the nipple so that any problem can be diagnosed and treated while it is entirely treatable . A form of breast screening, mammography, is more effective than self-examination but as it is not available to every woman, a routine of self-examination is most important.

It has been proven that if malignant lumps are found in the breast when they are small (less than 2cm in diameter) and new, the chances of survival are greatly enhanced. All breasts become lumpy in the week before menstruation. The tenderness of pre-menstrual syndrome may even become a permanent state of lumpiness. The breasts become heavy, enlarged and tender and the nipples may tingle if squeezed. The breasts feel as though they contain small orange pips. These are nothing to worry about. They are simply swollen milk glands which enlarge in the second half of the menstrual cycle.

How often should I do it?

You should therefore give yourself a regular breast examination at the same time every month so that you can become acquainted with the character of your own breasts at a given time in your cycle. Women of childbearing age should do this in the week after their period; after menopause try to do it on the same day every month.

WHAT MAY BE DETECTED THIS WAY

Lumps detected in this way should be reported to your doctor or family planning clinic. Depending on the findings of the examination you may be sent for further tests which include mammography or a biopsy where a small piece of tissue is removed for analysis. The lump will then be treated depending on what it is. While a malignant tumor indicating breast cancer is always a possibility when a lump is discovered, more than likely it will be one of the following:

- ◆ A symptom of premenstrual syndrome – the lumpy tender feeling in the breast experienced before your period may become exaggerated and remain throughout your cycle. This usually occurs after the age of 30 and is the result of your sensitivity to hormonal changes.
- ◆ A cyst that has developed in the milk-producing ducts or around the areola where the sebaceous glands keep the skin supple. If one of these ducts or glands becomes blocked, a fluid-filled cyst may develop. Treatment for a cyst is usually under a local anesthetic when a long needle draws off the fluid or by surgical removal of the cyst and if there is infection with a course of antibiotics.
- ◆ A fibroadenoma, where the milk-producing glands thicken and cause firm, painless lumps that seem to move about within the breast. These are harmless and don't usually require treatment. If they cause pain, your doctor may prescribe hormonal therapy to get rid of them.
- ◆ An abcess which may have resulted from infection of the milk duct. This is sometimes called mastitis. Infection enters through the nipple and the area will become red, swollen and tender. You may have a raised temperature and feel swollen glands in your armpit too. Cracking of the nipples during breastfeeding is a common cause of this complaint. Antibiotics and, in severe cases, drainage of the abcess effectively treats this problem.

You may prefer to do part of this examination in a warm bath when your hands are warm and slippery. If you feel unsure about what you are doing, ask your doctor to teach you to do it properly. Though 4 out of 5 lumps detected this way prove to be benign, breast cancer is the major cause of death for women aged between 35 and 55.

SEE ALSO:

BENIGN BREAST DISEASE
BREAST CANCER
BREASTS AND
 BREASTFEEDING
MENOPAUSAL PROBLEMS
NIPPLE PROBLEMS
PREMENSTRUAL SYNDROME

BREAST SELF-EXAMINATION

HOW IS IT DONE?

Breast self-examination is an important feature of health monitoring. Every woman is capable of examining herself once a month, in order to detect changes to her breasts not consistent with normal cyclical behavior. Any changes should be reported.

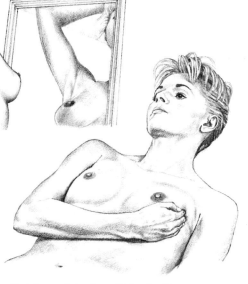

Stand before a mirror, stripped to the waist, and look at each breast carefully. Raise your arms above your head and turn from side to side so you can see each breast's outline. Check for any dimpling or puckering of the skin. Check your nipples carefully for any discharge or change in size, color or shape.

Put your hands on your hips or place them on your upper chest, exerting pressure to make your pectoral muscles stretch, and lean forwards.

Next, lie on a flat surface with the shoulder on the side you are examining slightly raised on the pillow. With the flat of your hand and your fingers straight, gently examine the outer edges of your breast moving in a clockwise direction (right hand left breast). Keep the other arm loosely by your side. Use your palms and straightened fingers.

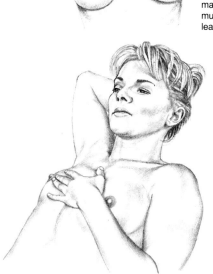

Examining larger breasts
If your breasts are very large, use two hands — one underneath to support the breast while the other examines the top surface, alternate to examine the lower surface.

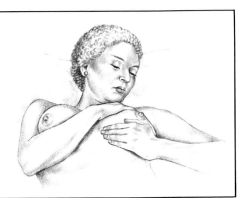

To examine the inner circle of the breast raise the arm not in use above your head. Feel the area along the top of the collarbone and in the armpit, too. Repeat the procedure for the other side.

BREASTFEEDING PROBLEMS

All breasts have the capacity to feed a baby. Any excuse for not feeding needs to be examined as there are probably deeper reasons for not wanting to do so. Some women find that breastfeeding is incompatible with the erotic role their breasts play, but most women enjoy knowing that they are able to provide not only the nourishment, but the intimacy that babies need.

Breastfeeding is entirely natural, and there are few problems, if any, that a mother experiences. However, one should be aware of possible complications.

ENGORGEMENT

During the first three days after childbirth, the breasts don't produce milk, they produce a light colored yellow liquid – colostrum. It is the perfect food for the first days of your baby's life. It contains valuable antibodies to protect your baby against diseases to which you have developed a resistance. It also contains a natural laxative which will get your baby's bowels going. After about three days the colostrum is replaced by mature breast milk.

It is usually the third or fourth day when the milk "comes in." This is also the time when the increased blood supply to the breasts and the onset of lactation causes them to become full, hard and sore and the nipple flattens out and disappears into the areola. (At this time, too, many women experience a feeling of sadness and anticlimax known as postpartum depression.)

What should I do?

The engorgement will worsen if the baby is unable to grasp the nipple and empty your breasts fully at each feed. If you feed your baby on demand, the principle of supply and demand will resolve the problem within two or three days. In the meantime, express a little before each feed so the areola is

softer and easier to latch onto (see index) and make sure both breasts are empty after each feed. Express milk if the baby doesn't fully empty your breasts. Hot and cold compresses help to ease the pressure and the pain. The easiest way to ease the engorgement is to soak in a hot bath and apply facecloths to your breasts. If milk does not spontaneously leak out after a few minutes, apply gentle pressure with your fingers above the areola.

LET-DOWN REFLEX

While milk is manufactured in the breast, it is only released or "let-down" when stimulated by a reflex. The stimulation can be anything from thinking about your baby's feed, to hearing a hungry cry, to the warmth and sucking of the baby at the breast. This reflex is set off by the pituitary gland which receives messages and releases a hormone called oxytocin. As the milk is already in the milk-producing cells in the breast, the oxytocin causes the muscles surrounding these cells

to contract, and the milk is emptied from the milk glands into the reservoirs behind the nipple.

What happens if the let-down fails?

The let-down reflex can be felt as a tingling in the breast. It may take up to two minutes to work so it is important that the baby keeps sucking. In rare cases there may be a failure to produce the oxytocin. Oxytocin nasal sprays can correct this problem. If you put the baby to your breast immediately after delivery this has been found to be the most satisfactory way of getting the let-down reflex established.

Some women are beset by doubt that they can't produce enough or the right milk for their babies. This is nonsense; every woman is physically capable of producing the right milk for her baby and to keep him or her nourished. However, if you are stressed or unhappy, the let-down reflex may be inhibited. This sets up a vicious cycle because the milk-producing glands aren't stimulated to produce more milk and the baby will be hungry and

The let-down reflex
When a baby sucks, the hypothalamus releases oxytocin which causes the milk to flow from the ducts into the nipples.

nerve impulses from nipple

prolactin and oxytocin

BREASTFEEDING PROBLEMS

act miserable.

Another reason for failure is if the baby is sleepy, perhaps because you had drugs during your delivery. If your baby doesn't suck energetically, the breasts won't be emptied at every feed and the milk will never build up sufficiently to satisfy the baby.

Perhaps your baby does not properly latch onto the nipple. The whole of the nipple and areola should be in the mouth, not just the nipple itself.

What should I do?
You have to have a positive frame of mind about breastfeeding and not be put off by old wives' tales, busy medical staff who won't let you finish a feed, and doubts about your adequacy. Take breastfeeding slowly. Try to get to know your baby and pick up signs so you can learn your baby's preferences. Don't be put off by one bad experience, be determined and carry on.

If things don't seem to be going very well, feed on demand to build up your milk supply and try to relax. Don't be disturbed by other mothers in the ward and their apparent ease. You are bound to feel happier when you get home. If relatives and friends put pressures on you, be resolute. Keep everyone away when you are feeding.

CRACKED NIPPLES

If you feel pain in your nipple when the baby is feeding, you may have a crack. This is usually because the baby is not properly latched on or the skin around the nipple has been too wet. You may find it impossible to continue feeding on the affected breast.

What should I do?
Stop immediately and express milk from the sore breast until the skin heals. It is fine to give your baby expressed milk from a spoon in this situation. The crack should heal

CARE OF YOUR BREASTS
You must be very careful with your breasts and nipples during the first few days because they are delicate and need time to toughen up. Two minutes on each breast at first is quite sufficient to give your baby a good feed. You can gradually build up to ten minutes each side by the fifth day.
- Wash your breasts in water only; don't use soap as it can defat the skin and cause unnecessary cracking.
- Always handle your breasts with care, never roughly. Don't rub them dry for example, pat them.
- Leave your nipples open to the air for a short time to prevent soreness and softening of the skin due to contact with a wet bra or pad. Change your pads frequently to catch any milk that leaks.
- You may avoid cracks if you apply a little lanolin, olive or peanut oil as often as you remember and certainly after feeding.
- At the first signs of soreness, give the breast a rest for a couple of days. Express the milk instead.
- At the end of a feed, don't break the suction by pulling away. Rather, insert your finger into your baby's mouth and then gently ease him or her off the breast by pressing down on the chin.
- Wear the best maternity bras you can afford. Wear them night and day for the first three months.

within two days. Reintroduce the baby slowly to the sore nipple. You can use a nipple shield which is placed over the affected nipple and the baby sucks on this.

BREAST ABCESS

If you notice a lump on your breast, this could be a blocked duct which, if it becomes infected, could result in a breast abcess. Massage it gently to get rid of it. Feed your baby to drain the block. Change to a less tight bra if that is the problem. You will know if there is infection because the lump cannot be massaged away or it becomes red and swollen and you have a temperature and feel as though you have the 'flu.

What should I do?
Don't offer the breast to the baby and consult your doctor immediately. The development of a breast abcess is not a catastrophe. It is painful and precludes feeding from that breast, but you must get

rapid treatment. Antibiotics will be prescribed in the first place with hot and cold compresses to relieve the pain but if these are not entirely successful, you may have to have the abcess surgically drained.

SEE ALSO:
BENIGN BREAST DISEASE
BREASTS AND
  BREASTFEEDING
NIPPLE PROBLEMS
POSTPARTUM DEPRESSION

BREECH BIRTH

This is a variation of the normal birth because your baby will be born buttocks first. Until the 32nd week of pregnancy, nearly all babies are in the breech position, but after this time most turn upside down so that their heads face the birth canal. About 5%, however, stay head upwards.

This is not a matter for concern. By far the majority of breech labors are smooth and the baby is normal. However, you will have to have the baby in a hospital.

What will happen?
At about 34 weeks, your doctor may try to turn the baby head down by manual massage known as external version. This is painless but often the baby springs back to its favorite upright position. You should never try to turn the baby yourself.

When you go into labor, you may find that it is longer than usual and you will probably have a bad back-ache. Kneeling on all fours will help alleviate this during the first stage of labor. You will almost certainly need an episiotomy as the head must be born quickly after the buttocks. You may also need forceps to protect the baby's head. While the body is being delivered, it is better to breathe through the contractions rather than push. Your doctor will direct you. The baby's weight will draw the head down into the vagina when the body is lifted to deliver the head. This is when the forceps may be used.

Are there any complications?
You may have some swelling in the genital region and your baby's buttocks and genitals will be bruised for a few days.

If your pelvic girdle is small or your baby is large, your doctor may elect to deliver the baby by Caesarean section. Talk this over with the medical staff. Many mothers deliver breech babies vaginally with no problems.

PRESENTATIONS FOR BIRTH

Some of the positions a baby adopts make a vaginal delivery unlikely, because the baby cannot negotiate the birth canal easily.

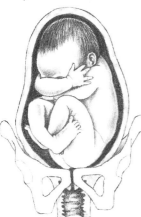

Full breech
The baby's flexed position permits maneuverability in the birth canal.

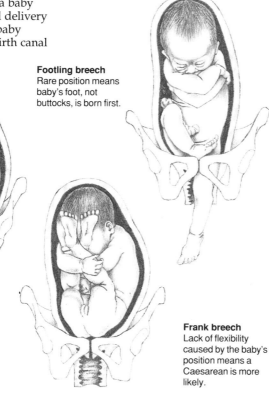

Footling breech
Rare position means baby's foot, not buttocks, is born first.

Frank breech
Lack of flexibility caused by the baby's position means a Caesarean is more likely.

SEE ALSO:

BACKACHE
CAESAREAN SECTION
EPISIOTOMY
LABOR

BULIMIA

Overeating is quite often one of the ways we meet the stresses in our lives. It is a comfort to many women; for some, it is a means of learning to cope with the world.

Of course, chronic overeating leads to weight gain and once women are overweight they may seek abnormal ways to control their girths. This may result in a psychological condition known as bulimia.

Because standard dieting measures inevitably fail with binge eating, some bulimics vomit back a meal immediately after eating it or abuse laxatives or diet pills and take excessive amounts of exercise to keep slim. To a certain extent, this mimics anorexia nervosa, another psychological disorder in which a young woman tries to control her life by controlling her eating habits and her shape and weight.

What happens to your body?
Bulimia is essentially a western disease. Much attention is paid to the overeating side of the syndrome, but the starvation side is just as important. When you starve yourself for a length of time, your body starts to crave food, so that when you eat something, your body demands more and more. Eating becomes uncontrollable and a response to a psychological need, not the physical one of hunger. However, because of the pressures in our culture to be slim, the compulsive eater at the same time wishes to control her weight. She still feels she can spoil herself by bingeing, and comes to rely on vomiting or purgatives to get rid of the food and keep her weight down.

In the middle of a binge, the desire for food is uncontrollable. Food is consoling, much as drugs are to an addict, and in most instances, the binges are carried out in secret so that friends and relatives are unaware of what is going on. The starve/binge pattern of eating, however, causes chemical changes in the body that make

bingeing almost inevitable. Starving induces a form of depression and bingeing relieves it.

Starving, vomiting, bingeing and purging is a dangerous way to live. Starvation and excessive use of laxatives lead to mineral and vitamin deficiencies, and vomiting wears down the teeth due to acid erosion. Many bulimics suffer from acid stomachs, gastric ulcers and mouth ulcers.

· S y m p t o m s ·

▲ Binge eating habits with extreme methods of dieting in between binges
▲ Secretive vomiting or use of purgatives
▲ Obsessional concern about weight and shape

Should I see the doctor?
It is very difficult for a bulimic to examine the problem of starvation and bingeing on her own, so you will need to make the first approach for treatment if you suspect it in a family member or friend. As with anorexia nervosa, many sufferers are adolescent girls.

If you are able to detect the syndrome before any of these physical symptoms occur, approach your family doctor for advice on where to go for counseling.

What will the doctor do?
Counseling by therapists with a good understanding of the disorder is the basis of treatment. Progress is nearly always slow with bulimics but self help groups have a good record of success. Family physicians and non-specialist psychologists are not, as a rule, able to treat bulimia successfully though they may be worth a try. They usually recommend hospitalization involving psychotherapy and anti-depressant drugs.

What can I do?
Many bulimics overcome their

cravings and compulsions to starve and can lead normal lives. The average time spent regaining normal eating habits is four years. Counseling and encouragement is needed to remove the central preoccupation with food and weight in these women's lives.

SEE ALSO:

ANOREXIA NERVOSA
EATING PROBLEMS
OBESITY

BUNIONS

A bunion is a bony protrusion at the main joint of the big toe where it joins the foot. Bunions are caused by an heredity weakness of the toe joints. If there is excessive stress and strain to this joint due to wearing high-heeled, ill-fitting shoes, the bursa, which is the soft pad that minimizes friction near the joint, may become inflamed and fill with fluid. This condition is known as bursitis. (If it occurs on the knee it is known as housemaid's knee.) The higher the heel, the less well distributed is your body weight and the more pressure is concentrated into the smaller area of the big toe joint. With very high-heeled shoes, this can be translated into weights as great as half a ton. It's not surprising therefore that the joint responds by producing fluid to cushion it from the jolting force of each step.

Initially the joint rubs against your shoes and forms hardened skin or calluses. If bursitis develops, the joint becomes tender, swollen and painful whenever you move. These symptoms settle down if you stop wearing high heels. If you continue to wear them over a long period, chronic changes take place within the joint so that the fluid never quite disappears and the bursa thickens. Inflammation in the bursa grumbles on and remains low grade and gradually the joint becomes deformed. This deformity is encouraged if narrow-toed shoes are worn so that the big toe is turned outwards.

· S y m p t o m s ·

▲ Protrusion of the bone where the big toe joins the foot
▲ Toughened skin over this joint
▲ Pain, swelling and tenderness whenever you wear shoes

Should I see the doctor?
If the bunion is giving you trouble because you can't find shoes to fit,
or calluses are developing over the joint, visit your podiatrist. The podiatrist will probably pare down any calluses and advise you to wear sensible shoes and leave your shoes off as much as possible or cut a hole in the side of your shoe until any inflammation dies down. If the bunion is severe and causing you pain, your podiatrist may advise you to visit your doctor in case surgery is the best option.

If you get an infection near the bunion, seek advice from your doctor. Infections of the feet take a long time to heal and you may need antibiotics.

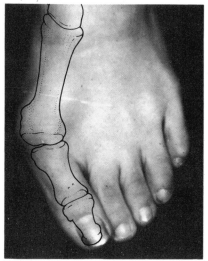

Bunion
The underlying cause of a bunion is an abnormal outward projection of the joint and an inward turning of the toe.

What can I do?
To prevent bunions it is important to take care of your feet at all times and to choose proper-fitting shoes:
◆ Wear high heels only inter-mittently.
◆ Wear flat shoes or go barefoot whenever you can.
◆ Don't pare down calluses or corns with sharp implements like scissors or razor blades; rub them with emery boards or a pumice stone.
◆ Exercises such as curling your toes over the edge of a book help to counteract the strain of wearing high-heeled shoes both on the bones, joints and muscles.
◆ After wearing high-heeled shoes for any length of time, a foot massage brings relief. Learn how to do this yourself or get your partner, friend or children to do it for you.

What will the doctor do?
Bunions can be realigned surgically without breaking the joint. Part of the protruding bone is cut away. This allows you to wear soft leather shoes again if your feet are so badly deformed that they are too wide for any shoes. With this operation, your feet will be bandaged or in a cast for a couple of weeks. If you have surgery to remove the bunions, you may not be able to wear normal shoes for perhaps six months. After this time, wear supple leather and open shoes until your feet feel normal again.

SEE ALSO:

FOOT PROBLEMS

CAESAREAN SECTION

It is sometimes necessary to deliver a baby through the mother's abdomen rather than the vagina. This is known as a Caesarean section and this surgical procedure can be elective, when your doctor decides in advance to deliver your baby this way, or an emergency when there is no other course of action.

The incidence of Caesarean sections is increasing, especially in North and South America, and there is a feeling that "fashion" and the convenience of the doctors may be contributing factors. However, depending on the circumstances, your doctor should allow you to undergo a trial of labor to see if you can progress to a normal vaginal delivery. A Caesarean can always be performed, if necessary, afterwards.

How is it done?

Caesarean section always used to be done under general anesthetic. Today, many women are able to have a Caesarean section with an epidural anesthetic so that they can remain awake and hold their babies immediately after birth and develop the vital bonding relationship.

Your pubic hair will be shaved and the epidural set up. An intravenous drip in your arm supplies you with fluids and a catheter empties your bladder. A screen is usually placed in front of you.

The birth of the baby will be quick – about 10-15 minutes. The incision is made through the abdominal wall just above your pubic hair line and into the uterus close to the cervix. The amniotic fluid is suctioned out – you will recognise this sound. The baby is then lifted out, head first, with the doctor pressing down on your abdomen to deliver the body. An injection of Pitocin may be given to hasten the expulsion of the placenta. Infants are often handed to the husband or partner to hold while the operation is finished. Stitching the wound is the longest part, taking about 30 minutes, because the uterine wall and abdominal wall have to be separately repaired.

You should be able to put your baby to your breast although the drip and catheter will remain in place for a few hours. Your partner should be allowed to remain with you throughout the operation.

What will happen after the operation?

You will be kept in bed for a day and you should use this time to get to know your baby and feed regularly to establish breastfeeding. You will be uncomfortable and this is one of the most difficult aspects of a Caesarean – the discomfort when feeding. The second day is when you should get up and start the essential postnatal exercises. There will be inevitable soreness around the wound and you may

WHY IS IT DONE?

A Caesarean will be performed in an emergency, whether or not you have gone into labor on your own if:
◆ The umbilical cord has prolapsed through the cervix.
◆ The fetus shows signs of distress when either the heartrate slows or dips or green meconium (the first bowel movements) stains the amniotic fluid.
◆ The cervix fails to dilate.
◆ The baby cannot be delivered by forceps.
◆ The labor is long and you become extremely tired and the baby shows signs of distress.
◆ You suffer convulsions due to eclampsia.
◆ The placenta detaches itself from the uterine wall – placenta abruptio.

A Caesarean will be planned and you will be prepared for the operation rather than allowed to go into labor naturally if:
◆ The placenta is sited in the lower segment of the uterus – placenta previa.
◆ The baby is extremely large – larger than the pelvic cavity.
◆ There is an active infection of the vagina such as genital herpes.
◆ There is Rhesus incompatibility.
◆ You have a sexually transmitted disease.
◆ There is a uterine infection.
◆ There is heroin or other drug addiction which would prevent a normal labor.
◆ The baby needs to be delivered early and induction and labor are considered to be an unnecessary risk for you or the baby.

◆ There is a maternal illness such as heart disease or high blood pressure.
◆ The baby is in the breech position. Delivery this way of breech babies is not strictly necessary and a trial of labor may be allowed.
◆ You have had a previous Caesarean section. This should not indicate that all your babies need be born this way. This is, however, a view held by some obstetricians. You should discuss your particular situation fully with your doctor.

HAVING A CAESAREAN

Today, many procedures are performed with the mother fully conscious and her partner present. Screened off from the lower part of her body and anesthetized, the mother hears first the surgeon sucking out the amniotic fluid and then, soon after, her baby's cry. She or her partner may hold the baby while being stitched up.

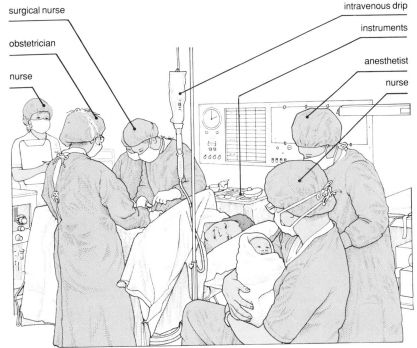

surgical nurse
obstetrician
nurse
intravenous drip
instruments
anesthetist
nurse

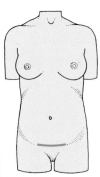

Types of incision
The preferred incision is horizontal and made low down near the pubic hair where a bikini could conceal it. Horizontal incisions are more stable than vertical incisions which are more often employed in emergencies.

Area of incision

have a headache from the epidural. Ask the hospital staff for painkillers. Most women feel back to normal after a week. You will be allowed home in five to eight days.

Even though your baby was born through your abdomen, you will have a blood-stained discharge (lochia) from your vagina for three to five weeks after the birth.

Pillows are a useful aid to finding a comfortable position for both feeding and sleeping. When you cough or laugh, hold your hands over the wound to give you confidence.

What can I do?
You may feel somewhat disappointed because you have been looking forward to a vaginal delivery. Whatever happens don't feel guilty and don't feel that you've let anyone down. Prepare yourself if you have a planned Caesarean by discussing the operation with other mothers who have had one and ask to visit the operating room and see a film if possible of such an operation.

Discuss the anesthetic and if you have an epidural make sure the hospital staff know that you want the baby handed to you or your partner immediately after the birth. If you are having a general anesthetic, giving the baby to your partner is an extremely important part of the bonding process for you all as a family. If the reasons for having the operation necessitate that the baby should be placed in intensive care immediately after birth, your doctors should alert you to this possibility so you can prepare yourself emotionally.

Will I need repeat Caesareans?
Depending on the reasons for having the Caesarean section, you may worry that all your babies will be born this way. Conditions may differ for a second or third baby so that another Caesarean won't be necessary. In some countries, however, doctors tend to do repeat procedures no matter what the circumstances.

By talking to other mothers, you can allay your fears. Self-help groups can put you in touch with midwives and obstetricians who have a more flexible approach to pregnancy and childbirth after Caesarean section.

SEE ALSO:
BREASTFEEDING PROBLEMS
EPIDURAL ANESTHETIC
GENITAL HERPES
PLACENTA PREVIA
RHESUS INCOMPATIBILITY
SEXUALLY TRANSMITTED
  DISEASES

CANCER

Cancer is a disease caused by the unrestrained growth and division of cells in a specific tissue. All cells have the potential to become cancerous and we believe that most cells would become cancerous were it not for chemical substances which restrain their growth. The immune system produces chemicals and cells which police the body, monitoring cell division and growth and keeping it normal. Any condition which injures the integrity of this system can result in tumors.

There are some general principles which apply to all malignant growths. As a rule, the younger the age of onset the more malignant the growth. The more primitive the cell type of the cancer, the more quickly it spreads and causes death. Tumors may grow from different embryonic types of cell: strictly speaking those which grow from the outermost layer of cells, the epithelial cells, are called cancers, and those which grow from the innermost cells, the endothelial cells, are called sarcomas. More often than not sarcomas are more virulent than cancers. Other tumors are known from experience to be slow or fast growing. For instance, cancers of the skin, except malignant melanoma (see *Skin cancer*), are known to be slow growing and therefore not dangerous, whereas cancer of the lung can be rapid (see *Lung cancer*).

The most common female-only cancers are *breast cancer* and *cervical cancer*. Wherever its site, cancer spreads in certain classical ways. All tumors enlarge by direct spread, simply by cells overtaking adjacent tissues. As most cancers are fragile, malignant cells can split off from the primary tumor and spill over into the bloodstream. If this happens, the cells will circulate in the blood until they are deposited in a distant organ where they form another cancerous tumor called a metastasis.

Cancer may also spread into the lymphatic system; cancerous cells become trapped in the nearest lymph glands which is why the glands affected by cancer become large enough to be felt. The enlarged glands are usually those which drain the area in which the cancer is situated. Therefore, it is the lymph glands of the armpit which swell with cancer of the breast.

The greatest chance of a cure is when the cancer is detected prior to spreading (metastasizing). It's possible for minute cancers to metastasize and so diligent screening to detect very small tumors is imperative. Early detection is the single most important factor in allowing curative treatment and so *breast self-examination, mammography* and regular *Pap smears* are mandatory health checks which all women should adhere to.

Prevention is always better than cure and as we know there are certain factors which promote cancerous change. The Western diet, high in animal fat and low in fiber, seems to be one. Stress plays some part, though we are not sure exactly what. The body's immune system is weakened by stress and it may be that lack of stress or relaxation techniques play a protective part.

There is quite a list of factors which are carcinogenic and may either trigger off cancer or promote the growth once cancer is formed. Obvious substances are the tars contained in cigarette smoke which promotes *lung cancer*; excessive exposure to sunlight which promotes skin cancer; smegma, the white waxy substance which collects under the prepucial skin in uncircumcised men has been implicated in cervical cancer. Women who suffer from genital warts have a higher incidence of cancer of the cervix than women who are free of the wart virus. A high number of sexual partners in teenage girls is thought to increase the risk of developing cancerous changes in the cervix (see *Genital herpes*).

Cancers of the female genital organs are often hormone related. The health of the genital organs depends on the presence of the female hormones estrogen and progesterone during a woman's fertile life. Should a cancer form in one of these organs, its growth can be stimulated by the presence of estrogen or progesterone. This is the case with cancer of the breast.

In general, treatment of a cancer can include surgical removal of tumors, *radiation therapy*, or chemotherapy, either as a single treatment or in combination.

CARPAL TUNNEL SYNDROME

This is a numbing disorder of the hand that rarely affects men but is fairly common in women, especially those who are of middle or advanced age, and during pregnancy.

At the wrist, the nerves that carry signals from the brain to the hand pass through a tunnel formed by fibers and the wrist bones (carpals) on their way to your hand. Although this carpal tunnel is rigid, if the space inside the tunnel becomes tight, this puts pressure on the nerves, leading to a feeling of numbness in the fingers and hand and a sensation of pins and needles down the arm. Sometimes the pain can be so severe that painkilling drugs are necessary.

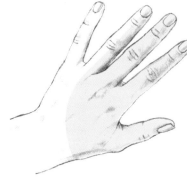

Affected area
Pressure of swollen tissue on the median nerve where it passes through the carpal tunnel can result in loss of sensation in part of the hand, thumb and next three fingers.

What is it caused by?
Carpal tunnel syndrome often makes its appearance around about the time of the menopause and it is thought to be a combination of factors which come together at this time. Frequently there are small joint changes with growth of new bone around the margins of the joints, making spaces between the joints smaller than they were. This is particularly so in the joints of the fingers, wrists and hands. There may also be a degree of water retention due to fluctuating levels of female hormones at the time of the menopause causing swelling of the tissues that surround the joints. This hormonal fluctuation is the reason for the symptoms during pregnancy. Both these factors can be aggravated when your body is warm and blood vessels expand, taking up more space. This is why carpal tunnel syndrome is more often a night pain with discomfort sufficient to wake you up and not allow you to go back to sleep without painkillers.

Carpal tunnel syndrome may also be sports-related, being brought on by activities that involve repeated or strenuous use of the wrists, such as tennis or handball.

· S y m p t o m s ·

▲ Numbness in the fingers and hands, one or both sides can be affected
▲ Pins and needles down your arm
▲ Severe pain, most commonly at night

Should I see the doctor?
If you can get no relief and the pain is sufficient to keep you awake at night and the self-help treatment (below) fails to bring relief, consult your doctor.

You should not rely on painkilling drugs in the long term. See your doctor if they are necessary for more than three nights in a row.

What will the doctor do?
Your doctor will treat the condition depending on its severity. To reduce the fluid retention, diuretic drugs may be prescribed or a steroid drug to reduce inflammation. However, the surgical treatment for carpal tunnel syndrome is extremely simple and effective. Under a general anesthetic, the constricting tunnel of fibers through which the nerve passes can be opened up with a small incision. This releases pressure, relieves the symptoms and leaves the function intact with no complications. The scar will be barely noticeable.

What can I do?.
As a temporary measure, you can raise your hands above your head so the fluid drains back down your arm and decompresses the tunnel through which the nerve is passing. Placing your wrists under a cold running tap or applying an ice pack will reduce swelling and relieve the symptoms.

If you are pregnant, be assured that the numbness will disappear after the baby is born.

SEE ALSO:

MENOPAUSAL PROBLEMS
PREGNANCY PROBLEMS
SPORTS INJURIES

CATARACTS

A cataract is a progressive clouding of the jelly-like substance which forms the lens of the eye. In severe cases the total lens may be affected, making the pupil appear white from the front. This obviously affects your vision depending on the extent and the location of the cataract. However, in all cases nearly all direct vision is blurred. Cataracts usually affect both eyes.

More women than men have cataracts because we live longer. If we all lived long enough, nearly all of us would develop cataracts. From the age of 40 onwards, most people need brighter light to read by.

Eventually, opacities in the lens render it no longer transparent and this interferes with the passage of light to the back of the eye onto the retina. Depending on the number and severity of the opacities, vision begins to blur and dim.

Cataracts, if removed, do not lead to blindness because they are so easily treated so they need never be severely disabling.

We now know that long exposure to bright sunlight encourages the formation of cataracts. So although aging is the most common cause of cataracts, excessive sunlight, diabetes and a congenital condition can also be causes.

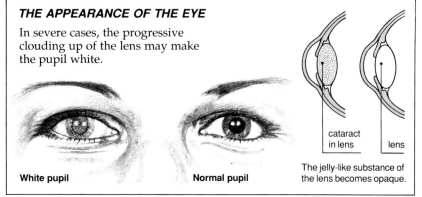

THE APPEARANCE OF THE EYE

In severe cases, the progressive clouding up of the lens may make the pupil white.

White pupil　　　　**Normal pupil**

cataract in lens　　lens

The jelly-like substance of the lens becomes opaque.

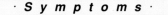

· S y m p t o m s ·

▲ Blurring and dimming of vision
▲ Opaque cloud over the eye, visible from the front when the cataract is in an advanced stage

Should I see the doctor?
If you experience any reduction of your normal vision, see your optician or ophthalmologist. If your optician suspects cataracts, you will be referred to your ophthalmologist.

What will the doctor do?
If your case isn't too severe, and particularly if only one eye is involved, eyeglasses may be all that is required. However, if your vision is limited, the lens and cataract will be removed in a safe and effective operation.

What is the surgical treatment?
The operation may be performed under a general anesthetic but is more usually done under a local in the form of drops which are put into your eyes and a local nerve block. Your eye and head are held still during the operation.

The lens is removed and your prescription lens implant, made from plastic, is inserted. If you don't have a new lens put in, because only one eye is affected or you are suffering from some other disease of the eye, such as glaucoma, you can have contact lenses or glasses fitted later.

What can I do?
Your eyes will hurt in bright natural or artificial light, so wear sunglasses inside and out for the first week or so until you feel better. You may be instructed to put pads over your eyes at night to prevent irritation.

Don't expect your vision to be completely normal. After the operation you may be farsighted, depending on whether you had a plastic lens implant, or cataract glasses or contact lenses.

Objects may appear magnified the closer they are. These changes can be adjusted to in time.

It is a good idea to wear sun-glasses in very bright light and wear prescription sunglasses if you're reading in sunlight.

As diabetes predisposes to the formation of cataracts, you should maintain regular check-ups with your eye doctor.

SEE ALSO:

DIABETES MELLITUS
EYE PROBLEMS

CERVICAL CANCER

Cervical cancer, while not as common as it used to be, is still certainly a cause for concern among women. The peak incidence of cervical cancer is, on average, at age 48. There is an infrequence of this cancer in young women but 7.4% of cervical cancers do occur in women below the age of 30. According to the American Cancer Society, white women with cervical cancer have a five-year survival rate of 67% and black women, who have a higher incidence of cervical cancer, have a 59% survival rate at five years. The slow-growing cervical cancer can be detected and treated by regular Pap smears. As the condition has no early symptoms it can only be detected by routine screening. Women's groups and concerned medical practitioners are constantly lobbying politicians to improve the screening facilities and co-ordinate an efficient call-up system to catch those women who are most at risk because they don't have regular Pap smears.

Cervical cancer has a pre-invasive stage during which time it may grow but not spread. As this pre-invasive stage may last for several years, any woman who has regular Pap smears should be identified early enough for the cancer to be totally removed by simply taking out the tissue from the cervix.

What causes it?
It is thought that sexual activity plays a part in causing cancer of the cervix because the lining cells are vulnerable during adolescence. Therefore frequency of intercourse during this period and with several different sexual partners may initiate the cancer process. The inference is that there is a virus passed during sexual intercourse. This would provide the reason for the higher incidence of cancer among women who started sexual activity at an early age and with several or more different partners. This is backed up by looking at certain religious groups such as Orthodox Jewish and

WOMEN AT RISK
Those women who are most at risk include:

Women who started sexual activity at an early age. Black women and women from lower socio-economic groups.

With pre-existing genital disease such as genital warts or herpes or other sexually transmitted diseases. Women who have antibodies to both these viruses have a higher incidence of cervical cancer.

Certain racial groups though these differ depending on the country in which the studies were carried out. In the U.S. these groups include Mexican, black and Puerto Rican women.

Moslem women. Cervical cancer is rarer among these women; their men are circumcised and the morals regarding extramarital

---

· S y m p t o m s ·

▲ Can be none at all
▲ Ulceration of the cervix, seen on vaginal examination using a speculum
▲ Inter-menstrual bleeding, spotting after intercourse or after the menopause
▲ Offensive vaginal discharge

---

intercourse are particularly firm. It follows that virgins and celibates are at low risk as well. On the other hand, women whose mothers took DES during pregnancy are among others with a particularly high risk (see box).

STAGES OF CERVICAL CANCER

Cancer of the cervix is divided into five stages. The reason for this staging is that it gives an indication of the expected cure rate after five years. The cure rate descends depending on the stage.
Stage 0: Pre-malignant cancer that has not spread below the first layer of cervical tissue.
Stage 1: Cancer that has invaded the cervix but has not spread beyond it.

Stage 2: Cancer extended outside the cervix either into the tissues adjacent to the cervix or to the upper two-thirds of the vagina, but not to the walls of the pelvis.
Stage 3: Extended out to the lateral walls of the pelvis or to the lower third of the vagina, or has obstructed one or both of the ureters.
Stage 4: The cancer has directly invaded the bladder or rectum or there are distant metastases.

What is the medical treatment?
The treatment you receive will be determined by the stage of your cancer. Whether you have a Pap smear as a routine or symptoms caused you to be referred for one, the results are classified into four or five categories. Negative gives you the all-clear, some mild dysplasia means you may have some infection and should be screened more regularly, and a positive Pap smear, though not always indicating cancer, means there is a detectable change in the cells necessitating further investigation.

If some abnormal cells were discovered, the first examination may be with a colposcope to give a clear magnified view of the suspect area and to remove cells for more laboratory tests. Sometimes abnormal cells may be treated with a laser at the same time. If, however, colposcopy reveals cancerous cells but does not determine their extent, a biopsy will have to be done.

What is the surgical treatment?

A cone biopsy can offer treatment as well as investigation if the entire layer of suspect cells is removed. This may be done with a scalpel or a laser beam. Only after the tissue is examined microscopically can doctors determine if you require any further treatment. Depending on the stage, this may involve radical surgery for the removal of the uterus, ovaries and fallopian tubes as well as the upper part of the vagina. Certain muscles and glands from inside the pelvis may be taken away.

Other surgical methods include intense cold cryo-surgery or intense heat electro-coagulation to destroy cancerous tissue.

What other treatment is available?

Nearly half the cases of cervical cancer are treated with radiation therapy. The aim is to give a fatal dose of radiation to the center of the cancer. Radiation also kills those parts of the growth that were invading other areas. It is interesting to note that comparing women who had radiation therapy with those who had radical surgery, after five years, the survival rate was about the same. Therefore, discuss the options fully with your doctor.

What can I do?

You will be required to have regular checks over the next five years or so to make sure the cancer spread has been stopped. You will almost certainly not be able to have any more children and if you had your ovaries removed, you will go through a premature menopause. If this causes you to suffer unpleasant symptoms, see your doctor for treatment. If you maintain regular appointments for Pap smears, any cancer will be caught at a time when chances of a

cure are high. Even if cancerous cells are found, you should take an interest in the disease and co-operate with your medical advisers to fight it. Cancer cures do depend to a certain extent on the interest of the sufferer in beating the disease.

PAP SMEAR RESULTS

Tissue removed from the cervix is examined microscopically to note any changes to the cell and particularly its nucleus. These changes determine the future treatment.

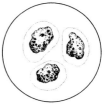

Negative or Normal
Can include mild inflammatory changes present in nearly all smears.

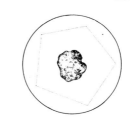

Severe inflammatory changes
A larger than normal cell nucleus is apparent. There may be no symptoms, or a vaginal discharge or irritation. A repeat smear is sometimes recommended.

Mild abnormality
The nucleus here is large with irregular outlines and contains heavy clumps and strands. This stage can be present for years or revert to normal, or get worse. Frequent tests will be advised and colposcopy may also be recommended.

Severe abnormality
The cells are smaller with irregular outlines and large nuclei. They contain very coarse lumps and strands. These cell changes indicate cancer that may be pre-invasive or invasive. Cone biopsy is normally carried out.

CERVIX PROBLEMS

The cervix is the neck of the womb and connects the vagina with the uterus. It is an active sex organ and responds to the cyclical secretion of the female sex hormones, estrogen and progesterone. It secretes mucus which changes in character during the menstrual cycle, and a study of these changes will delineate when ovulation takes place. In the second part of the cycle, the thick mucus is hostile and impenetrable to sperm and this effect of progesterone is the theory behind the progesterone-only mini-pill. By taking a small dose of progesterone every day, the cervical mucus is rendered hostile to sperm, which cannot penetrate the cervical canal and reach the ovum to complete fertilization. This is a highly efficacious form of oral *contraception*.

Under ordinary circumstances, the healthy cervix is firm and feels almost like cartilage. Under the influence of the pregnancy hormones, and particularly those produced by the placenta, the cervix swells, softens and changes color. Its characteristic purplish, plush appearance is a confirmatory visual pregnancy test for the doctor during a *pelvic examination*. As pregnancy progresses, the cervix becomes plumper and softer and much more elastic so that during labor it can stretch easily and the baby's body can be expelled. Its contractility and resilience is such that it can retract to its normal size in a few days.

By far the most serious condition affecting the cervix is cancer. Fortunately, *cervical cancer* is a treatable and curable condition if it is picked up in its early stages. When it first develops, it is non-invasive and does not spread. If regular *Pap smears* are performed, tumors can be caught and dealt with long before they are worrying, without radical surgery. Very early tumors, for instance, can be treated by a *cone biopsy*.

Cervicitis
Inflammation of the cervix can be caused by a sexually transmitted disease such as *gonorrhea* or *chlamydia,* or be of unknown origin. The main symptom is a vaginal discharge of mucus and pus, and pelvic pain, backache and painful intercourse may also be noticed. Abnormal inflammatory tissue may

have to be removed by cryosurgery, cauterization, laser therapy or cone biopsy.

Incompetent cervix
Occasionally, when a woman experiences several miscarriages, it is found that the cervix is incompetent, meaning that the cervical opening into the vagina is slack and loses its firmness. (This weakness may result from an inexpert abortion or from a previous rapid birth.) This type of miscarriage only occurs after the uterus has enlarged somewhat and the developing baby becomes heavy enough to press the cervix open. Once it is opened, there is the possibility that labor will start and the pregnancy will miscarry. Cervical incompetence can be treated easily; one of the simplest methods is to tie the neck of the cervix closed and tighten it very much in the way that you can tighten the strings of a purse. The stitch is cut at about the 38th week when labor is imminent. At the six-week postnatal check, damage to the cervix is specifically looked for so that it can be spotted early and treated promptly.

Cervical erosion
Occasionally during pregnancy, due to the action of the female hormones, the interior lining of the cervix swells so that it covers the external opening. (Some women are born with this phenomenon.) This type of tissue is mucus-producing so there may be a heavy vaginal discharge, and as it is relatively delicate tissue, there may also be a bloody discharge, particularly after intercourse. While it is advisable to have a pelvic examination if symptoms are noted, cervical erosions are rarely treated unless symptoms are extremely troublesome.

Cervical polyps
Small, tear-shaped, fragile growths that dangle on a stalk may develop from the mucous lining of the cervix. They are simply outgrowths of glandular cells which are almost always benign. Because their surface is delicate, they may bleed easily and cause spotting after intercourse or mid-period. They can be treated simply with electrocautery, usually at your doctor's office.

CHILD ABUSE

Child abuse covers physical as well as sexual violence against children. With growing public awareness of the widespread incidence of child abuse in our societies, and the fact that most abusers are known to the children, it is important to acknowledge any suspicions you might have regarding your children or those in your family or community.

In the case of pure physical abuse, men and women are implicated, but in sexual abuse, women rarely are. Women hardly ever engage in sexual activities with their own or other children. Sexual abusers are quite often men, but women must play a special role in being on the look-out for tell-tale signs, of meeting the situation head-on and not silently colluding with the abusers, and reporting their suspicions to the right authorities, thus stopping any abuse.

A woman who suspects child abuse within her family faces great difficulties. The abuser may not always be the father but perhaps an older, trusted relative, friend or neighbor who enjoys a good relationship with her children. There are obvious pressures for that woman to stay silent . But there is absolutely no excuse for a woman outsider, who with good evidence, suspects that child abuse is occurring in a family she knows or is acquainted with, to stay silent. In that instance, her duties are absolutely clear: she must in no circumstance let her suspicions go unreported. While a friendship may be lost if investigation reveals nothing, a great deal more is lost if a case goes undetected. The emotional and psychological trauma inflicted on abused children is well documented. We know the effects may continue throughout their lives and prevent them forming close relationships.

How can this be detected?
Children are sometimes more prepared to confess to a neighbor or a relative that an adult, often trusted and loved, is sexually interfering with them. Be on the alert for any small hints or attitudes which lead you to believe that a child is being sexually abused. If you feel that your suspicions are well founded, then take action early.

Sometimes a child may simply express the desire not to see, visit or go out with a certain relative. If they do this more than once, you should question them at a convenient moment to see what their feelings are for this relative. You must keep the channels of communication open with these children. Although children rarely confide in other adults, always listen to them. Be gentle and understanding so that the children feel free to tell you things that they might not tell other people. Two crucial areas of questioning are whether any adult has asked them to keep secrets and whether they feel any adult is touching them in a special way. If you do suspect that a child is being abused, don't hesitate to report the possibility to someone.

Who should I talk to?
Speaking to your own family doctor may be all that you have to do and then he or she will take up the case for you through the correct channels. Ask for a confidential interview with the social worker or counselor you have been advised to contact. Report what you have noticed or found out in conversations with the child in as much detail as you can. Be prepared to act as a witness at any inquiry which should ensue.

It's very important to take this step. Most abused children feel that their experiences are entirely their fault, that in some way they are unworthy, unclean or that they encourage the adult to abuse them sexually. Most abused children never confess to the incidents of abuse until they are much older; some carry the secret with them for the whole of their lives.

To make matters worse, medical experts often seem to disagree about whether child abuse took place or not. As most diagnoses of child abuse involve intimate physical examinations, we must question whether the physical examination of young children is enough to confirm that abuse has taken place. That could inflict its own kind of abuse on children.

PARENTAL BACKGROUND
Physical abuse has always been seen in a different light from sexual abuse and quite rightly so. There can be physiological reasons for the absence of mother love – one of the precipitating factors for child abuse. Mother love is thought to be almost entirely under hormonal control. It follows that if the correct hormones are not secreted in the proper balance then mother love could be interfered with and even stunted. It is very rare but occasionally it does happen that a mother and a child simply do not get on and do not like each other. More commonly, some women who suffer from pre-menstrual tension become barely in control of their actions when the tension is at its worse.

The background of parents can partly determine their behavior to their own children. Many parents who beat their children were beaten themselves when they were young or were deprived of normal parental affection and care. The environmentalists would say that this mitigates against the crime of physically abusing children.

In a child who is not physically very active, repeated bruises, scratches, cuts and grazes are signs to look out for. A child flinching when one of the parents simply raises his or her hand or arm could be interpreted as a warning sign.

It might be possible to tackle the problem of child abuse in a different way from simply taking the child into care. Instead of removing the child from the family, which brings its own traumas, we should consider taking the abuser away from the family and leaving the child and the family otherwise intact.

CHLAMYDIA

Chlamydia is the most common sexually transmitted disease. However, at any given time, most women affected with chlamydia will have no symptoms. Women with untreated infections risk losing their fertility, hence the alarm caused by this once little-known disorder. Although easy to treat, chlamydia is difficult to diagnose because the symptoms are usually slow to develop, mild or non-existent. But as long as there is awareness of the possibility of the disease, modern tests and treatments can eradicate it before any serious consequences develop.

Theoretically, chlamydia can infect the linings of the vagina, the mouth, the eyes, the urinary tract or the rectum but in women, the infection is usually confined to the cervix, leading to an offensive yellow-colored discharge. The worrisome effect is that a third of cases with chlamydia can go on to pelvic inflammatory disease which damages the fallopian tubes and causes infertility.

It may also be responsible for ectopic pregnancy which is potentially life threatening and could result in infertility due to tubal blockage or scarring. During childbirth an infected woman may infect her baby, who will have conjuctivitis and, rarely, develop pneumonia.

· S y m p t o m s ·

▲ An unusual cervical discharge
▲ Abdominal pain and fever
▲ Partner has pain or urinary problems

Should I see the doctor?
If you have any symptoms of unusual discharge, or more likely your sexual partner has the symptoms, see your doctor or go to your nearest sexually transmitted diseases clinic.

What will the doctor do?
At one time it was necessary to take a specimen of the vaginal secretions and culture chlamydia in a laboratory. This meant waiting at least 48

WOMEN AT RISK

Any sexually active woman runs the risk of contracting chlamydia; there are certain groups, however, who should have regular checks as a precaution.

 With multiple partners
Among sexually active teenagers, for example, the rate may be as high as 20%,

hours for the result of the tests. However, new laboratory tests have been devised which can give results in 30 - 60 minutes, therefore permitting immediate treatment.

What is the medical treatment?
Chlamydia is simply and completely cured with a course of antibiotics. It is essential to take the medication exactly as prescribed and to complete the full course. Do not stop taking the pills simply because the symptoms disappear; chlamydia could return. If you develop side effects while taking the pills, do not stop the course; contact your doctor. It is essential that your partner is treated at the same time.

What was once diagnosed as non-specific urethritis was probably chlamydia. If the diagnosis is wrongly stated as gonorrhea, the treatment will not cure the chlamydia. Therefore, as many cases of gonorrhea also have chlamydia, and penicillin is not adequate, tetracyclines or sulphon-amides are used for the treatment.

What can I do?
If you have many sexual contacts, all of them must be informed of the infection and screened and treated if necessary. To prevent re-infection use barrier contraceptives such as condoms and diaphragms with spermicidal creams.

thereafter the risk gradually diminishes. It is estimated that between five and 10% of college aged women now have chlamydia.

 Pill users
The pill may increase a woman's susceptibility to chlamydia, though these reasons are not understood.

SEE ALSO:

CONTRACEPTION
ECTOPIC PREGNANCY
GONORRHEA
INFERTILITY
PELVIC INFLAMMATORY
 DISEASE
SEXUALLY TRANSMITTED
 DISEASES
VAGINAL DISCHARGE

CHORION BIOPSY

Also known as chorionic villus sampling (CVS), this is a new technique which can diagnose certain genetic disorders earlier in pregnancy than amniocentesis. The test, which was pioneered in China in the early 1970s, can be done as early as eight weeks after the first day of the last menstrual period and give the results within 5-12 days. This avoids the agonizing delays that are at present experienced by women who undergo amniocentesis and means that if a termination is indicated, it will not be as difficult and painful as an induced labor in the second trimester.

Why is it done?
Many genetic disorders can now be diagnosed during pregnancy and a termination carried out if necessary, or if desired by the parents. The risk of carrying a Down's syndrome baby, for example, rises steeply with maternal age. Therefore any woman over 35 or a woman who has previously given birth to an abnormal baby should be offered this test.

How is it done?
The entire procedure is monitored simultaneously on an ultrasonic scan. Most commonly, under a local anesthetic, the doctor inserts a needle through the abdominal wall into the placenta, which is located by ultrasound. Then a sample of the chorion, the membrane surrounding the embryo, is withdrawn into a syringe. Alternatively, using no anesthetic, the doctor inserts a small catheter into the vagina to take a sample of the chorion.

The cells in the chorion have the same genetic make up as the embryo so an examination of them reveals whether the embryo has a particular genetic disorder.

Because the sample of chorion is quite large compared to the cells found in the amniotic fluid, the chromosome count can be carried

HAVING A BIOPSY
Chorionic sampling allows for an accurate diagnosis of certain genetic disorders very early in pregnancy. However, because it carries some risk of miscarriage, it should only be carried out when genetic disease is a real possibility.

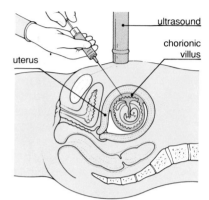

A small piece of membrane, the chorion, which surrounds the developing embryo, is removed via suction through the abdomen. The genes contained in it are identical to those in the embryo.

out right away with no delay for culturing cells.

What are the risks?
At the present time, CVS is still somewhat in the experimental stage. It is still not known whether there is a higher rate of miscarriage and other complications than amniocentesis. When the catheter plucks at the fronds on the uterine wall, some damage may be done. At present women who have had an abnormal baby should be offered this test if they want it, after counseling about the possible risks.

Although the test is like a routine Pap smear, it can cause abdominal aches and cramps for the next few days.

CHROMOSOMAL PROBLEMS

Each cell in the body has 23 pairs of chromosomes, 46 in all; each parent donates half. The chromosomes, which are formed from thousands of genes, determine all the characteristics of the body – the physical, the anatomical, the physiological and probably the emotional characteristics, too. The genes are responsible for traits. A trait can mean tallness or shortness, blondness or darkness. A trait can be dominant or recessive; tallness happens to be dominant and will always "dominate" the opposite gene for height, that is shortness. Darkness is dominant and will mask the opposing gene for blondness. So two very tall parents are unlikely to have a small child or two dark parents to have a blond baby.

Most serious genetic disorders are caused by a single defective gene which is usually recessive. Such a disorder will therefore only occur if both parents possess the defective gene. In the general population, the chances of two people who choose to have a child together carrying a defective gene for, say, cystic fibrosis, is slim, and the chance of their child inheriting this defect is about 1 in 400, though of course, once a single child is affected, they are more likely to produce other affected children. Even if the child does not suffer from the disease, he or she may carry it to the next generation without realizing it. In such cases, the child has only inherited one abnormal gene; the normal one dominates.

Our sex is determined by the two sex chromosomes, X and Y. Women genetically are XX and men are XY. Because there are two identical X chromosomes in women, an abnormal gene on one X chromosome is completely masked by the normal gene on the other X chromosome. This explains the "carrier" state of some women, for example, those carrying hemophilia. Hemophilia does not show up in women because the hemophilic X chromosome is neutralized by the normal X chromosome. If, however, the hemophilic X chromosome is passed on to a boy, the disease must show up because the Y chromosome does not match and cannot cancel out the trait for hemophilia.

Similarly, if certain diseases are carried on the Y chromosome they will always show up in men

CHROMOSOMAL PROBLEMS

because there is never a normal Y chromosome to neutralize the abnormal one. An example of this is color blindness which is exhibited in more men then women because it is carried on the X chromosome.

Sometimes a particular pair of chromosomes may be abnormal, one of the commonest being the appearance of an additional chromosome. This is called "trisomy" and it most commonly affects the 21st pair of chromosomes, resulting in Down's syndrome.

Genes account for all the normal body processes. There is a separate gene for every anatomical structure, every reaction and every process in the body. A gene may be responsible for an enzyme which affects a crucial chemical reaction within the body. An abnormality of the gene can lead to something such as an abnormal body fluid and this is exactly what is found in fibrocystic disease. There is an abnormality of the mucus secreted by the glands in the lungs, in the pancreas and elsewhere, leading to the classical signs of chest disease and malabsorption syndrome. *Chorion biopsy* may display this abnormal enzyme before the baby is born so that appropriate measures can be taken in the first few days of life.

Some abnormalities can be detected in utero with a number of tests, and if the test is positive, a woman is given the opportunity to consider a termination. She and her partner will be offered *genetic counseling* to help them make the decision. Genetic counseling is there for anyone or any couple who is carrying any kind of chromosomal abnormality or may suspect from their family history that there is an abnormal gene running through the family. Any woman over the age of 35 may seek genetic counseling, preferably before she conceives.

Some conditions where genetic counseling may be helpful would be conditions where there is an abnormality in the blood such as sickle cell anemia and thalassemia. A counselor may suggest that a wide variety of tests be done during pregnancy in order to confirm or reject a genetic abnormality, including *amniocentesis*, *chorion biopsy*, *ultrasound* and *fetoscopy*. The whole process should be integrated with your *prenatal care*.

COLD SORES

These are tiny blisters that form around the nostrils and lips but they may extend further on to the cheeks. They are caused by a virus, herpes simplex I. Once the virus is transmitted to the skin, usually by kissing an infected person, it lies dormant in the nerve endings in the skin. A rise in skin temperature, which may be due to a variety of factors such as a common cold, direct sunlight or a fever, even the rise in body temperature that occurs around ovulation, then triggers off the virus.

Once the virus becomes active, the skin overlying the virus becomes hypersensitive, tender and tingling. Within hours a swelling occurs which becomes a small blister. Within 24 hours, the blister enlarges, bursts and crusts over. The sore itself takes between 10 and 14 days to heal over completely.

The other herpes virus, herpes simplex II, causes genital herpes and it is thought that about 10 percent of cases of genital herpes are caused by simplex I, probably from oral sex.

· S y m p t o m s ·

▲ Raised red area around the nostrils, mouth or cheeks which tingles and feels itchy
▲ Tiny blisters form within hours
▲ Weeping blister that crusts over

Should I see the doctor?
Consult your doctor if the cold sore appears anywhere near your eyes. This can cause ulcers to form on the front of the eyeball. If the self-help treatment fails to reduce the discomfort, or if the cold sore becomes infected, see your doctor right away.

What will the doctor do?
If the virus has affected your eye, your doctor will refer you to an ophthalmologist.

Your doctor may prescribe an anti-viral agent in ointment form. If it is applied locally to the area when the tingling starts, you may be able to abort or limit an attack next time. Application of the cream should be repeated every 30 minutes to prevent blisters forming. Special ophthalmic drops can be used in the treatment of herpes infections of the eyes.

What can I do?
Everyone has their own personal way of treating a cold sore and limiting its irritating and temporarily disfiguring effects. While it is open, before it crusts over, it is highly infectious, so avoid kissing and sexual contact. Some people prefer to keep the skin well lubricated and flexible with Vaseline; others like to dry it out by applying alcohol, though this method stings a great deal. Because the cold sores are caused by a virus, it must run its course and, once established, nothing will alter this. So prepare yourself for 10 to 14 days of feeling self-conscious and uncomfortable.

Once you have an attack of cold sores, try to avoid a recurrence by wearing sunblock on your lips when you go out in the sun or wind. If you keep an anti-viral agent in the house, you can apply it whenever you feel the tingling sensation.

Make sure you wash your hands after applying the medication. The virus can be easily spread.

SEE ALSO:

EYE PROBLEMS
GENITAL HERPES
SKIN PROBLEMS

COLORECTAL CANCER

Colorectal cancer is a portmanteau term for cancer of the large intestine, the colon and the rectum, and it is second only to lung cancer in the total number of new cases reported and the number of deaths caused by it. The high fatality rate associated with colorectal cancer is partly because symptoms are not dramatic, or if they are noticed, they are ignored and neglected. This is largely because cancer of the bowel is considered a taboo subject and many people believe the myth that it is not curable. The vast majority of colorectal cancers can be detected at an early and curable stage if you are observant about certain symptoms. Colorectal cancer should not be an unmentionable cancer; it is on the increase and it is important that we overcome any hesitation or embarrassment in talking about it with doctors.

· S y m p t o m s ·

- ▲ Dark brown or tarry stools
- ▲ Flecks of blood in stools
- ▲ Changes in bowel habits, such as difficulty passing stools
- ▲ Abdominal pain or perhaps vague indigestion
- ▲ Tiredness and lethargy

Should I see the doctor?
There are very few early warning signs. By the time rectal bleeding becomes obvious, the growth may be large. Small flecks of blood in the stool should always be heeded and a specimen of stool taken along to the doctor for examination.

If you notice a stool which is dark brown or tarry colored, you should also ask your doctor to examine it for "occult" blood tests. An occult blood test can pick up microscopic quantities of blood in the stool and three consecutive stools with positive occult blood tests necessitate further investigation by a specialist.

If you have any change in your bowel habit from a previously regular

DIAGNOSTIC TESTS
If your doctor suspects any kind of growth in your large intestine, you will be admitted to hospital for a diagnostic procedure such as:

Colonoscopy
This is a relatively simple technique for viewing the whole length of the large intestine without recourse to surgery. You are not usually given an anesthetic, just a sedative so that you relax. Your bowel will need to be clear of fecal matter.

The colonoscope is a flexible tube with a light source, magnifying eyepiece and tubes for blowing air in to inflate the bowel and suck back mucus and other secretions and to perform a biopsy if necessary. Colonoscopy usually follows a

daily motion to constipation or watery diarrhea, this should also alert you to the possibility of a colonic growth. A well-formed stool which suddenly becomes thin and pipe-like might suggest a stricture of the bowel caused by a scarring cancer and you should discuss this with your doctor. Any persistant abdominal discomfort or pain needs investigation.

What will the doctor do?
Your doctor will carry out a rectal examination in which a gloved, lubricated finger is passed into your anus to feel for growths or irregularities. You may then be referred to a specialist clinic for investigation of the bowel symptoms.

A barium enema may be performed when a radio-opaque fluid is injected into the rectum and colon and an X-ray picture taken to show up any irregularities in the walls of the intestine, indicating a tumor.

The wall of the bowel may be examined directly by use of a sigmoidoscope which can be passed into the bowel so that the tumor can be visualized, assessed and even biopsied.

barium enema if any irregularity was shown up on the X-ray picture.

Sigmoidoscopy
The other non-surgical means of diagnosing colorectal cancers is sigmoidoscopy. This is a wider tube to view the lower part of the large intestine. The air is used to expand the bowel and make insertion easier. This can cause cramping pains and you may feel the urge to pass a stool. It is important to relax; breathe through your mouth. It only takes about 15 minutes and when the instrument is withdrawn, the cramping pain will disappear. The main problem with these investigations is the feeling of indignity.

What is the medical treatment?
Cancer of the colon or rectum is nearly always treated by surgery.

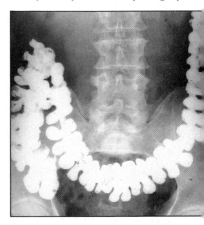

Barium enema
The human colon is revealed by X-ray. A tumor would be seen as a dark mass.

Although it is difficult to recognize at first, it is slow to spread and there is good chance of recovery. A section of the bowel containing the tumor is excised and the healthy ends of the intestine reunited. This is known as an intestinal resection. If it isn't possible to keep a passageway for food, an opening in the wall of the lower abdomen (a stoma) allows for a colostomy or bag to catch the undigested material. Surgery is often followed with anti-cancer drugs or radiation therapy if the cancer has spread. Very early cancers which have not yet pierced the wall of the intestine can be completely eradicated by surgery.

What can I do?

Most medical authorities agree that attention to diet may help. A regime which includes wholegrain breads or cereals, extra bran every day, and reduced quantities of animal fat may play an important protective role.

◆ Cut down on fried foods.
◆ Use low fat milk and substitute low fat yogurt for sour cream.
◆ Make stews and soups ahead and cool them so that fat may be removed easily.
◆ Serve more poultry, fish and less red meat; when you serve red meat trim off the fat and broil, don't fry.
◆ Serve high-fiber baked goods like wholewheat bread.
◆ Use as many of the cabbage family vegetables as you can and other stringy root vegetables.
◆ Serve high-fiber cereals and choose more high-fiber vegetables, especially legumes and fruits.
◆ Stir-fry vegetables and meat.
◆ After the age of 50, at least once a year, ask your doctor to perform a digital rectal examination and if anything untoward is discovered to perform a sigmoidoscopy. If you have any bowel symptoms at all which might be referrable to a tumor, request an occult blood test on your stools and if one comes up positive, follow up with further tests.

SEE ALSO:

CANCER
DIGESTIVE PROBLEMS
RADIATION THERAPY

COLPOSCOPY

This is the procedure that usually follows first if a Pap smear shows up any abnormal cells. The colposcope is a device with a light and powerful binoculars which allows a doctor to get a clear, magnified view of your vagina and cervix.

Why is it done?

When the results of a Pap smear are known, the action taken will depend to some extent on your doctor. If there is only mild dysplasia, your doctor may keep you under surveillance and do a smear every few months. If your doctor decides to use a colposcope, that may reduce the worry for you and even avoid the need for a biopsy which means going into hospital.

The colposcope doesn't offer a treatment, but it can determine the next stage; that is whether you have a cone biopsy or whether no further treatment is necessary because the abnormal cells can be explained as cervical erosion, for example.

How is it done?

This test can be performed in your doctor's office because it requires no anesthetic. A speculum is introduced into your vagina as for a Pap smear. The vaginal mucus is then wiped away and the colposcope placed at the vaginal entrance – it never actually enters the vagina. The doctor looks closely to try to identify the precise area of abnormal cells. A Pap smear only shows that there is some change but cannot pinpoint where. The doctor will then remove the speculum slowly so that the vaginal walls can be inspected too.

The whole procedure takes about 15 minutes. Sometimes the doctor may take a sample of the abnormal tissue with a curette. This will be sent to the laboratory for examination. If a sample is taken, you may experience some bleeding, but there should be no other side effects.

A COLPOSCOPIC EXAMINATION

Colposcopy has come to play an increasingly important role in the prevention and treatment of cervical cancer. It is a non-invasive way of viewing any changes to the tissue which will have been picked up by a Pap smear.

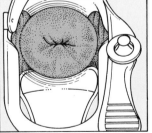

During colposcopic examination, a speculum is used to hold the vaginal walls apart and give a clear view of the cervix.

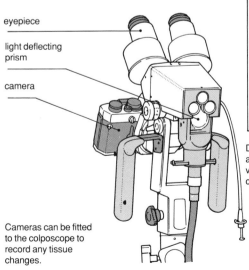

eyepiece

light deflecting prism

camera

Cameras can be fitted to the colposcope to record any tissue changes.

SEE ALSO:

CERVICAL CANCER
CERVIX PROBLEMS
CONE BIOPSY
PAP SMEAR

CONE BIOPSY

A cone biopsy, or conization, is one of the methods used to remove suspect tissue from the cervix for investigation or treatment. Colposcopy is the less invasive method of diagnosis and, where available, is preferable for investigating and diagnosing any changes to cervical tissue.

Why is it done?
A cone biopsy is performed if one or more Pap smears indicate dysplasia or the presence of cancerous cells in the cervix.

Dysplasia (cell abnormality) occurs if the skin on the outside of the cervix changes. This is symptomless and presents no risk to health, although in some cases, cancer develops after a long period of time. It is detected as the result of a routine Pap smear when some change in the cells is noted.

Cone biopsy is also used if colposcopy has failed to pinpoint the diseased cells. This is most likely to be the case for women over 35, as less of their cervical tissue can be seen on inspection due to retraction caused by age, or when the full extent of suspicious cells cannot be determined.

How is it done?
A cone biopsy is usually performed under a general anesthetic. The entire area of affected tissue, usually cone-shaped, hence its name, is removed using a scalpel or laser beam. Often a D & C will be performed at the same time to check the lining of the uterus for any spread of cancer. The area will be stitched to reduce bleeding, although cautery or freezing can also be used. The tissue is then sliced and examined microscopically to confirm the diagnosis.

Although used as a diagnostic tool for cervical cancer, a cone biopsy can result in successful treatment if the entire cancerous area is removed. If this is not so, further surgery or radiation therapy will be required.

What happens afterwards?
You will remain in hospital for two or three days and although there won't be much discomfort, the major problem may be your anxiety about the outcome of the biopsy.

You will probably have some bleeding and this may be staunched by packing gauze into your vagina or if it is light, by a sanitary towel. If the bleeding recurs, consult your doctor for treatment.

You will still require regular Pap smears to check if the cancer has spread.

Are there any risks?
There is some risk to the cervix with this procedure; the cervical canal narrows, bringing reduction in fertility. Any future births may have to be delivered by Caesarean section.

About 10 percent of women undergoing cone biopsy suffer a considerable blood loss. Carbon dioxide laser has recently been introduced as another means of removing tissue for analysis. The risk of bleeding and other complications is reduced with this method and it can also be performed on an outpatient basis.

HAVING A BIOPSY

If a woman has recurrent abnormal smears and colposcopy cannot reveal the entire area of suspicious cells, cone biopsy is done to remove a sufficient sample of tissue.

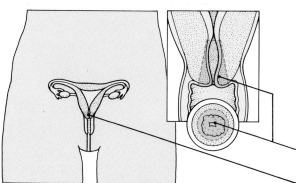

Under a general anesthetic, a cone-shaped piece of cervix containing the area of abnormal cells is removed with a scalpel, and the resulting crater is repaired by stitching flaps of tissue over the wound.

cone of cervix tissue

affected area of cervix

SEE ALSO:

CERVICAL CANCER
COLPOSCOPY
DILATATION AND
    CURETTAGE
PAP SMEAR

CONSTIPATION

The precise definition of constipation is hard, infrequent stools. Infrequent means less than every three or four days, and hard means pebble-like and painful to pass. Out of a thousand cases of constipation, only one or two are likely to be due to underlying disease. The majority of cases are caused by the wrong diet, insufficient exercise, lack of fluid intake and obsessive fussiness about daily bowel movements. There's hardly a bowel that doesn't respond to a natural purgative such as figs or prunes.

Paradoxically, chronic purgation can lead to constipation because the healthy bowel comes to rely on the purgative medicines. It ceases to react to natural reflexes and comes to rely on the purgatives completely. An unhealthy, lazy bowel may develop diverticulitis in which small growths develop on the colon and become inflamed, causing the individual severe pain and discomfort.

Constipation can also result from anxiety about pain if you have hemorrhoids or an anal fissure (a small ulcer in the anus); these make passing stools very painful.

· S y m p t o m s ·

▲ Infrequent stools
▲ Hard, pebble-like stools
▲ Red blood from the anus with pain

Should I see the doctor?
If you think that constipation is a symptom of a disorder, particularly if you suffer pain or notice any bleeding when passing stools, consult your doctor.

If constipation continues for a week or so and you previously had no problem with your bowels, particularly if you are over 50 years of age, see your doctor.

What will the doctor do?
Your doctor will question you about your diet, perhaps prescribe a

CONSTIPATION IN PREGNANCY

Progesterone is one of the hormones released in large quantities during pregnancy. It relaxes smooth muscle to enable the baby's head to pass out through the birth canal. The muscles in the bowel also relax and this can lead to constipation.

In late pregnancy, the pressure of the uterus on the bowel can aggravate the condition. As long as you eat a good high-fiber diet and get plenty of exercise, the constipation shouldn't become chronic. Avoid taking any laxatives without your doctor's approval.

---

gentle bowel softener and advise you to change to a high-fiber diet. You will probably be examined to check for hemorrhoids or an anal fissure if there is pain.

If there is no obvious reason for the constipation, you may be referred to a specialist for blood tests and perhaps a barium enema which helps to show up any problems in the bowel on X-ray.

What can I do?
Test yourself to see if poor diet is your problem. Eat 12–14 prunes or 6 figs one morning, and if your constipation corrects itself within 24 hours, this is proof that you need to change your diet to include more fiber. High-fiber foods are particularly useful as fiber holds water in the stools and this makes them soft and easy to pass. The fibrous foods that help correct bowel movements are any root, green or raw vegetable, any form of fresh fruit (make sure you eat the skins of apples and pears), high-fiber cereals, bread and cakes. Avoid eating too much of one item such as bran for example. This can deplete certain essential minerals in your diet.

You should try to drink at least $1^1/2$ liters (3 pints) of liquid per day. If you don't get enough liquids, the bowel, which is a water-conserving organ, will draw out the moisture from the stools and they will become drier and harder.

Exercise on its own can help reduce constipation. The pelvis and

intestinal muscles respond to any exercise. You may be leading too sedentary a life.

Don't take unnatural purgatives. Stop worrying about the frequency of stools. It's not unhealthy to empty your bowel once every three days.

Start listening to your bowel reflexes. If you lead a busy life, you may be forgetting to try to pass stools before you rush out in the morning. Retrain your bowel by giving it a chance to empty every time the reflex occurs.

Be sensible. If you've been ill, or off food for any other reason, or if you are in a hot climate and sweat a lot, don't expect your bowel movements to be normal. Most people suffer from mild constipation after a high fever, for example. Fever allows the evaporation of a great deal of sweat which renders the body relatively short of liquid and so the body attempts to conserve liquid by taking moisture out of the stools. This transient constipation will revert to normal when you resume your normal diet or drink plenty of water.

SEE ALSO:
DIGESTIVE PROBLEMS
HEMORRHOIDS
PREGNANCY PROBLEMS

CONTACT LENSES

Contact lenses may be hard or soft. Generally speaking, soft lenses are better for the eyes because they allow oxygen to pass through the contact lens and reduce risk of corneal abrasion. Hard lenses are not worn much longer than 12 hours per day; soft lenses can be worn for longer periods.

The newer, softer materials permit "extended" wear, but even so, most eye doctors recommend that they are not worn at night. Both hard and soft lenses improve visual acuity equally efficiently, but many wearers prefer soft lenses because they can be worn for long periods. Both types come in various colors such as blue, turquoise, green and violet, which can enhance the color of your eyes. Soft lenses are usually more than 70% water and therefore must always be kept wet in a saline solution; if they dry out they crystallize and crack.

Can I wear contact lenses?

The next time you visit your eye doctor ask if your visual defect could be corrected with contact lenses. If it can, the only way you can find out if your eyes will tolerate lenses comfortably is by trying them. A good eye doctor will fit you with trial lenses and suggest that you wear them for an hour or so, then come back for further examinations to report how you got on with them.

Very few people have such persistent difficulties that it's impossible to wear contact lenses, though they may be uncomfortable at first. Usually it takes no longer than a couple of hours to get used to how they feel and then the benefits are enormous. There are some instances when they aren't so convenient.

How to use contact lenses

Your eye doctor will give you your contact lenses in a kit which provides the contact lens holders and the cleaning and storage solutions. He will want to watch you putting the lenses into your eyes and taking them out and make sure that

HOW TO PUT THE LENSES IN

Make sure your hands are clean and your lenses thoroughly rinsed before inserting them in your eyes.

For your left eye place the lens the right way up on the top of your left index finger. With the fingers of your right hand, lift the left upper eyelid as high as you can, exposing the eyeball.

With the middle finger of your left hand, pull down the lower eyelid. Look downwards and place the lens on the eyeball.

Blink your eyes in front of a mirror and make sure that the lens is centered on your iris. Repeat the operation in reverse for the right eye.

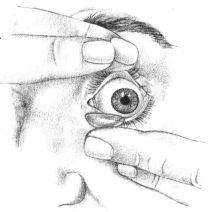

you are confident about handling them before allowing you to take the lenses home.

What are the complications?

Most problems result from poor standards of hygiene or leaving the lenses off for a time for some reason. If when you look at lights you see a halo, take the lenses out immediately. This could mean that your cornea is short of oxygen and is swelling up (corneal edema). Late intolerance can also occur after years of trouble-free wear. Contact your optician if this happens. Usually the problem is resolved if you change the material that your lens is made from.

One of the first symptoms that something is wrong is edema. This is painless but your vision may be somewhat foggy. Many women retain fluid pre-menstrually and this can cause increased pressure inside the eye, slightly altering its shape. Some women may find that contact lenses become slightly more uncomfortable at this time. Check with your eye doctor. Women on the pill may experience the same problems for the same reason. If you are on the pill always tell your eye doctor before contact lenses are fitted. You may be unsuitable for wearing contact lenses.

Avoid greasy makeup products as they can run and cloud the lenses.

Avoid mascara with "bits" in it as these can get into the eye, under the lens and scratch the cornea.

Always be meticulous about the hygiene and cleanliness of your lenses and the cleanliness of your hands. Any makeup or grease which get onto the lenses will hurt your eyes and blur your vision. Certain manufacturers have special lines of eye makeup for contact lens wearers.

Start wearing your contact lenses in easy stages, don't rush it. Most eye doctors would recommend two hours on the first day, four hours on the second, eight on the third and not longer than 12 for a week.

If the lenses hurt for any reason – remove them. The cause is usually a scratch of the cornea by the lens or a piece of grit has found its way underneath. You need to maintain high standards of cleanliness when handling your lenses, even after years of wearing.

SEE ALSO:

CONTRACEPTION
EYE PROBLEMS
PREMENSTRUAL SYNDROME

CONTRACEPTION

Preventing conception is a very old idea. The Egyptians used chemicals and plant extracts, both to prevent pregnancy and to procure an immediate abortion. Barrier methods of contraception using such methods as lemon rind, lamb skin and silk squares have been known for centuries.

Contraception has separated sexual intercourse from procreation so that while once women avoided sex because of a fear of unwanted pregnancy, this is no longer the case. It also enables women to face up to their own sexuality and take on the role of initiating sexual experiences. It puts women in the position of being free to explain to their partners what they prefer and what they find enjoyable.

Contraception, in contrast to the past, and because it is more in a woman's interest, has become the woman's responsibility, though ideally it should be a dual responsibility. However, this is changing again. With the advent of AIDS, the simple condom is coming back into fashion, forcing men to take back some of the responsibility.

What is the most effective means?
If you require near 100% efficacy of your contraceptive method, without resorting to sterilization, there is only one choice – the combined contraceptive pill. This prevents ovulation so that pregnancy cannot occur. The morning-after pill, as long as it is taken right away, can be 100% effective, too.

The second most effective means is the mini-pill or progestogen-only pill. Next there are the intra-uterine devices, followed by the various barrier methods. The more efficient the adherence and care taken with these methods, the more effective they can be. This is why effectiveness can be judged by two criteria: theoretical and actual. Invariably, the latter has a higher failure rate because of the human element. The least effective, largely because of

human error, are the so-called natural methods, ones that rely on determining safe periods and abstaining from intercourse during that time.

The greatest risk of contraception is getting pregnant. As all the medical complications of pregnancy outweigh those medical complications in women who take the combined pill, it therefore follows that the greatest risk is with those methods that have the lowest efficiency rate.

Methods of contraception
Your choice of birth control will probably change during your fertile years. No one method is ideal for this length of time, punctuated as it may be by planned pregnancies and changes in sexual partners. You need to think about and consider all the forms of contraception and match them to your personality, sexual practice and stage in life.
For example:
Are you forgetful?
Do you dislike touching your own genitals?
Would you be prepared to have a baby if your method failed?
Do you have to practice "safe sex?"

All methods do have their advantages and disadvantages and it is sensible to discuss them with your doctor or at a family planning clinic.

NATURAL METHODS

These include the oldest forms of contraception and are of three main types – periodic abstinence, breast-feeding and coitus interruptus.

Periodic abstinence
Abstaining from intercourse during the time of ovulation is based on calculations using the calendar, the rise and fall of the woman's body temperature and the appearance of vaginal secretions. Using these indicators, you can, with the co-operation of your partner, abstain from full intercourse for the period during which the egg is released and

the sperm can survive to fertilize the egg.

All natural forms of contraception attempt to pinpoint the time of ovulation accurately. The calendar or rhythm method requires you to chart your cycle and abstain from intercourse during the fertile days between the last day of your period and the expected first day of your next. This method relies almost entirely on a regular cycle.

The sympto-thermal method is more accurate. It involves taking your temperature and observing the consistency and color of your vaginal secretions. By taking your temperature with a very accurate thermometer at the same time every day (preferably first thing in the morning), you should be able to notice a rise of a fraction of a degree during the second half of your cycle, providing you are not suffering from an infection. This is because the hormone progesterone is secreted at the time of ovulation. It is capable of raising the body temperature by about .6°C (1°F) and keeping it at this level until the next menstrual period.

The second part of the routine is known as the Billings method. Your vaginal secretions also change during your cycle. Immediately after menstruation, you will be comparatively dry. Then as the mucus builds up, you may notice it as thick, cloudy and sticky. This changes to clear, stretchy and abundant about the time of ovulation. Shortly afterwards it reverts back to thick and cloudy until your next period. The safe period here is when there is no mucus following your period, and then not again until the mucus reverts to thickness after being thin, indicating that ovulation has occurred. The problem is that semen can mask the true nature of your vaginal secretions.

What are the risks?
This method is hopeless for women with irregular cycles and it requires a strong commitment from both

partners which is a positive advantage. However, there are no risks to health but there may be to relationships and, with the comparatively high failure rate, problems of unwanted pregnancy. The techniques need at least six months to become established and for you to gain a clear idea of what is normal for you.

Some research into more effective methods for pinpointing ovulation precisely is being done to make periodic abstinence more successful as a means of contraception.

Breastfeeding
This is a well-established method in the third world and works well for those women who choose to feed their babies for more than three months. Breastfeeding over a 24-hour period changes the levels of hormones and prevents ovulation. However, it is not a reliable means of birth control and becomes particularly unreliable once you offer the baby solids and the 24-hour feeding regime is reduced. Just because you don't have a period during breastfeeding does not mean you are not producing eggs. So although breastfeeding can work for individual women, it is not a reliable option

without taking other precautions, such as the low-dose mini pill or barrier methods. You must also think of your new baby and the risk of having another too quickly.

Coitus interruptus or withdrawal
This is another ancient method where the penis is withdrawn just before ejaculation. It is still popular amongst those who are jointly happy about it – the woman must have great confidence in her partner's ability to withdraw in time. It removes the need to organize and discuss methods and means with doctors and at clinics and requires no financial outlay. It also leaves much of the responsibility with the man. But it has a high failure rate.

BARRIER METHODS

These methods physically block the sperm from reaching the ovum or chemically inactivate them. They include condoms, the diaphragm and cervical cap, contraceptive sponges, and spermicides. Even in the present sexual climate when people are less likely to have unplanned sex due to the number of sexually transmitted diseases, they

are less bothersome than in the past. A diaphragm or cap can be inserted several hours before intercourse may take place and spermicides can be "topped up" quickly and unobtrusively.

Condoms
The condom is a latex rubber or plastic sheath that is placed over the erect penis before penetration. It should be lubricated and freed from air so it doesn't burst inside the vagina. It comes in different sizes, textures and colors. It works by preventing the sperm from entering the vagina.

Although the condom has been easily available for years, its popularity declined with the advent of the pill and IUDs. However, it is now back in use even where another form of contraception is practiced because of the increased incidence of sexually transmitted diseases and especially AIDS. I would therefore advise all women who have not been engaged in monogamous relationships for over five years to insist on their partners using condoms.

The diaphragm and cervical cap
The diaphragm is a cone of rubber with a coiled metal spring in its rim. This is made in different sizes depending on a woman's internal shape and size. It fits diagonally across the vagina and is used with a spermicidal agent and must be left in place for six hours after intercourse.

The cervical cap is smaller and more rigid than a diaphragm and fits over the cervix where it is held in place by suction. Some resemble over-sized thimbles. They are used by women whose internal anatomy makes the diaphragm difficult to retain. It must also be fitted to size and used in conjunction with a spermicidal agent. Although not readily available in the U.S., the cervical cap is presently distributed by a limited number of clinics on a trial basis.

NATURAL METHODS

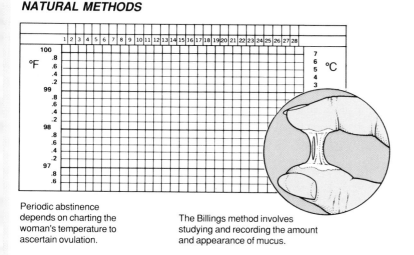

Periodic abstinence depends on charting the woman's temperature to ascertain ovulation.

The Billings method involves studying and recording the amount and appearance of mucus.

CONTRACEPTION

BARRIER METHODS

These include a number of different devices and/or chemicals which block or otherwise prevent sperm from reaching the ovum. Spermicides should be used with devices for maximum protection.

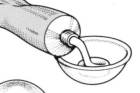

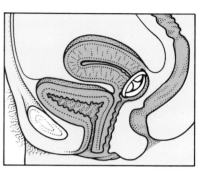

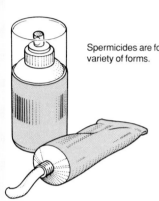

Spermicides are found in a variety of forms.

A diaphragm fits diagonally across the front wall of the vagina with the top part of the rim up behind the cervix. The smaller, more rigid cervical cap fits tightly over the cervix itself.

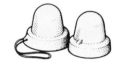

Types of cervical cap

Condoms

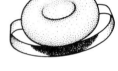

Contraceptive sponge

The diaphragm and cap work by preventing sperm reaching the cervix. Their most important function, and probably the reason for their effectiveness, is that they act as receptacles for spermicides. They make intercourse less messy during menstruation, too.

The diaphragm or cap must be fitted regularly, particularly if your internal shape changes because of childbirth or weight gain or loss.

Contraceptive sponge

This is an old form of contraception updated with more contemporary materials. These days it is usually made of polyurethane foam and is impregnated with spermicide. A loop is attached which is used to remove the sponge. The sponge is moistened with water to activate the spermicide and left in place for six hours after intercourse.

Spermicides

The use of a spermicide is essential with these barrier methods to ensure their effectiveness by blocking and killing the sperm; they are not effective on their own as they must be at the cervix, not just somewhere in the vagina. They come in many forms, including aerosols, suppositories, foams, film and creams. This means that the manufacturer's instructions must be followed carefully. For example, some should not be used with a rubber cap; some need to be inserted 15 minutes before intercourse. The spermicide should not be washed away for at least six hours after intercourse to catch any sperm.

Spermicides would seem to be an added protection against contracting sexually transmitted diseases.

What are the risks and problems

These methods may interfere with spontaneous lovemaking. The degree of planning means that they are more suitable for well-organized people, or those in an established relationship. However, they are effective and relatively cheap and, unless you are allergic to the spermicide or the rubber, present no risk to health. Some men do say that condoms reduce their sensations and cystitis is more common among diaphragm users.

HORMONAL METHODS

These methods use hormones to suppress ovulation. They alter the hormonal balance so the ovaries do not produce eggs. In fact, they convince your body that you are already pregnant, and interfere with the cervical mucus, making it thick and impenetrable to sperm and thin the uterine lining so the egg cannot attach itself there. The forms include the combined pill, the low-dose mini-pill, hormonal injections and implants, and the post-coital pill.

Combined pill

This uses synthetic progestogen and estrogen to suppress ovulation. It must be taken for the full course of either 21 or 28 days to be effective.

Low-dose mini-pill
This pill contains progestogen only. It is slightly less reliable because ovulation may occur but the other factors still apply. Estrogen is implicated in some of the side effects of the combined pill because of its effect on the circulatory system.

Hormonal injections and implants
While not yet approved for general use in the U.S., hormonal injections and implants are currently available through research programs established to investigate this revolutionary method which has proved quite successful in Europe. Most injectable contraceptives contain only progestogens and they are administered every two or three months. They have the same make-up as the mini-pill but are injected rather than swallowed. They are ideal for those women who have difficulty remembering to take the pills. Implants are usually inserted under the skin of the upper arm and remain active for five years. Both these methods are relatively free from side effects because of the lack of estrogen, and they are extremely effective because motivation by the user is not a problem.

The return to fertility is sometimes slow after an injectable contraceptive but usually quite soon after an implant is removed. There may be breakthrough bleeding.

Post-coital methods
There are two means of preventing conception after intercourse and they must be started within 24-72 hours after unprotected intercourse. These are usually reserved for rape victims and for unprotected intercourse when the woman may have been ovulating. This is not recommended as a routine form of birth control.

The hormonal method involves a five-day course of estrogens or a short high-dose course of the combined pill. The doses are similar to those used in the 1960s when the pill was first introduced and present no danger if used rarely. They may cause nausea and vomiting. It is not entirely clear how this method works in preventing pregnancy.

For women who cannot take the high-dose pill, a copper-bearing IUD can be inserted within five days of unprotected intercourse; this prevents a possible pregnancy.

What are the risks?
These hormonal methods are the most effective because they act on the reproductive cycle in the same way as our natural hormones do. However, there lies the difference. They are synthetic hormones (the natural form is destroyed by our gastric juices) and for a lot of women the idea of taking drugs for many years when you are otherwise healthy is not a pleasant prospect.

Before the pill is prescribed, you will be examined to determine whether taking the pill endangers you or not. It will not be suitable for women who are overweight; those who smoke; are over 35; suffer from diabetes, high blood pressure, a heart condition, deep vein thrombosis, or certain forms of migraine headache.

New methods under investigation
Research is continuing all the time into new methods of contraception, including the male pill. New research includes the use of luteinizing hormone-releasing hormone which regulates the release of the other hormones during the ovulatory cycle. This is being investigated as a nasal spray which works only on the

HORMONAL METHODS
These are made of synthetic progestogens, sometimes combined with synthetic estrogens.

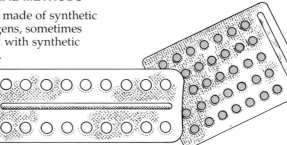

Advantages
The mini-pill is more advantageous for breastfeeding women (estrogen inhibits milk production), young women or those over 35 who want to continue to use the pill. All contraceptive pills
- regulate menstruation and reduce pain and bleeding
- reduce chance of developing anemia
- reduce effects of premenstrual syndrome
- reduce incidence of benign cysts and ovarian cancers
- are highly effective against pregnancy
- are easy to use

Disadvantages
These mainly consist of increased medical risks and include
- greater risk of thrombosis
- chance of increasing blood pressure
- increases breast size
- reduces libido
- results in slower return of fertility
- requires motivation to take it at the same time every day
- breakthrough bleeding with some forms

CONTRACEPTION

pituitary gland and ovaries and not on other parts of the body, an obvious advantage over the pill.

There is an anti-progesterone being developed. This would stop production of progesterone in the second half of the cycle, thus preventing implantation of any fertilized egg in the uterus.

Various devices impregnated with hormones are being developed for insertion into the vagina or the uterus to release the progestogens slowly and to act directly on the reproductive organs.

INTRA-UTERINE DEVICE

This is a device inserted into the uterus and left there. It probably works by preventing the fertilized egg from implanting itself on the uterine lining by creating a hostile environment. They are immediately effective in preventing pregnancy and do not interfere with breast-feeding or the natural hormonal balance. They are generally best for women in stable relationships who have already had children.

There are many different shapes and sizes of IUDs. Most have a tail for easy removal and as a quick check that they are still in place.

Risks and disadvantages

While the IUD continues to be a popular contraceptive option throughout the world, in the U.S., medical problems associated with the IUD have given rise to safety concerns. Fears were particularly triggered in late 1973 by the Dalkon Shield, a plastic IUD which was linked directly to septic midtrimester spontaneous abortions, pelvic infection, sterility, and even death. The device was withdrawn from the market and these findings led to large scale reduction in IUD manufacture throughout the 1980's.

Currently, only one IUD, the Progestasert, is readily available in the U.S., although many women continue to use IUDs prescribed to

INTRA-UTERINE DEVICES

Made mainly of plastic, these devices are left in the uterus but can be removed readily by a doctor.

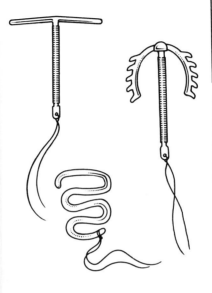

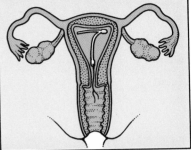

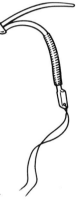

Some IUDs may have copper or a female hormone (progester-one) added to reduce side effects. All contain a string for checking that they are still in place or for removal.

them before the reduction in IUD manufacture. However, improved IUDs are now in the research stage and should be available soon. But, the risks associated with IUD use are still quite real and should be thoroughly discussed with your health care professional. If, for some reason, you have a Dalkon Shield in place, you should immediately visit your physician to have it removed. IUDs are not ideally suitable for young women who have not had children. IUDs have been implicated in cases of perforation of the uterus, septic abortion, pelvic inflammatory disease and ectopic pregnancy. They may increase bleeding and pain during menstruation so they are not suitable for women with heavy periods. Expulsion of the devices is not uncommon and they are painful to insert in some cases.

SEE ALSO

ABORTION
AIDS
BLEEDING
CYSTITIS
DEEP VEIN THROMBOSIS
ECTOPIC PREGNANCY
HYPERTENSION
PELVIC INFLAMMATORY
   DISEASE
PREMENSTRUAL SYNDROME
STERILIZATION

COSMETIC DENTISTRY

Cosmetic dentistry includes all those treatments that improve the appearance of your teeth. This ranges from whitening or repositioning the teeth, to complicated techniques like crowns and bridges. A skilled cosmetic dentist can alter the look of your teeth or your smile as well as the set of your mouth and therefore to some degree can alter your facial expression. In conserving teeth, dentists and oral hygienists are our best friends. A six-monthly visit to a dentist for check-ups and minor repairs can obviate the necessity for fillings, crowns and radical dental work. Regular visits to the hygienist are even more important because with ultrasonic instruments, it's possible to remove plaque from between teeth carefully and painlessly. With three-monthly visits, plaque never builds up and is never able to damage the gums; more people lose teeth through gum disease than for any other reason.

Quite a number of dentists specialize in cosmetic dentistry and can perform a variety of dental operations which can make an enormous difference to the way we look and vastly improve our appearance.

WHITENING THE TEETH

Toothpastes can make the teeth "appear" whiter. A pink-colored toothpaste can create an optical illusion; the teeth look white in comparison to the pink gums. Another method is to add abrasives to the toothpaste. These are generally thought to be too harsh to be used in preparations for teeth because they may scratch the surface of the enamel which may then become damaged or worn away by the prolonged use of such toothpastes.

The best and safest way to give your teeth a new look is to visit a dental hygienist who will remove plaque from between the teeth and will de-scale them and give them a good polish to remove surface stains. This makes everyone's teeth look several shades whiter, particularly smokers'. The teeth darken with time, however, as the outer enamel thins, revealing more of the darker inner dentine.

Discolored teeth – this is usually because the pulp is dead or has been removed – can be bleached by painting them with an oxidizing agent, and then exposing them to a special light.

RE-POSITIONING THE TEETH

If teeth are malaligned, this can lead to tooth decay because you can't clean them properly. This problem can be solved with orthodontics which should ideally be started before the age of 14 by a pediatric orthodontist who will use braces and wires to pull badly positioned teeth into alignment. This is because the jaw and teeth are still growing and developing.

Buck teeth can be treated in adulthood by the use of crowns. The malpositioned teeth are filed away and the crowns are fitted to follow the normal line.

CROWNS

A broken, ugly or severely malpositioned tooth can be given a new appearance by crowning or capping (the two terms are synonymous). This is usually done by filing the tooth away to form a peg onto which the crown is cemented. Even a tooth that has snapped off or has had to be removed at the line of the gum margin can be crowned. In such cases, the tooth is trimmed to the gum margin and the pulp removed. This space is known as a root canal; it will be cleaned out and one post, onto which the crown can be fixed, is drilled into it.

Crowns are hollow shells made of a variety of materials; the good modern ones are composed of porcelain. This can be matched to the color of the teeth so that the finished crown won't be noticed as different to the rest of the teeth. The crown can be made in any shape to conform to the size and contour of the mouth. Crowns for back teeth have to be stronger; these are made from gold, or porcelain bonded to gold or some other metal.

BRIDGES AND DENTURES

A bridge is an artificial tooth (or teeth) that fits permanently into a gap between existing sound teeth. This is done by crowning the teeth on either side of the gap. A bridge can consist of as many as four teeth.

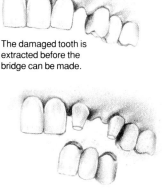

The damaged tooth is extracted before the bridge can be made.

The healthy teeth either side are shaped to take crowns.

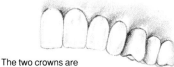

The two crowns are cemented in place and "bridge" the gap.

Dentures replace many missing teeth and unlike crowns are removed for cleaning. The requisite number of false teeth are secured in the appropriate places on the plate. The plate slips easily into place and is held snugly in the mouth by wires that fit around existing teeth. It can be removed for cleaning either with sterilizing solution or with a brush.

COSMETIC DENTISTRY

Replacement of all your teeth is by means of a full denture. This stays in place by suction with the base plate resting on the gums.

BONDING

This is a technique which can be used in preventative dentistry as well as for cosmetic reasons.

Preventative dental bonding uses sealants to protect teeth from decay and sensitivity. It is a plastic coating, usually applied to the back molars. For example, young children have their teeth sealed routinely at around age 10. This is known as fissure sealing.

Cosmetic bonding involves attaching plastic or porcelain to the surface of the tooth. This can be used to level off chipped teeth, to fill in spaces between teeth, to correct malformations and to provide a key for veneers. The technique is sometimes called acid-etching. The liquid bonding material or resin is then applied to the surface of the tooth to fill the chip or space, and shaped on the tooth and allowed to harden.

For front teeth, veneers made from porcelain or acrylic can be bonded to the surface of the tooth. The enamel is acid-etched and an adhesive resin attached. Then the pre-shaped veneer is placed on top of the resin.

Bonding procedures last on average about five years, so they will need redoing. However, they are painless because they require no drilling or anesthetic. Bonded materials aren't as strong or durable as crowns, however, so problem back teeth are better replaced with crowns. Other drawbacks of bonding on front teeth include, firstly, that certain foodstuffs can stain the veneers, and secondly, that the veneers are more likely to chip.

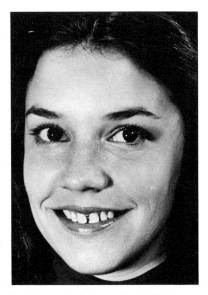

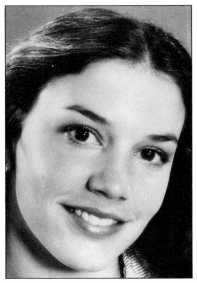

A painless and effective method of filling the gap between the two top front teeth is with bonding materials. Here natural ceramic facings were bonded to the two front teeth and extended slightly to fill the gap. These materials may chip or discolor, however.

SEE ALSO:

DENTAL PROBLEMS
GUM DISEASE

COSMETIC OPERATIONS

With modern operations and new techniques of cosmetic surgery, it is possible to re-contour almost any part of the body if you are unhappy with the shape you've got.

However, there is a price to pay over and above the cost of the surgery. There is no question that extensive cosmetic surgery of this kind leaves scarring although many women are happy to put up with this. What you have to weigh up is the trade off: are you the kind of woman who wants to look good in clothes or do you wish to be free from scars when you are naked? If you want the former then cosmetic surgery is an option. If not, then you would be advised not to consider it.

ABDOMINOPLASTY

This is the removal of folds of fat from the lower abdomen, sometimes called apronectomy. This operation is done for cosmetic reasons, or if you have been grossly overweight and, after dieting, have lost so much weight that the loose skin of your abdomen forms tucks of redundant skin.

Doctors are unwilling to perform an abdominoplasty until you have completed your family, because new fat and stretchmarks might occur with a pregnancy.

How is it done?
You will have to go into hospital for about seven days. Under a general anesthetic, the incision is made along one of the body lines across the lower abdomen and the fat removed. The site of the scar means it is barely visible afterwards. The operation lasts about two hours and you will have a drainage tube in the wound for about three to five days.

The stitches will be removed after two weeks, but for the first three to five days you will have to maintain a position with your body bent so that the wound isn't stretched. Your general mobility will be restricted for up to three months.

BUTTOCKS, HIPS AND THIGHS

These can be completely reshaped by removing fat and skin. Your doctor may insist that you diet to try to lose as much weight as possible before the operation.

How is it done?
Under a general anesthetic, incisions are made along natural body lines. These are known as Lange lines and are used by cosmetic surgeons. Slices of skin and fat are removed in an operation lasting between two and three hours, depending on the complexities of the fat removal. You will suffer only mild discomfort for the first two weeks and will need to limit sports-type activities for about a month. The results of this operation are good though there will be some visible scars.

THE UPPER ARMS

It is possible to remove loose fat and skin from the upper arms in a simple and straightforward operation. You should only need to be in hospital for 48 hours. There will be hardly any discomfort and you can undertake stretching movement after two weeks. There will be scarring along the underside of the arm afterwards.

TOTAL BODY LIFT

This operation is rarely done in one go. It involves the removal of sagging skin from the abdomen, buttocks, thighs, arms and neck. Each stage requires a hospital stay on different occasions. You will be asked to lose as much weight as possible with diet and exercise prior to surgery.

LIPECTOMY

The aim of lipectomy or fat aspiration is to flatten or reduce unwanted curves. It is said to be particularly effective for "jodhpur" thighs.

How is it done?
This is the most modern technique of localized fat removal. Under local anesthetic, a fairly wide tube (diameter 1cm – $^3/\sin$) is placed inside the skin in the subcutaneous fat. The fat is then drawn off using vacuum suction. Quantities of up to one liter (2 pints) can be drawn off at one treatment.

What are the results?
Sometimes the results can be unsatisfactory because it is impossible for the operator to draw fat from a particular spot and so the treated area may be abnormally dented following treatment.

There is also a medical hazard involved with this technique. Body fat is in biochemical equilibrium with blood and bone fats. Removal of a sizeable amount will inevitably interfere with this delicate balance. As no scientific studies have quantified this effect, lipectomy should be treated with caution and only performed by a skilled medical practitioner.

Afterwards there is quite a lot of pain when walking.

SEE ALSO:

FACE LIFT
OTOPLASTY
RHINOPLASTY

COSMETIC SURGERY

Plastic surgery was a speciality which started during World War II because of the necessity to repair the disfiguring injuries sustained by pilots. Even in recent wars, because of the pressure on surgeons to be ingenious and innovative, the field of plastic surgery has advanced in leaps and bounds with this essential part of war work. Over the past 25 years, popular attitudes to this form of surgery being used for cosmetic reasons have changed substantially. At one time *facelifts* or *rhinoplasty* used to be considered frivolous. Today, any cosmetic surgery for a condition which has proven to be emotionally traumatizing, such as rebuilding a breast after *mastectomy*, can be performed to a high standard. If breasts are embarrassingly pendulous, they can be reduced (see *Breast operations*); if a chin is disfiguringly undershot or a nose too long, it can be augmented or shortened. If ears protrude, they can be pinned back through a simple procedure known as *Otoplasty*.

If you seek cosmetic surgery not merely to transform your face or body but to transform your life, then you are doomed to disappointment. Never decide on cosmetic surgery immediately after a crisis such as a divorce or a bereavement. You should opt for cosmetic surgery when life is going well and not when you are feeling lonely, guilty or disorientated.

Re-shaping various parts of the body has become now almost a universal option with the advent of lipectomy. In this operation, fat is sucked under vacuum from those parts of the body where there are unsightly bulges, such as at the top of the thighs and the arms (see *Cosmetic operations*).

Most of these cosmetic operations are done in the hospital, under general anesthetic, with a minimum stay of 48 hours, considerably longer for the more complicated operations. After most of the operations you will feel some stiffness for several days until you get the parts working again, but usually in about two months everything is back to normal and there will be no residual stiffness.

The majority of the operations are very effective and give results with which patients are highly delighted. A very small number do go wrong and it is as well that you prepare yourself for that eventuality. It's unusual for any patient to be worse off than they were before, but the effect may not be exactly the one you desired. If your cosmetic surgeon is any good, you should be told of this before the operation and have discussed a course of action should it occur. Most surgeons will be happy to re-do the operation though you may not feel like taking another chance. Some of the worst results in the past were where implants were used, particularly silicone in the breasts. It was thought that this and other substances used as implants would stay exactly in place and be ignored by the body. Both of these things proved not to be the case. Implants did slip, and some of them became very hard when they were invaded by body cells and turned into scar tissue. Though rare with modern materials, you should discuss these possibilities with your cosmetic surgeon before undergoing treatment.

While most operations are effective, they don't last forever. A "face job" would not be guaranteed for longer than eight years. The operation can be repeated, but for how long? If you are obsessed with looking youthful, one face lift can follow another with your skin getting tighter and your smile more fixed. You should examine your attitude to getting older rather than consider another face lift.

To have the best chance of a satisfactory result, choose a good surgeon. Avoid a surgeon who is willing to perform exactly the operation you want and offers no professional opinion as to what you "need." A good surgeon will try to do the operation that gives you the best result and should certainly offer suggestions about what should be done. If you are offered a 100% guarantee of success, leave the office. A realistic surgeon will always discuss what might go wrong and will never guarantee anything.

Other non-surgical means of improving your appearance include *dermabrasion* and *facial treatments* such as chemical skin peeling. These are particularly useful for scarring after bad *acne*.

COUGHING

Coughs are unproductive when they are dry and seem to have no obvious cause, or productive when they produce phlegm. The cough is the body's way of reacting to an irritant in the throat or lungs, or it is a symptom of an illness. Though coughs are irritating they are not usually serious on their own.

If you buy proprietary cough mixtures, make sure you choose the correct sort for your cough. For example, if you are coughing up phlegm, do not use a cough suppressant medicine. Only use this if the cough is dry and troublesome.

If you have an irritating dry cough which keeps you awake at night, and if it is accompanied by a sore throat, prop yourself up with pillows and gargle with a soluble aspirin to reduce the pain or take a hot lemon drink to soothe your throat.

Although we all have coughs from time to time, a persistent cough that suddenly gets worse may indicate a serious problem in your lungs. It could be a symptom of lung cancer, particularly if you are a smoker.

If you are unable to make a diagnosis from this information, consult your doctor.

NATURE OF COUGH	PROBABLE CAUSE
It produces phlegm and you also have a fever	This could be bronchitis, an infection of the lungs or pneumonia. Consult your doctor right away.
You have difficulty in breathing	This could indicate a serious condition. Your doctor can diagnose the cause for you.
You have a runny nose and/or sore throat	This is a common cold. Treat yourself symptomatically and prop yourself up at night so the postnasal drip doesn't irritate your throat further and cause more coughing.
The cough is recurrent, dry and getting worse over several weeks	This may be an allergy, or the result of smoking. However, it could also be a symptom of a tumor on your lungs, so consult your doctor (see *Lung cancer*).
The sputum is yellow/green	This could be a lung infection such as chronic bronchitis or pneumonia. You probably need a course of antibiotics. See your doctor.
There are streaks of blood in your sputum	This may be the result of a burst blood vessel caused by constant coughing or vomiting. However, a more serious lung condition may be present, so see your doctor.
The cough is accompanied by wheezing where you have difficulty breathing	This may be an asthma attack or an infection in the lungs. See your doctor.

CYSTITIS

Cystitis is an inflammation of the bladder. The inflammation may be caused by an infection or by mechanical trauma and bruising. Nearly all infections which reach the bladder are due to bacteria entering the urethra from the outside; they spread upwards from the vagina, the anus and the skin of the perineum and inflame the bladder lining.

If the infection spreads from the bladder to the kidneys and causes pyelonephritis, the pain may radiate round into the flanks. If a fever is present, there may also be nausea and vomiting.

A strong yellow to orange-colored urine, even one with a strong smell, is not indicative of an infection. Both of these can occur simply because you do not drink enough fluid or you may be dehydrated due to vomiting or sweating profusely. Also, you may have eaten some food, asparagus is one, that can cause urine to change color, if eaten in large quantities.

If you experience a burning feeling when you pass urine, this may be urethritis, inflammation of the urethra. If you also have severe pain, and this pain is nearly always worse when urination is completed, this is cystitis. The inflamed walls of the bladder contract down to extrude the last few drops of urine, squeezing the inflamed tissues as they do so.

Cystitis is very common, annoying and inconvenient, but it does not endanger general health. Most women have it at some time in their lives. It is particularly common during pregnancy, especially in the first few months. Pregnancy is a predisposing factor, not because infections are more common, but because the urethra relaxes under the influence of the pregnancy hormone progesterone and therefore infections ascend more easily. Later on in pregnancy the pressure of the enlarging uterus may cause a small amount of residual urine to remain in the bladder after urination. The urine becomes stagnant and lack of flow may encourage bacterial multiplication.

· Symptoms ·

▲ The urgent need to pass urine frequently though only a small amount of urine may be passed each time
▲ A severe dragging-down pain, usually in the front of the abdomen but quite often radiating up the flanks and to the back
▲ A burning or stinging sensation when passing urine
▲ A severe pain on passing urine
▲ The passage of blood in the urine which may be pink, red or simply streaked with blood
▲ The necessity to get up several times in the night to empty your bladder even though there may be very little urine present

---

What causes it?

The commonest infecting organism is E.coli which is a bacterium living normally within the bowel and around the anus and usually causing no problems. The bacterium spreads from the rectum onto the perineum and up the female urethra, which is much shorter than the male urethra, into the bladder.

Mechanical trauma such as strenuous sexual intercourse is another common cause of cystitis (honeymoon cystitis). If sexual intercourse brings on an attack of cystitis, this is also known as urethral syndrome. During the Second World War, land army girls riding on the unsprung seats of tractors also complained of cystitis due to the bumpy ride. In more modern times, the advent of nylon panty hose and very tight jeans has given rise to cystitis because of pressure on and even bruising of the urethra.

In older women, prolapse of the front of the vaginal wall, causing kinking of the urethra, may be associated with cystitis because of poor urinary flow and a possible ascending infection.

Occasionally, cystitis can be caused by the use of antiseptics in bath water or the over-zealous use of vaginal deodorants. Vaginal douches can also cause cystitis. As women get older and reach the menopause, a shortage of the female hormones, estrogen and progesterone, can lead to thinning and loss of integrity of all the genital organs and the perineum and in some unexplained way this can contribute to a menopausal type of cystitis.

If for any reason a woman needs an in-dwelling catheter, as she might if she is suffering from incontinence due to a disease such as multiple sclerosis, for example, then an infection may occur. However, the chances are reduced if a sterile technique is assiduously employed when the catheter is passed.

Contrary to popular belief, dirty toilet habits do not per se cause cystitis, not unless there is another predisposing factor, although you should always wipe yourself from the front back towards the anus.

Should I see the doctor?

If self-help measures don't bring relief and ease the pain, then seek help from your doctor quickly. Cystitis needs antibiotic treatment so you should get in touch with your doctor and make an early appointment. By far the greatest pain relief comes with taking antibiotics. Some women report that as soon as the antibiotics appear in the urine, which is about half an hour after taking them, pain is relieved.

What will the doctor do?

Before prescribing antibiotics your doctor should take a specimen of urine for bacterial culture to see which bacterium is causing your symptoms and to find out its sensitivity to a range of antibiotics. As soon as the specimen has been taken, however, your doctor can start you on a course of antibiotics. This is usually in the form of a sulphonamide drug or a penicillin derivative.

It's absolutely essential that you take a full course of treatment even

CYSTITIS

though your symptoms may have subsided completely within 24 hours. If you do not do so, the infecting organisms may become resistant to antibiotics and your cystitis become chronic. If this happens, it is exceedingly difficult to eradicate, so doctors usually recommend that cystitis is treated by a full seven, or ten day course of antibiotics.

If the cystitis proves to be intractable, it is essential that you have a full hospital investigation to see whether or not there is any predisposing internal cause. Tests may include a cystogram where a radio-opaque dye is passed into the bladder and you are X-rayed while passing urine so the doctor can observe your bladder reflexes.

If investigation shows no trace of a bacterium, you may be suffering from an irritable bladder which is often caused by emotional factors.

What should I do?

Drink plenty of fluids at the first sign of the symptoms. It's important to get urine flowing fast so drink plenty of water. Thereafter, try to drink the equivalent of a glass of water or fruit and vegetable juices every half hour.

Make the urine alkaline. An alkaline urine discourages bacterial growth. As urine is usually acid you can render it alkaline by adding a little bicarbonate of soda to your drinks. You will find that this eases bladder pain quite considerably.

For pain relief, take acetaminophen every four hours. A warm pad or hot water bottles on the front of the abdomen may relieve pain.

How can I prevent a recurrence?

◆ Drink plenty of water at all times.
◆ At the first symptom, increase your water intake and alkalinize the urine by adding a little bit of bicarbonate of soda to your drinks. Don't continue this for too long or you'll have unpleasant side effects, such as wind.
◆ If you are having very frequent intercourse, "cover" it by drinking a lot of fluid and keeping the urine flowing. Pass urine before and after sexual intercourse.
◆ Use tampons instead of sanitary towels as they are less likely to allow the bacteria to thrive; some women find, however, that tampons irritate the bladder further.
◆ If you suspect that wearing a diaphragm is a contributory cause, ask about another form of contraception.
◆ Wear cotton panties or cotton liners.
◆ Don't use antiseptics in the bathwater, vaginal douches or vaginal deodorants.
◆ Don't be obsessive about washing the perineum with soap and water too frequently.
◆ Depending on the drugs prescribed by your doctor, you can help them be more effective by adjusting the acidity or alkalinity of your urine. Ask your doctor what your antibiotic is. For example, tetracycline will be made more effective if you have an acidic urine, so drink plenty of cranberry juice.

MALE AND FEMALE URETHRA

The female urethra is short, allowing offending organisms easy access to the bladder and, in severe untreated cases, to the kidneys. In men, an enlarged prostate can lead to cystitis.

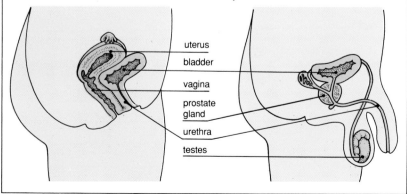

uterus
bladder
vagina
prostate gland
urethra
testes

SEE ALSO:

CONTRACEPTION
INCONTINENCE
MENOPAUSAL PROBLEMS
PAINFUL URINATION
PROLAPSE
URINARY PROBLEMS

DANDRUFF

Dead keratin cells are shed constantly from the surface of the skin. The outer layer of the skin of the scalp is composed of these dead cells and they can accumulate if they are trapped by the presence of hair until they show as tiny white flakes. This is dandruff. It is not a disease; it's simply a variation of normal skin growth. If the skin of the scalp is irritated in any way, by vigorous combing, brushing, massage or shampooing, it responds by increasing the production of keratins and producing dandruff.

Should I see the doctor?
Dandruff is not serious although it can be embarrassing, but there is no reason to see your doctor. Don't confuse dandruff with seborrheic dermatitis which produces red, inflamed, scaly, weeping patches in any area of the skin where a large amount of grease and sebum is produced. It affects the scalp and the folds around the nostrils, eyebrows, and ears. You should see your doctor if this is the condition on your scalp as you require anti-inflammatory skin creams.

· S y m p t o m s ·

▲ Flakes of tiny, white particles present on the scalp, they are seen when you brush your hair and on your shoulders

---

What can I do?
Dandruff should be treated gently. Too vigorous brushing may make it worse. But, in some cases, frequent washing (four to six times a week) with a mild shampoo may keep the scalp free of dandruff. Many people, however, find a medicated shampoo to be more effective.

Medicated shampoos usually contain active ingredients such as tar, sulfur or salicyclic acid which soften the dead scales and make them easier to remove.

Shampoos that contain zinc

AGE AND DANDRUFF
At certain times in your life, you may notice that dandruff is more bothersome than at other times.

Teens
Hormonal changes during puberty can affect hair resulting in dandruff. Altering your diet so that junk foods are eliminated and adding more foods containing Vitamin B may help.

Middle age
Interruption of the hormonal balance can cause scalp dryness resulting in dandruff. Using a shampoo for dry hair may help, as may massaging your scalp as you lather. Your head must be throughly rinsed after washing.

Old age
Dandruff at this time could be due to less efficient circulation. Massaging your hair while shampooing and cutting down on hair spray so that your hair can be brushed through may also help.

pyrithione, chloroxin or selenium sulfide are often effective for more severe cases. These reduce the formation of dandruff by slowing down the growth of skin cells. They also have a mild anti-fungal action. (Some doctors believe that yeast infection is a cause of dandruff.)

Anti-dandruff shampoos containing selenium should be treated with particular caution. If it is applied more frequently than once every two weeks, selenium may act as an irritant to the scalp.

Dandruff is not infectious so there is no need to use a medicated shampoo. Most cases of dandruff respond to frequent gentle washing with a mild shampoo, such as baby shampoo.

Apply a diluted measure of the shampoo to your hair once you have throughly wet it. Bring gently to a lather and leave the shampoo on your hair for half a minute or so and rinse off thoroughly. Don't wash your hair twice; this is unnecessary with modern shampoos.

DEEP-VEIN THROMBOSIS

A thrombosis is when a blood clot forms, blocking a blood vessel. If this happens in the larger, deeper veins, this is called deep-vein thrombosis. It usually occurs in veins in the legs, though sometimes veins in the abdomen may be affected. If part of the blood clot breaks away and passes through your circulation, it may cause damage elsewhere. This breakaway part is called an embolus.

What is it caused by?
The most common cause of deep-vein thrombosis is immobility. Following surgery or childbirth, if you are immobile for several days due to enforced bedrest, this can cause the blood to stagnate in the veins in your legs.

Deep-vein thrombosis is not as common today because of greater awareness. Many surgeons now insist that surgical patients wear thigh-high support stockings throughout the post-operative period. Early mobilization is common following surgery and childbirth where once patients were encouraged not to move. If bedrest is mandatory for any reason, special exercises and physical therapy to the lower legs with an emphasis on relaxation and contraction of the calf and thigh muscles keeps the venous blood pumping back to the heart, thus preventing stagnation in the feet and legs. Women are also advised to come off the contraceptive pill months before surgery to reduce the risk.

The major risk with deep-vein thrombosis is when a large embolus breaks away and reaches the lungs. This can cause a life-threatening pulmonary embolism. An artery within the lungs may become blocked, reducing the volume of blood returning to the heart.

· S y m p t o m s ·

▲ Tenderness in the calf of the affected leg
▲ Pain when the calf muscles are stretched
▲ Swelling (edema) of the foot, ankles and lower leg

Should I see the doctor?
If your leg is tight and swollen, try to pull your toes up towards your knee. If this is very painful and when you press your thumb firmly but gently into the swollen skin for 10 seconds, the pit mark left is clearly felt, then see your doctor.

What will the doctor do?
The examination will be concentrated around your heart and lungs as the doctor will be checking on your circulation system. If your doctor is unsure, you may be referred for tests, such as venography (when dye is injected into the vein and X-rays taken to confirm the blockage) and ultrasound, to pinpoint the site of the thrombus.

What is the medical treatment?
As soon as the condition is diagnosed, anti-coagulants will be given to reduce the clotting time of the blood and prevent the blood clot extending in the leg veins. Medication with anti-coagulants will continue until the danger period is passed. Analgesics will also be given to relieve the pain.

What can I do?
Any swelling in your legs can be relieved by raising the leg and allowing the fluid to drain away. The affected leg will always have a tendency to swell after a long day on your feet and in hot weather. Therefore rest it as much as you can and keep your foot on a stool whenever possible

Wear good quality support stockings and try to be as active as possible if you are overweight.

A severe deep-vein thrombosis may affect the venous drainage of the leg permanently. There is the possibility that you will develop varicose veins. Be on the lookout for these and consult your doctor if they appear. If they do and they go untreated, you run the risk of developing a varicose ulcer.

If you were on the pill, you will be advised not to use it as a means of birth control.

WOMEN AT RISK
Although this is a relatively rare disorder which may affect anyone who is immobile for prolonged periods, those particularly at risk include

 Post-operative patients who cannot get up and move about after surgery

 Contraceptive pill takers who have been taking the estrogen contraceptive pill for five years or more.

 Overweight women The risk for these women is fourfold if they are over 35 and smoke as well and there is a family history of thrombosis.

 Hormone therapy patients especially if they smoke

SEE ALSO:

CONTRACEPTION
HORMONE REPLACEMENT
  THERAPY
PHLEBITIS
ULTRASOUND
VARICOSE VEINS

DENTAL PROBLEMS

Your most important concern about your teeth should be to conserve them and this is something that is within your control. You should take care of the gums with proper use of a toothbrush and judicious use of dental floss. Teeth are conserved with a proper diet low in sugar, good cleaning and fluoride, either in the diet or painted on the teeth.

Teeth can't be healthy if the gums are unhealthy. When gums are infected or swollen with plaque, the alveolar margins no longer adhere to the teeth which may become loose, making chewing difficult; they may even fall out (see *Gum disease*). It's essential, therefore, that we take care of our gums by preventing the formation of plaque. Plaque is a hard, calcareous substance, deposited around the edges of the teeth from certain chemicals in the saliva and food. Sugary, sticky food encourages bacteria to grow and invade the margins of the gums. Plaque can be prevented by twice-daily toothbrushing. If it builds up it must be removed by scaling, a process carried out in a dentist's office. Regular six monthly checkups will help prevent destructive plaque buildup.

If you have a problem with plaque or with inflammation of the gums, consider buying a water-pick which forces food particles from between the teeth with a fine jet of water under pressure. This is entirely non-traumatic and doesn't hurt or damage the gums at all.

Halitosis or bad breath is a not uncommon form of *body odor* though its cause is always difficult to track down. Occasionally, aphthous ulcers occur as the result of trauma from the sharp edge of a tooth or from stress (see *Mouth problems*).

Tooth abscess

A tooth abscess may form at the root of a carious tooth. The treatment is to let out the pus either by making a small nick in the gum over the swelling or by drilling into the tooth and draining it through the root. A root canal treatment to take out the nerve from the tooth is usually necessary (see *Cosmetic dentistry*).

DEPRESSION

Women are particularly vulnerable to depression because of their physiology. The way that hormones affect our moods and the change in the level of circulating hormones during the menstrual cycle, for example, can cause women to suffer bouts of depression before each period, with the cessation of menstruation at the menopause, after the birth of children or after a miscarriage or termination (abortion). One in ten of the population will suffer depression at some time in their lives, but one in ten women will suffer a depressive illness.

Why does it occur?
Depression may arise from two main sources; it may result from a reaction to events past or present such as a death in the family, isolation caused by a difficult marriage or unemployment, or severe financial worries. This is termed exogenous depression. The other reason for depression has no obvious source, though there may be a physiological cause such as fluctuating hormone levels or the aftermath of a viral infection such as hepatitis or glandular fever, when it is known as endogenous depression.

Everyone feels depressed at some time; during the winter when there is prolonged cold, wet weather a higher instance of depressive illness is reported. But a full-blown depressive illness produces definite psychological symptoms.

In part, depression is the result of modern times and the pressures of our way of life. Women today are encouraged to have higher expectations, to take advantage of opportunities, and to improve their social and legal standing. When aspirations go unfulfilled, depression may be the natural result. Of course, these aspirations may be socially-dictated anyway, and so a woman's combined role as wife, mother and worker can in many instances be an impossible illusion and not what she really wants at all. Discrepancies between a woman's traditional role and the way she is seen outside the home may lead to conflict from within and result in low self-esteem.

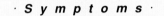

· S y m p t o m s ·
▲ Weepiness
▲ Mood shift in the direction of sadness, despair, misery, gloom and blackness
▲ Decrease in feelings of love and affection
▲ Loss of self-esteem
▲ Lethargy, slovenliness and apathy
▲ Insomnia
▲ Loss of touch with reality and aberrations such as shoplifting, nymphomania
▲ Indigestion, headaches and sweating

Should I see the doctor?
See your doctor at once if you feel depressed and suffer any of the symptoms listed above. Don't hesitate and run the risk of seriously disrupting your life just because there is no obvious physical illness and you feel you will be labelled neurotic.

What will the doctor do?
Your doctor will examine you and question you about your feelings and any physical symptoms. If the cause of your depression is related to hormonal levels, hormone therapy may be prescribed. Treatment with progesterone, for example, may be used for depression associated with premenstrual tension.

The mainstay of medical treatment for exogenous depression is usually anti-depressant drugs. Often these are prescribed in an unsubtle way and statistics show that middle-aged depressed women are the heaviest drug takers in our society. You must tell your doctor all about your feelings so that any specific elements can be distinguished and some cause or trigger found so that the appropriate treatment can be given.

What types of drugs can be prescribed?
If one of your symptoms is insomnia, you will be prescribed sleeping pills on a short-term basis to get you over the bad patch while

---

MARRIAGE AS A POSSIBLE CAUSE OF DEPRESSION

Marriage on the whole can be bad for women. Research has indicated that the mental health of married women is often worse than that of single women and married men. Marriage is often a shock to a woman; it causes serious disruptions, changes and discontinuities. With childbearing, an enjoyable job and pleasant workmates are left behind. Isolation often ensues, though today more and more women are taking maternity leave and returning to work.

Domestic chores are boring and repetitive and the loss of certain legal and financial rights lowers a woman's status at marriage. Many women are besieged by feelings of inadequacy and feel unable to make the adjustments necessary to keep their marriage smooth and happy. Intellectually a woman may have to make many adjustments to make her marriage work – concessions, submissions and changes in her level of expectations to suit her husband's wishes. Not surprisingly, married women suffer more mental distress than married men, have more phobic reactions and suffer more depressive illnesses.

leeping patterns are re-established. Sleeping pills should not be taken in the long term; withdrawal from them results in worsening insomnia and dependency.

Anti-depressants usually result in some improvement of a mild depression within a month. Your doctor might refer you to a psychotherapist to help you try to reduce any internal conflict which precipitates depression.

Is there another form of treatment?

In really severe cases, particularly if there is a risk of suicide, you may need hospital admission for psychiatric help. This can also be arranged on an informal daily basis. Remember that mental illness is just as real as a physical illness and the unfortunate reputation of mental hospitals must not prevent you from accepting this treatment if it is necessary. Electroconvulsive therapy (ECT) is still occasionally used with cases of severe depression for those who don't respond to other treatments. In special cases it is now used with remarkable success.

What can I do?

If you are feeling unhappy, if work helps you to forget and stops you brooding, increase your work load. If this isn't true for you, try to keep as normal a routine as possible or change your environment for a while. Go on a vacation or resolve any conflict you feel may be precipitating the crisis. Any kind of activity helps to reduce sadness and will bring the pleasure of achievement. Finishing something develops a sense of worth which is an antidote to depression.

Good wholesome sex makes all aspects of life brighter, so if your libido is not depressed, speak to your partner about mutual enjoyment of your sex life.

You mustn't hesitate to lean on people. Join a self-help group and get help dealing with the problems of everyday life. Don't be afraid to approach therapy groups. Try helping other people and if you ever contemplate suicide, talk to someone or contact a suicide hotline right away. Avoid being alone and be with people you like.

Even though cyclical events may bring on a depression for the first time, there is no guarantee that it will not recur. Depression unrelated to illness or hormonal changes often recurs, so at the first sign of a worsening mental state, get in touch with someone who knows your mental history before your normal life is affected.

ELECTROCONVULSIVE THERAPY

Electroconvulsive therapy is a form of treatment for depressive, psychiatric illnesses in which an electric shock is passed through the brain for a few seconds.

Why is it done?

In the past, it was used as a first-line therapy but gradually fell into disrepute as it was felt to be brutal. The electric shock was large and the resulting "convulsion" could be quite severe. Today, ECT is reserved for those patients with an illness that is resistant to anti-depressant drugs. The procedure has now been refined though there is still controversy surrounding it.

How is it done?

Now, a patient is given a general anesthetic and a muscle relaxant before two padded electrodes are applied to the temples, one on each side or both on the same side. A controlled electrical pulse is delivered to the electrodes from a small machine until the patient has experienced a brain seizure. This is deduced by a brief muscular rigidity followed by slight twitching of the limbs and eyelids.

A course of treatment normally consists of six to 12 seizures at the rate of two or three per week.

How does it work?

No one knows quite how ECT works. In observations of patients with epileptic fits, the brain was observed to be affected by spontaneous shock waves so that an altered state of consciousness and tranquility follow on from the interference.

In some cases, drowsiness is experienced after a session of ECT and there may be some loss of memory of recent events. However, there is no pain, although there are the after-effects of the general anesthetic. Patients often improve quite dramatically after the third treatment.

SEE ALSO:

ANXIETY
DRUG DEPENDENCY
INSOMNIA
MENOPAUSAL PROBLEMS
MOOD CHANGES
PHOBIA
POSTNATAL DEPRESSION
PREMENSTRUAL SYNDROME
SEXUAL PROBLEMS

DERMABRASION

Cosmetic surgery is used to improve a person's appearance by removing embarrassing or unwanted imperfections. Other means, such as dermabrasion and chemical skin peel, rejuvenate areas of skin by non-surgical methods. It is essential that a skin test is done before any of these methods is widely applied.

Dermabrasion involves abrading the skin with a rough surface to remove the upper layers, rather like sandpapering. It is chiefly used to treat skin conditions on the face where a generous supply of hair follicles and sebaceous glands allows the skin to regenerate quickly without scarring. If hair follicles and sebaceous glands are destroyed, then the skin doesn't recover and scars will result.

Depending on the condition being treated, and the skill of the operator, abrasion may continue until the entire epidermis is removed. This leaves a raw, weeping and bleeding surface.

Great advances in dermabrasion have been made in the last 25 years due to the use of high-speed rotary drills and better cooling techniques. In its less radical forms, where only the top layer of skin is removed, dermabrasion is used in many cosmetic and beauty clinics.

Why is it done?
Dermabrasion is a technique used to remove the pitted scars of bad acne, or to treat large birthmarks and disfiguring scars resulting from car crashes – scars that have not been driven deep into the skin. It can give good results for stretchmarks and fine lines around the mouth. It can also be used to remove unwanted tattoos.

How is it done?
The patient is sedated or tranquilized and the area of skin to be treated is cleansed and any vulnerable parts of the body nearby are protected such as the eyes, nose, and hair if treatment is being carried out on the face and neck.

A stream of cold gas is usually used to freeze the skin and then the high-speed drill abrades the skin to the required depth.

The time this takes depends on the rate at which the skin thaws and recovers its sensitivity.

Dermabrasion should only be performed by medically trained and qualified personnel under sterile conditions. The degree of freezing and drilling is learned from experience and there are refinements too in the angle of the drill head and the direction and extent of the abrasion.

What happens afterwards?
The skin usually bleeds for 15-30 minutes and then a non-adhesive dressing is applied. This is removed a day later. The crusts which form separate after about a week and the wound heals quickly when left open and dry.

The same area can be treated again after four weeks if the technician has chosen to treat a little area at a time rather than adopt the radical approach of removing too many layers of skin at once.

The skin will be much pinker than the surrounding untreated skin.

What can I do?
Sunlight and cosmetics can cause mild irritation, so you should avoid strong sunlight and makeup for several weeks. Always use a sunscreen before exposing your treated skin to the sunlight.

What are the risks?
As with any treatment, there is always the risk of infection. Any redness or pussy areas of skin should be seen by your dermatologist immediately. There may be persistent redness, brown pigmentation or lumpy scars on the skin where the treatment was carried out. In this case you may consider the treatment a partial success only, and you may need to wear a heavier makeup or repeat the treatment.

Dark skinned people may develop patches of lighter skin but this is nearly always temporary.

SEE ALSO:

ACNE
BIRTHMARKS
COSMETIC SURGERY
FACE LIFT
FACIAL TREATMENTS
WRINKLES

DES

Diethyl-stilbestrol (DES) is an artificial estrogen which was used up until 1971 to prevent miscarriage in early pregnancy. It was administered to those women who had already experienced early miscarriage. However, doctors found that there was a higher incidence of cancer of the vagina in the daughters of mothers who had received DES when carrying them than in the rest of the population. Nine out of ten of these daughters had abnormal growth of the glandular tissue in the cervix and vagina. More recently, it has been discovered that about 75% of women exposed to DES in utero have abnormalities of the uterus and a higher incidence of incompetent cervix during pregnancy.

Should I see the doctor?
If you or your mother were given DES during pregnancy, it is essential that you see your doctor for referral to a gynecologist who is familiar with DES-induced changes.

What will the doctor do?
All children of women who took DES should be followed up and monitored regularly. You and your daughters should visit the gynecologist for regular check-ups. After menstrual periods begin, annual internal examinations with Pap smears, occasional biopsies of the vagina and cervix and colposcopy will need to be carried out.

As certain genital abnormalities such as cysts, small testicles and a low sperm count have been detected in boys whose mothers took DES, they should also have an annual examination.

What can I do?
Even though your children may be declared fit, don't neglect an annual check-up. New methods of prevention and detection are being introduced all the time and you should not become complacent.

Stay in touch with your gynecologist so that immediate action can be taken if he or she thinks fit.

Recent research has indicated that the women who took DES may themselves be at higher risk of developing breast cancer, so be assiduous with your monthly breast self-examinations and make sure your doctor treats you as a high-risk patient .

SEE ALSO:

BREAST SELF-EXAMINATION
CERVIX PROBLEMS
COLPOSCOPY
PAP SMEAR
UTERINE CANCER

DIABETES MELLITUS

This is the result of a deficiency or the loss of effectiveness of a hormone called insulin. Insulin is produced by the pancreas and it controls the passage of glucose (extracted from carbohydrates and starches in our diet) from the blood into the liver and muscles. Without insulin, glucose rises to frightening levels in the blood and the body cells are deprived of energy. The body then turns to fats and proteins as its sources of energy. When these are burned up, they produce poisonous waste products called ketones. If treatment is not given, the sufferer will fall into a hyperglycemic coma, becoming dehydrated, drowsy and eventually unconscious.

What happens to your body?

There are two main forms of diabetes: the first begins in childhood or early adulthood and the second occurs in older, obese people – more often women. In the former, the insulin-dependent form of the disease, there is a severe deficiency of insulin and sufferers depend on daily doses of insulin throughout their lives. In non insulin-dependent diabetes, which usually develops gradually, there is no true lack of insulin; the pancreas is healthy and produces insulin, but too much carbohydrate and starch is taken in from the diet. There is not sufficient insulin to cope, and so the body becomes relatively deficient in it. In some milder cases, therefore, it is just a matter of cutting back on carbohydrates and starch in the diet. In other cases drugs stimulate the pancreas to produce more insulin or lower the blood glucose levels in tandem with dietary measures.

Pregnancy can precipitate the onset of diabetes (see box). Diabetic women are more at risk with certain hormone therapies such as the contraceptive pill and hormone replacement, so always tell your doctor that you are

· Symptoms ·

▲ Profound thirst due to excessive urination

▲ Itchiness of the vulva, soreness, inflammation, redness and even pussy spots in the genital area because of glucose in the urine

▲ Loss of weight because the fats are used for energy

▲ If ketones are produced this leads to breath that smells like pear drops, dehydration and changes in mineral metabolism which can affect cardiac and kidney function and lead to coma and death

pancreas

diabetic if you have a consultation for any other reason. You are also more likely to suffer with vaginal and urinary tract infections because of the presence of glucose in your urine.

Should I see the doctor?

Diabetes often runs in families so be on the alert in case you notice some of the symptoms. If you think you might be suffering from diabetes, see your doctor about having a urine test.

What will the doctor do?

Glucose and ketones in the urine indicate the presence of the disease. You may then have a blood test to

confirm the diagnosis and be referred for a full examination before treatment is worked out. Non insulin-dependent diabetes is, in many cases, controlled by diet and weight loss alone but the dependent form will require daily doses of insulin. Once the dose is decided it must be taken regularly as instructed. You will be taught how to give yourself injections – insulin is destroyed by the digestive juices and cannot be absorbed in tablet form.

What can I do?

You will probably have to test your urine regularly for glucose to check that insulin levels are correct.

Infection and excessive exercise, for example, can alter your insulin requirements. As well as the insulin therapy, you will be on a strict diet for life to maintain the glucose in your system at steady levels throughout the day.

Many people feel that the diagnosis of diabetes is a stigma or a death knell; it used to be a fatal disease and even though there is no cure, modern treatment means you can lead a normal life provided you maintain the strict regularity of your treatment. Don't slip back into bad habits; you will be monitored with blood tests to make sure that you have normal levels of blood glucose. If you suffer from the non insulin-dependent disease, diet should control it in mild forms, but you may need regular tablets and eventually insulin injections. Keep your medical appointments; constant checking is vital in the management of this disease.

It's a good idea to have a bracelet or neck disc identifying your condition in case you become ill.

DIABETES IN PREGNANCY

Pregnancy often unmasks diabetes when glucose appears in your urine during a routine prenatal test. This doesn't necessarily mean that you are suffering from true diabetes. It may simply mean that your kidneys' threshold to glucose has been lowered and more glucose is excreted. You will need to have a blood glucose level test to confirm the diagnosis. Your doctor will keep a regular check on your glucose levels after pregnancy to make sure diabetes is not developing.

Hidden diabetes may show itself if you give birth to a very large and heavy baby. If your first baby is over 5 kg (11 lbs), and there is a family history of the disease, be on the alert for the symptoms of diabetes, particularly if you become pregnant again.

A diabetic women who becomes pregnant is given preferential treatment and very special care during her pregnancy. Pregnancy can tip diabetes out of balance. This is not surprising as your baby is now drawing on your blood glucose too so your dose of insulin will need to be varied. Don't be concerned about this chopping and changing. It is very common in pregnancy and your doctor will take good care of you. You may be admitted to hospital towards the end of your term. Babies of diabetic mothers may outgrow the food supply from the placenta in the last four weeks and it may be necessary to induce you early; this is routine management of diabetic pregnancy.

The baby probably will be over-weight and may need some special care in the first weeks of life. There is a higher risk of perinatal mortality with diabetic pregnancies, but with good prenatal treatment and pre-term delivery, this risk is greatly reduced.

TESTING YOUR URINE

Diabetics should test their glucose levels at least twice a day. Do-it-yourself kits are readily available at pharmacists.

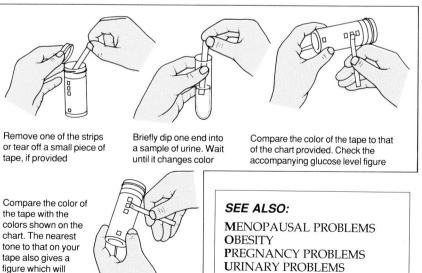

Remove one of the strips or tear off a small piece of tape, if provided

Briefly dip one end into a sample of urine. Wait until it changes color

Compare the color of the tape to that of the chart provided. Check the accompanying glucose level figure

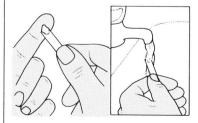

Draw a large drop of blood from your fingertip edge and wipe it onto the tape. Wait for one minute, then wash the blood off for a few seconds. Blot the tape on a lint-free paper towel.

Compare the color of the tape with the colors shown on the chart. The nearest tone to that on your tape also gives a figure which will indicate the level of sugar in your blood.

SEE ALSO:

MENOPAUSAL PROBLEMS
OBESITY
PREGNANCY PROBLEMS
URINARY PROBLEMS
VAGINAL PROBLEMS

DIARRHEA

This is the passage of frequent, loose, watery stools. It is rarely cause for concern and as long as you take in plenty of fluids to prevent any dehydration, you should recover within 48 hours.

In cases of acute diarrhea, you will need to look for a source. This could be either a virus, bacteria or as the result of a reaction to drugs. The drugs that most commonly cause loose stools are antibiotics such as tetracycline, laxatives and some antacid medications.

Chronic diarrhea, which will be accompanied by weight loss and lethargy, could be a symptom of a serious disease of the large intestine. There are even stress-related disorders that cause diarrhea.

The most common treatment after laboratory examination of the stool is to replace lost fluids and essential minerals. Investigations to find the underlying cause include a barium enema where a dye is injected into the large intestine through the rectum and its progress shown up on a series of X-ray pictures. A barium meal is taken by mouth and investigates the upper part of the digestive tract.

If you are unable to make a diagnosis from this information, consult your doctor.

NATURE OF THE DIARRHEA	PROBABLE CAUSE
Sudden onset and you have eaten in the last 2-4 hours	You may have eaten something which is spoiled, or to which you may be allergic; this could be food poisoning. Eat nothing and drink water or diluted fruit juices. Don't take any medication, especially not aspirin. If the symptoms persist for 48 hours, consult your doctor.
You are taking antibiotics or another drug as medication	This may be a side effect of your medication. Call your doctor to check if that could be so.
You have had attacks of diarrhea interspersed with constipation	This could be a disease of the bowel, diverticulitis, or it could be an irritable colon, a stress-related disorder (see *Digestive problems*).
There is red blood in your feces	This could indicate something as minor as *hemorrhoids*, or as serious as ulcerative colitis or *colorectal cancer*.
The loose motions are accompanied by gripping pain and vomiting and they continue for more than 48 hours	You could have a bowel infection, such as dysentery. This is only likely if you have travelled abroad recently, but consult your doctor and keep up the fluids to prevent dehydration.
You have been suffering with diarrhea for some time and your weight is down and you feel tired and feeble	This could be a symptom of a serious disorder of the large intestine (see *Colorectal cancer*).
You also have aches in your limbs and a sore throat	If you have influenza, this can affect your bowel and cause mild diarrhea with cramping pain.

DIGESTIVE PROBLEMS

The digestive problems described here are not exclusive to women but they may be more commonly experienced at certain times, particularly during pregnancy.

Many digestive problems have features in common. For example, hiatus hernia, heartburn and indigestion (sometimes called dyspepsia) are usually secondary to the production of too much acid in the stomach. Indigestion, heartburn and flatulence are quite often the result of eating too much at one time. Gallbladder disorders arise after eating meals containing too much fat. Most of these digestive problems can be dealt with by dietary means, and medical treatment is rarely necessary.

HEARTBURN

The tendency to produce too much acid in the stomach is often inherited. You can't do anything about it, but you can alleviate the discomfort by eating small meals and avoiding rich foods. Eating small, non-rich meals quite often neutralizes the acid and nearly always relieves pain because pain due to excess acid is often worse when the stomach is empty. Heartburn has nothing to do with your heart.

What can I do?
Avoid rich, fatty foods and spicy meals and large meals. Take small meals instead – a snack every two hours or so. Prop yourself up in bed and take a glass of milk with you to sip during the night. Antacid medication works for some people, but during pregnancy don't take too much. Antacids limit the absorption of iron so if you are pregnant or anemic, this could be detrimental to your general health.

IRRITABLE (OR SPASTIC) COLON

One condition that is more than twice as common among women is an irritable colon. Symptoms include both diarrhea and constipation because the passage of food along the intestine is disturbed. In a normal intestine, the food is pushed along by regular contractions. With an irritable colon, the disturbance sets up problems further down the intestinal tract. Because of this irregular flow, there is distension and pain felt low in the abdomen. The pain eases with the passing of stools.

In some cases, the disorder may be the result of an allergic reaction to certain foods.

What can I do?
It appears that emotional stress may be the root cause of this complaint, so even with drugs to limit diarrhea, laxatives to ease constipation and tranquilizers for the stress, the best treatment is to reorder your life to limit stress and emotional upheaval. A high-fiber diet also regularizes the activity of the intestine.

If you can find no relief from the abdominal pain, try an exclusion diet. Ask your doctor to recommend how to do this or to put you in touch with a dietitian. You will probably be required to note the occurrence of the symptoms and then, without depriving yourself of essential nutrients, stop eating suspect foodstuffs (such as those containing artificial additives, smoked and preserved meats and fish, foods high in fat, citrus fruits, cow's milk and other dairy products, alcohol and caffeine beverages). After three days, foods are reintroduced one at a time and the symptoms noted. In this way you may be able to isolate the food that causes the problem.

HIATUS HERNIA

The esophagus or gullet passes through a hole (hiatus) in the diaphragm on its route to the stomach. A hiatus hernia occurs when the opening of the gullet is no longer tight and part of the esophagus and stomach protrudes back through the hiatus. This hernia can cause food to reflux from the stomach into the gullet if pressure inside the abdomen is raised. This happens when we cough or strain when opening our bowels. In early cases this may not be felt at all or produce a sensation which we call heartburn. Sometimes as with heartburn, acid may regurgitate into the mouth.

If hiatus hernia becomes severe, quite a lot of the stomach contents can reflux into the esophagus and

DIGESTIVE PROBLEMS IN PREGNANCY

Heartburn is a problem in pregnancy because the valve at the entrance to your stomach relaxes because of the effects of the hormone progesterone which relaxes many muscles in preparation for childbirth. Small amounts of acid may reflux into the esophagus, the tube running from your mouth to your stomach. Soreness or a slight discomfort is felt behind the lower end of the breastbone and sometimes acid regurgitates into the back of the throat and mouth. In late pregnancy, the enlarged uterus presses on your stomach and the heartburn may become worse. It should disappear after the birth. Follow the treatment, above.

Flatulence is also common in pregnancy because the intestine is more sluggish, and it is more difficult to get rid of any wind. Try to avoid those foods which produce wind, such as fried foods, onions and legumes. Peppermint drinks are helpful.

DIGESTIVE PROBLEMS

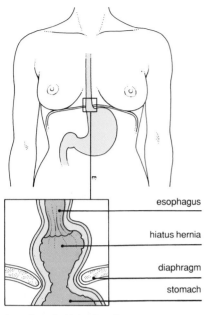

Location of a hiatus hernia
It occurs where part of the stomach protrudes back through the diaphragm opening into the esophagus.

esophagus

hiatus hernia

diaphragm

stomach

this can cause permanent pain, very like that of a duodenal ulcer or gallbladder disease pain.

Because the esophagus is not protected against the action of acid from the stomach, it quickly becomes inflamed, swollen and may even ulcerate. If the condition progresses to this extent, the inflamed and ulcerated area must heal before the condition can be repaired surgically.

What is the surgical treatment

Repair of a severe hiatus hernia is a simple operation. With fancy needlework, it is possible for the surgeon to narrow the gap between the entrance to the stomach and the exit from the esophagus. Normally, there is a valve which prevents food being regurgitated. Most surgeons can repair a loose or destroyed valve – even refashion a new one with simple surgical techniques.

What should I do?

Losing weight will nearly always cure this condition. Obesity is one of the commonest causes of hiatus hernia. Even if dietary or surgical means cure the hiatus hernia, it will probably recur if you become overweight again.
- Avoid rich fatty foods and eat small meals often rather than two large meals a day. The condition is relieved if there is some food in the stomach.
- Don't smoke or drink alcohol; this aggravates the condition.
- Raise the head of your bed about 4 inches or use at least four pillows to prevent reflux when you are asleep.
- Use commercial antacid tablets. These neutralize the acids in your stomach and consequently protect the lining of the esophagus from the effects of this acid.

GASTRIC ULCER

This is also known as a peptic or stomach ulcer. It is a raw spot on the lining of the stomach. It is caused by an excess of gastric acid. This could occur as a result of an inherited characteristic or because you just have more acid cells thereby creating a relative excess of acid in your stomach. If there is too much acid for your stomach to cope with, a gastric ulcer can result.

Acid doesn't burn the stomach as it does the duodenum and the esophagus. The stomach is completely coated with a layer of protective mucus which doesn't allow the acid to penetrate down to the sensitive cells. The ulcer, however, allows the acid to burn through the stomach lining and if left untreated, the acid may eat its way through to the pancreas.

Symptoms arise when the stomach is getting empty and the level of acid is building up. The pain may last for 30 minutes or some hours and usually is related to food;

it may be worse in the early morning when the stomach is comparatively empty.

These ulcers are equally common among men and women but they are more common among smokers, people who take a great deal of aspirin and rush their meals.

What can I do?

The pain will increase until something is taken to neutralize the acid in the stomach. Many individuals react with the secretion of acid to certain foods. Harmful foods would include anything containing fat, vinegar, spices or cream, undercooked food and part cooked stringy vegetables. Foods which are bland will nearly always neutralize stomach acid. These include milk, bread (without butter or margarine), steamed fish or chicken, cereals and mashed potatoes.

What will the doctor do?

Your doctor will be interested if there is a family history of such a digestive disorder. You will be advised about a suitable diet and to eat little and often so your stomach is never empty. You may be referred for a barium meal X-ray to confirm the diagnosis. Any surgical remedy is quite radical and doctors will be loathe to do this and will try diet and antacids first.

A gastric ulcer usually heals within a month if you follow the dietary guidelines. Stop smoking, don't drink coffee, tea or alcohol and rest as much as possible. If the pain returns, see your doctor again. You may be given drugs this time but if the ulcer recurs, surgery could be the only option.

SEE ALSO:

GALLBLADDER DISEASE
OBESITY
PREGNANCY PROBLEMS

DILATATION AND CURETTAGE

This is a fairly common surgical procedure for women that is used for a number of conditions involving the uterus. It is a diagnostic device as well as one of the methods employed to terminate pregnancy.

Why is it done?

- To procure a termination of pregnancy, usually over 12 weeks gestation. A dilatation and evacuation is more common before this time as it does not require a general anesthetic
- To treat and diagnose heavy menstrual bleeding and other menstrual irregularities
- To clean out remnants of a retained placenta after labor or an incomplete abortion (or miscarriage) and prevent infection
- To investigate the reasons for infertility
- To diagnose cancer of the uterus or the fallopian tubes
- To investigate bleeding with an ectopic pregnancy, for example
- To clear uterine adhesions
- As a routine procedure after certain operations such as sterilization

How is it done?

This operation can be performed on an in- or out-patient basis. Under a local or general anesthetic a series of metal rods are inserted into the vagina to dilate or stretch the cervix. A spoon-shaped curette is then inserted, under direct vision using a speculum, to scrape out the uterine lining. The endometrial tissue will be sent off for laboratory investigation. The process takes about 10–20 minutes. You may experience cramps and some bleeding afterwards.

Are there complications?

This is a simple operation and although it carries a slight risk of perforation of the uterus with heavy

HOW IS IT DONE?

The procedure can be carried out under a local or general anesthetic. Occasionally, a suction curettage technique is employed to remove tissue. Suction is thought to be safer for early pregnancy termination and miscarriage, but the curette is preferred for diagnostic procedures.

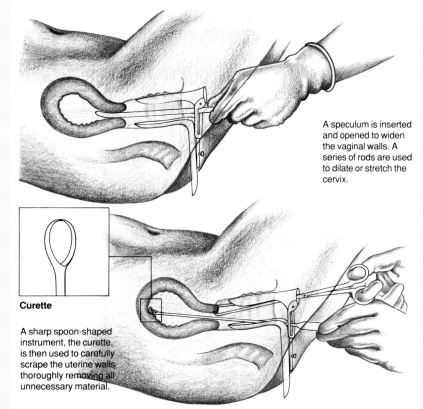

A speculum is inserted and opened to widen the vaginal walls. A series of rods are used to dilate or stretch the cervix.

Curette

A sharp spoon-shaped instrument, the curette, is then used to carefully scrape the uterine walls thoroughly removing all unnecessary material.

bleeding if inexpertly performed, it is a valuable diagnostic procedure and positively beneficial if you have been suffering heavy bleeding because the lining of your uterus has been too thick.

SEE ALSO:

ABORTION
ECTOPIC PREGNANCY
ENDOMETRIOSIS
FIBROIDS
LAPAROSCOPY
MENSTRUAL PROBLEMS
MISCARRIAGE
STERILIZATION
TERMINATION OF PREGNANCY
UTERINE PROBLEMS

DOWN'S SYNDROME

Down's syndrome is the most common chromosomal abnormality. Children with Down's syndrome have 47 chromosomes instead of the normal 46. The presence of the extra chromosome 21 can be detected by means of a karyotype when the third number 21 can be clearly seen. The extra chromosome usually, though not always, comes from the mother's egg. This occurs about once in every 600-800 births but the real instances are probably twice this because more than half the affected fetuses are spontaneously aborted early in pregnancy.

There is a high correlation between maternal age and the abnormal 21 chromosome. For mothers aged 20, the condition occurs in about 1 in every 2,000 births. But for women over 40, the risk is about 1 in 100 births (see above). In fact, the risk of having a child with any chromosomal abnormality, is higher after 35.

There is evidence that the chromosomal abnormality could be paternal in origin in approximately one third of cases. This is a much higher frequency than had been thought hitherto. These cases are independent of maternal age.

Other correlations have been made with exposure to X-rays of the abdomen. There have been clusters of Down's babies following epidemics and infectious hepatitis; this could show a viral factor at work.

Over-ripeness of the ovum due to delayed fertilization because of a decreasing frequency of intercourse has also been suggested as a reason. The assumption being that older women have intercourse less frequently.

What characterizes the disorder?
A child with Down's syndrome has obvious observable physical characteristics:
◆ the bridge of the nose is wide and the eyes have an upward slant
◆ the hands are short and broad and there is a single deep crease running across the middle of

Estimated rates of Down's Syndrome (New York state study)	
Maternal age	Estimated rate
20	1/1925
25	1/1205
30	1/885
33	1/590
35	1/365
36	1/285
38	1/175
40	1/110
45	1/32
49	1/12

the palm
◆ there is a large gap between the first and second toes
◆ the tongue is large, seemingly too large for the mouth, and protrudes from it
◆ a 50% chance of having a heart defect
◆ some degree of mental retardation
◆ the possibility of an intestinal blockage

What can you do?
If either you or your husband are over 35, or there is any history of Down's syndrome in either family, you should request amniocentesis to see whether or not your baby is affected. For women and men over 40 or with a Down's child already, chorionic villus sampling (CVS) may be requested as this brings the results a lot sooner, between weeks 8 and 12.

To help you make any decisions about Down's syndrome, you should seek genetic counseling to weigh up the risks and formulate your response if the tests prove positive.

Amniocentesis or CVS will provide some of the baby's cells for analysis. If the condition is diagnosed, you can then choose to have your pregnancy terminated.

What can be done for these children?
If you decide to go ahead and have the child, you will find that attitudes of doctors and society have changed

considerably in the last decade. At one time, these children were labeled mentally retarded mongols and were treated accordingly. We now know that with proper stimulation and parental support and encouragement, Down's children can develop and thrive almost as well as children with no mental defect. The intellectual potential of Down's is nowhere near as low as w previously thought. Therefore early stimulation in the first year of life and thereafter is crucial for the Down's child. Careful nursery schooling means that these children can develop alongside normal children and be accepted by them and the community as a whole.

Many Down's children need help with dressing and feeding but others are quite capable of holding responsible jobs. What they need is the chance and encouragement. As parents you will need to help your child overcome the social stigma and to put an emphasis on what your child is capable of doing rather than on what he or she cannot.

SEE ALSO:
AMNIOCENTESIS
CHORION BIOPSY
CHROMOSOMAL PROBLEMS
GENETIC COUNSELING
PREGNANCY PROBLEMS

DRUG DEPENDENCY

When you become dependent on a drug the way you react to that drug changes. The most important change is that you no longer have the ability to choose when and where to take the drug. You have lost control over the power to decide and you have lost control of yourself. You are addicted or enslaved to the drug.

If the dependency worsens, your life may be given over to securing the drug and you will take the drug in order to maintain the artificial feeling of well-being it induces. After prolonged use of a drug, there will be withdrawal symptoms when it is stopped and very often, if the drug was being used in the first instance as a treatment, these symptoms will be similar to the symptoms that the drug was used to treat. This is a psychological dependence. For example, withdrawal from sleeping pills will bring back the insomnia. However, there are drugs that produce these withdrawal symptoms, but the person may feel no compulsion to start using the drug again.

Addictions to other substances such as alcohol, caffeine or nicotine also can cause serious damage to your physical health.

How does it happen?
There are two elements involved – the personality of the person and the type of drug.

Studies show that addicts have widely different reasons for using and becoming dependent on a drug. There may be a sense of inadequacy and low self-esteem, or hostility and depression. However, not all addicts can be described as having an inadequate personality; nicotine addiction through cigarette smoking is widespread and doesn't appear to produce personality disturbance, for instance.

Research has shown that certain drugs have the tendency to produce addiction in their users while others do not. Into the former group go narcotics, alcohol and barbiturates. More recently tranquilizers have been found to share this activity.

There is still no certainty as to why some individuals react to certain drugs while others do not and why some become psychologically dependent on that drug.

Years of research have found no obvious reason why certain people seek out and use illegal drugs and court addiction, knowing the physical and social consequences, while others

DRUGS
Drugs that are commonly prescribed but can cause dependence include:

Benzodiazepines
These include diazepam (Valium) and are prescribed for anxiety and insomnia. They can cause withdrawal symptoms sometimes after only a few weeks of use. Doctors, therefore, don't usually prescribe them continuously for longer than two weeks without review.

Barbiturates
These are stronger sleeping drugs which are not so frequently prescribed. They have largely been replaced by benzodiazepines because the side-effects of the latter are less severe. The barbitu-

do not or are able to stop using them.

Should I see the doctor?
Be honest and admit your addiction. Talk to somebody – your doctor, a friend or a self-help group. You need to want to overcome the dependency to succeed. Dependence develops insidiously with a gradually increasing need for escalating doses of a drug. This may be recognized first by your doctor or a member of your family. Be open-minded if someone mentions their fears to you; listen to them.

What will the doctor do?
Medical treatment is either in hospital or in self-help groups and depends on the addictive drug. Hospital treatment involves long periods of hospitalization or short sessions in special units with teams of doctors, psychiatrists, psychologists and social workers working as a team to give emotional support after the withdrawal of the drug. Medication helps with withdrawal symptoms and depression and group therapy and psychotherapy help in mental rehabilitation.

Self-help groups use counselors

rates include Nembutal, Seconal and Amytal. They are much more likely to cause tolerance, that is, the need to take increasing doses.

Antidepressants
Usually diagnosed for a specific depressive illness, these drugs don't work immediately and the course should be followed. They shouldn't be stopped suddenly. Most of them have some sort of sedative action.

Painkillers
The only painkillers to present problems of dependence are those that contain narcotics. These are only prescribed regularly for terminal illness or severe pain.

who are often ex-addicts because their programs depend on mutual support with shared experiences. The addict is also expected to help others. Self-help groups also give training in self control, social skills, relaxation and self assertion. These skills help you cope with your own problems and help others. One of the lynchpins of this type of therapy is the encouragement to develop strong bonds with the community by relearning to communicate.

What can I do?

Many women report success if they make a radical change in their lives such as forming new friendships, changing jobs or working in the community. Try to invest your energy in something that gives you a sense of usefulness and worth. The turning point will come when the reasons for kicking the habit are stronger than the reasons for continuing.

The greatest difficulty once you have got over your dependency is to avoid a relapse. Often a relapse is precipitated by a crisis. A crisis can be an emotional change or events. It is therefore important to try to avoid such a relapse by turning immediately to someone who is aware of your past problem and who can help you.

Another cause of relapse, particularly for those whose addiction involves illegal drug taking, is the presence of the drugs, the users and the culture surrounding it. This increases the craving. It is therefore important to avoid these acquaintances and prevent yourself re-entering the drug culture. Aftercare and support is vital in the short and long term for any addict to be able to remain cured.

TRANQUILIZER ABUSE

More men than women take drugs illegally. Legal drugs such as benzodiazepines, however, are overwhelmingly abused by women. In the U.S., nearly 98 million prescriptions for Valium are written annually. This is primarily prescribed to relieve anxiety. Though known as one of the minor tranquilizers, this is misleading. After taking the drug for as little as a few weeks, women report symptoms of depression, drowsiness, altered sex drive, sleep problems, constipation and confusion when they stop taking it.

Unfortunately, if a woman is prescribed benzodiazepines by her doctor to help with mental or physical problems, and she reports the same symptoms time and again and expects medication, she may be seen as addicted, and her doctor may refuse to renew the prescription without counseling. In such a case, a woman may go elsewhere to maintain her habit rather than admitting dependence.

SEE ALSO:

ALCOHOLISM
ANXIETY
DEPRESSION

DYSMENORRHEA

This is a menstrual period when cramps are extremely painful. It is known as primary dysmenorrhea if painful periods start within three years of the onset of menstruation. In these cases there is usually no underlying disease to account for it and it would appear that painful periods only occur when an egg is produced so it is a sure sign that you are ovulating.

Secondary dysmenorrhea is a symptom of some underlying condition, such as endometriosis or fibroids, which causes the pain; this usually arises after menstruation has been established for more than three years. About one third of all menstruating women suffer some form of dysmenorrhea. The primary form is most common in women under 25, though it may continue after childbirth and into the mid-thirties.

What causes it?

Research has shown that women suffering from primary dysmenorrhea produce excessive quantities of the hormone prostaglandin at the time of menstruation and are extremely sensitive to it. Prostaglandin is one of the hormones released during labor and is in part responsible for the uterine contractions. Dysmenorrhea can therefore be seen as a mini-labor with the prostaglandin causing uterine muscle to go into spasm producing cramp-like pain.

Should I see the doctor?

If you have recently begun to menstruate, don't tolerate this pain and inconvenience; visit your doctor if painkillers in moderate quantities are not sufficient to dull the pain and you need to spend at least a day in bed each month. Your work and normal family life should not be so affected.

If you have been menstruating for at least three years and the blood flow and pain increases, visit your doctor to confirm that there is

---

· S y m p t o m s ·

▲ Violent abdominal cramps lasting up to three days
▲ Diarrhea
▲ Frequency of urination
▲ Sweating
▲ Pelvic soreness with the pain radiating down into the upper thighs and into the back
▲ Abdominal distension
▲ Backache
▲ Nausea and vomiting

---

no underlying disorder which is responsible for the sudden change in menstrual behavior.

What will the doctor do?

Don't be deterred by the belief that dysmenorrhea is a common gynecological complaint that will pass as you get older or if you have children. Some doctors may even indicate that the pain is a neurotic ailment. Insist on a trial of anti-prostaglandin drugs. These are pills which need only be taken just prior to and for the first two to three days of menstruation. Frequently the contraceptive pill is prescribed because it inhibits egg production and alters hormonal balance; however, this carries its own risk and should not be considered for a young girl as there are increased risks of circulatory problems and because it could mean many years of exposure to estrogens.

If you have developed painful periods after years of predictable menstrual characteristics, your doctor will examine you and recommend treatment according to the diagnosis.

What can I do?

Most of us have our own methods of relieving this sort of pain: hot water bottles, hot baths and bed rest all contribute to some degree of comfort. Aspirin is thought to impede the production of prostaglandins so it is the best

painkiller to take. Experiment with herbal teas that reduce spasmodic pain such as mint or chamomile infusions. Relaxation or special yoga-type exercises can also relieve the pain. For example, the cobra and the bow positions may help (See index).

SEE ALSO:

ENDOMETRIOSIS
FIBROIDS
PELVIC INFLAMMATORY
 DISEASE
PREMENSTRUAL SYNDROME

EATING PROBLEMS

Women's attitudes to food and eating are extremely complex. Many women are obsessed by food, turning to food as comfort when depressed, and for solace when in need of affection. Some young girls exercise a form of control by refusing to eat (see *Anorexia nervosa*). Others binge to find comfort and then purge themselves in disgust (see *Bulimia*).

Obesity is almost a natural consequence of the Western diet, with its concentration on animal protein and processed carbohydrate. The diet of meat and two vegetables twice a day could not be more unbalanced, but we are gradually turning to a healthier diet with an emphasis on complex carbohydrates, fiber and less red meat, dairy products and fats.

Because of *digestive problems* not all of us are able to enjoy the food that we eat and for some, each meal presages discomfort. The onset of indigestion in an otherwise healthy person after the age of 35 should always be investigated. Fatty foods can cause severe indigestion for anyone suffering from *gallbladder disease*. In the large bowel, diverticulitis can be the result of too little fiber in the diet and can lead to troublesome *abdominal pain* and bouts of diarrhea. Irritable colon, thought to be more of a nervous disorder than an organic one, can mimic this condition.

Cancer of the lower bowel, the colon and rectum is the second most common cancer in the overall population (see *Colorectal cancer*). It usually shows up as a sudden change in bowel habit. Someone who has been quite regular with a daily bowel motion may suddenly notice *constipation* and then perhaps an attack of watery diarrhea and possibly streaks of blood in the motion. The sudden onset of such symptoms should always be investigated rapidly so urgent medical consultation should be sought.

Constipation seems to be a modern disease and is largely due to eating too little fiber; 99.9% of cases of constipation can be corrected, not by resorting to proprietary laxatives, but simply by adding fiber to the diet. A bowel which learns to rely on laxatives becomes lazy, necessitating the need for more laxatives. Busy lives make us ignore the body's reflexes which keep the bowels efficient.

ECTOPIC PREGNANCY

When a pregnancy develops in an organ other than the uterus, it is known as an ectopic pregnancy. The most common site is in a fallopian tube, but the fertilized embryo can be implanted and attached to various organs within the pelvis, though this is extremely rare.

The egg is usually fertilized by the sperm in the fallopian tube, and if the tube is damaged or abnormal in any way, for example due to an IUD-induced infection, the egg may become stuck there and not make its way to the uterus.

Ectopic pregnancies occur in 1 out of every 100 pregnancies and are more common in first pregnancies, if you have an IUD, are taking the progesterone-only contraceptive pill, and with post-coital contraception.

Is it serious?

An ectopic pregnancy is always serious. This is because the end result is inevitably that the fetus outgrows its surroundings and bursts through the fallopian tube. this leads to hemorrhage, shock, pelvic infection, peritonitis and if untreated, collapse and death.

Should I see the doctor?

If there is any chance you could be pregnant, and you are suffering pain in either the right or left side of your lower abdomen, consult your doctor immediately. Women with a history of pelvic inflammatory disease are particularly at risk and should ensure that a possible ectopic pregnancy is not diagnosed as PID.

Home pregnancy tests are not reliable in tubal pregnancies, so don't hesitate even if you had a negative result on the test.

What will the doctor do?

It is possible that your doctor will be able to feel the pregnancy by examining your abdomen externally. You will probably be given a pregnancy test if there is any doubt. Ultrasound scanning is also used as a diagnostic procedure.

· **Symptoms** ·

▲ Missed period, nausea and tiredness
▲ Colicky type of abdominal pain
▲ Unexpected vaginal bleeding, which could be mistaken for an early miscarriage
▲ Pallor, sweating and faintness if you have internal bleeding
▲ Sharp shoulder pain
▲ Shock; hot and cold flushes and dizziness

Once implanted in a fallopian tube, the fertilized egg starts to grow and sends out tendrils of placental tissue which rupture into blood vessels during the first six to eight weeks of pregnancy.

If a pregnancy is detected, you will need surgery. A specialist will probably perform a laparoscopy prior to removal of the pregnancy. The developing embryo, placenta and any damaged tissue will be removed. If the ectopic pregnancy has burst, salpingectomy, removal of the fallopian tube will need to be carried out, and the hemorrhage staunched to prevent infection. Your ovary may also have to be removed.

Are there any complications?

There may be. Even if the surgeon is able to save the fallopian tube it may heal with scar tissue, become distorted and/or blocked and further pregnancies may be prevented on that side. The

chances of conceiving are reduced slightly if you have one fallopian tube removed.

The condition of the remaining fallopian tube should be assessed, if possible, at the time of the procedure, as it may also be affected by conditions which brought about the present ectopic pregnancy.

SEE ALSO:

CONTRACEPTION
INFERTILITY
LAPAROSCOPY
PELVIC INFLAMMATORY
  DISEASE
PREGNANCY PROBLEMS
ULTRASOUND

ENDOMETRIOSIS

This disease, which affects the pelvic organs, starts before you are born, while you are developing in your mother's body. Tiny little balls of endometrial cells "stray" into the pelvis – the ovaries, tubes and even the bladder. Here they form tiny cysts. After puberty, with each period, the cysts behave like the rest of the uterine lining, the endometrium, and bleed. They become stretched, swollen and enlarged because the blood cannot escape. After ten to fifteen years, they are large enough to cause pain although this pain bears little relation to the extent of the disease. It is often called the career woman's disease because of the two unrelated statistics that the disease usually starts in the late twenties and tends to be most common among women with no families.

· Symptoms ·

▲ Cramping pains during menstruation, becoming severe and like labor contractions on the last day
▲ Dysmenorrhea
▲ Pain on intercourse
▲ Sub-fertility if the fallopian tubes are involved

Should I see the doctor?

If you are in your late twenties and have been unable to conceive, or suffer crippling pain with your periods, or during intercourse you feel pain deep in your pelvis, you should see your doctor as soon as possible.

Make sure you tell your doctor your menstrual history. If you have never suffered from dysmenorrhea before, it is unlikely it would start in your late twenties without some major reason. Don't be fobbed off with pain killers.

What will the doctor do?

Endometriosis can only be diagnosed for certain if the blood-filled cysts are seen directly. This will be done by laparoscopy under a general anesthetic. The cysts may be anything from a pinhead to the size of a walnut and they vary in number from two to nearly 100. They may be confined to a local area or scattered through the pelvic organs.

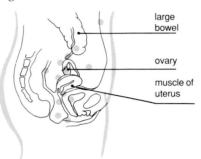

Common sites of endometriosis
The abnormal patches of endometrial cells migrate from the uterus to other parts of the abdominal cavity.

Once the diagnosis of endometriosis is confirmed, treatment will depend on your symptoms and the number and spread of the cysts. If it is widespread, it cannot be satisfactorily treated by removal of the cysts.

Obviously, the immediate problem is solved if you stop menstruating. This can be achieved by conceiving, and in some cases this clears the condition. If you don't wish to have children, hormones will be prescribed to simulate a pregnancy. The most popular hormone treatment is with the drug Danazol. This acts on the pituitary to prevent ovulation and menstruation. However, it has unpleasant side effects such as oily skin, acne, hairiness and weight gain. The side effects disappear after the drug is stopped.

If there are only a few cysts, most of the abdominal and menstrual symptoms will be relieved by surgical removal of the cysts. They can be scraped off by a surgeon to free the tubes and ovaries and increase fertility. Hormone treatment will usually follow to prevent any more growths.

If the condition is extensive, or your symptoms are extremely severe, you may opt for a permanent cure in the form of a hysterectomy, though this obviously prevents you having any more children.

What can I do?

Join a self-help group where you can share your experience with other women and discuss the latest treatments and the side effects of the hormone treatment.

SEE ALSO:

DYSMENORRHEA
HYSTERECTOMY
INFERTILITY
LAPAROSCOPY
MENORRHAGIA
MENSTRUAL PROBLEMS
PAINFUL INTERCOURSE

EPIDURAL ANESTHETIC

This is a method of pain relief which is used mainly in childbirth. It has been called the Rolls Royce of anesthetics because it is effective, safe and has the least side effects. Epidurals are sometimes used in the first days after major abdominal surgery. The patient is relaxed and free from pain during the time when postoperative discomfort is at its worst.

For many women it is the perfect answer to the question of how to have a baby because pain is relieved but you remain alert, fresh and able to experience the whole of the birth. It is even used with Caesarean section.

You should have discussed your labor with the medical staff during your prenatal clinic visits and specified whether you want pain relief during childbirth or not. If you initially decide against an anesthetic but change your mind during labor, it can still be possible to have an epidural.

Why is it done?

◆ Offers complete pain relief without dulling your mental faculties so you can enjoy your experience of childbirth and be an active participant.

◆ You will feel fresh and alert having been spared the hard work and effort of normal childbirth.

◆ You will need no other anesthesia in case of forceps, vacuum extraction or an emergency Caesarean section.

◆ It is a simple matter to increase the anesthetic if your labor goes on longer then expected, or to allow it to wear off when you push your baby out during the second stage.

◆ As it lowers blood pressure, it is ideal for women who suffer from high blood pressure or toxemia of pregnancy.

◆ It reduces the amount of work your organs and muscles need to do and is excellent if you have any lung or heart disease or diabetes.

What are the disadvantages?

You will be having a medically managed birth. You will need a drip to feed fluids intravenously in case your blood pressure falls and there will be a fetal heart monitor as you won't be able to sense the oncoming contraction and push during the second stage. You may feel dizzy and nauseous because your blood pressure is lowered and you may have a headache for the first few hours after delivery. There is also a greater possibility of forceps and episiotomy. You may need to have a catheter passed into your bladder in case you can't feel to pass urine. If your blood pressure drops severely, the amount of blood to the placenta may reduce oxygen to the baby. This will be carefully monitored and intravenous fluids given immediately to raise it.

SEE ALSO:

CAESAREAN SECTION
FORCEPS DELIVERY
TOXEMIA
VACUUM EXTRACTION

HOW IS IT DONE?

You will be asked to lie on your side and pull your legs up to your stomach. Your lower back will be washed with cold surgical soap and there will be an injection of local anesthetic. A tiny hole is then made in your back with a solid needle, then a hollow needle is inserted in its place. This hollow needle carries the catheter which is threaded into the epidural space, leaving a length protruding from your back. This is secured along your back with paper tape to keep it safe and still. The anesthetic is injected through the catheter. The initial procedure takes about 10–20 minutes before you feel the effects. More anesthetic will need to be given every two hours, depending on the length of your labor.

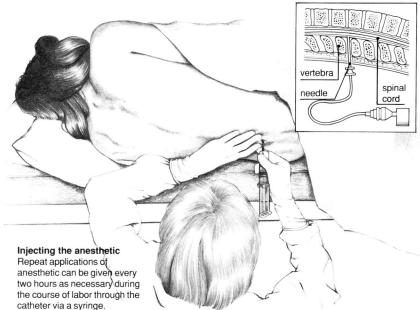

Injecting the anesthetic
Repeat applications of anesthetic can be given every two hours as necessary during the course of labor through the catheter via a syringe.

EPISIOTOMY

Normally performed at the end of labor to allow the baby's head to pass through the vaginal opening, this is a cut made between the vaginal opening and the anus if the doctor thinks the perineum will not stretch sufficiently to let the baby's head through without tearing the skin. The area, already numbed by the pressure of the baby, is injected with a local anesthetic before the cut is made. Until recently, an episiotomy was standard practice and was performed at most first births.

In the last five or so years, there has been a general reduction in the intervention from doctors during childbirth. However, episiotomies are performed in nearly 62% of all deliveries. It now becomes a woman's right not to have it done if she doesn't want to, so discuss the matter with your doctor. If you have a preference, have this recorded in your notes. Request that you be asked if and when the doctor at your delivery thinks it is necessary to have a cut made.

Why is it done?
Doctors and midwives use their judgements about whether an episiotomy is needed or not. The baby's head is its largest diameter and once the head is through the vaginal opening, the rest of the body doesn't stretch the vagina very much. The accepted belief was that a tear involving the perineum and underlying muscle healed badly and left weaknesses possibly creating a tendency to prolapse. Recent research, however, has shown that tears heal more quickly and less painfully than cuts. In addition, episiotomy involves a higher risk of infection and does not prevent prolapse.

How is it done?
As the head is crowning and the vagina is stretched to its maximum, the local anesthetic is injected into the perineal tissue and the cut is made with scissors at an angle away from the rectum. It is done either

REASONS FOR HAVING AN EPISIOTOMY

In some instances, a surgical cut may be unavoidable and you should take the advice of your doctor or midwife if:
▲ There is a need for a speedy delivery because of maternal or fetal distress
▲ The baby is in the breech position

▲ Forceps or vacuum extraction is necessary
▲ You have an epidural anesthetic; the sensations are reduced and you may not be able to control the birth of the baby's head
▲ The baby has a large head

on the midline or on a diagonal.

Once the baby and placenta have been delivered, the cut is stitched. This takes a while because the stitching is done in layers; the deeper muscles are stitched first and then the superficial muscles separately from the skin and other tissue. The sutures (or stitches) are usually soluble and will dissolve in 5–6 days. The degree of discomfort depends on the skill of the person who performs the cut and stitches you up. In a teaching hospital, this is often done by students.

What can I do?
Natural childbirth positions help reduce the need for an episiotomy. If you are standing, on all fours or propped upright, the perineal tissues will thin out more gradually.

There are useful exercises you can do during your pregnancy to learn to relax the area and help the vaginal area to bulge out easily without straining and pushing. If you are lying flat on your back, the strain of pushing the baby "uphill" will put extra pressure on your perineum, causing it to tear. The time when the baby's head crowns is the time to relax those muscles and let the baby emerge slowly and gradually. Your midwife will be able to help you by talking you through the delivery of the head and prevent you pushing too hard at the wrong time.

Stitches always cause some discomfort so be prepared for pain when sitting down, passing urine or moving your bowels. Sit on a rubber

ring and have plenty of warm salt baths to prevent infection and soothe the area. Dry your perineum with a hair dryer and change your sanitary pads frequently so the area doesn't become soggy and damp. If you feel sore and swollen, an ice bag or a sanitary pad soaked in witch hazel may give relief.

The discomfort may continue for weeks and prevent intercourse. Don't let the pain interfere with your sex life in the long term. If you keep putting it off there is a possibility that you will shrink from sexual relations later on.

If you had an episiotomy and you had problems with the stitches and pain, mention this at your next labor. Ask for the best surgeon to stitch you and correct any problem.

SEE ALSO:

EPIDURAL ANESTHETIC
FORCEPS DELIVERY
LABOR
PERINEAL TEAR
PROLAPSE
SEXUAL PROBLEMS
VACUUM EXTRACTION

EYE PROBLEMS

Eyes are self-cleansing organs. They are bathed by the tears, which contain chemicals that kill bacteria. Eyes left alone should come to little harm.

Infections occasionally occur. The most common being conjunctivitis with swollen, painful red eyes. Conjunctivitis needs treatment with antibiotic eye drops and this treatment should start the same day as the symptoms appear. No over-the-counter products should be put into the eyes.

An infection of one of the eyelash follicles is called a stye. It is a self-limiting condition in that pus forms in the hair follicle, comes to a head and bursts. If the eyelash is loose, removing the eyelash will let out the pus and relieve the pressure, bringing immediate relief. If not, bathing with a hot, salt-water solution should help to bring the stye to a head. If the stye is painful, consult your doctor.

Some skin conditions may also affect the eye. Seborrheic dermatitis is a condition where there is eczema in greasy areas such as the eyebrows (known as blepharitis), the folds of the nostrils and in the ears. The skin around the eyelashes has a red, scaly appearance.

Allergies often appear very dramatically around the eyes. In hayfever the eyes are itchy, sore and weepy. With angioedema, the upper and lower eyelids puff up and swell so the eyes may become two slits or even close altogether. This kind of severe allergic reaction requires prompt medical treatment.

There are two major ways in which the eye changes shape as we get older. It may flatten from top to bottom, in which case we become farsighted, or from back to front when we become nearsighted. Appropriate glasses correct these defects. Such changes are so common as to be seen as a normal part of aging. *Cataracts* are opacities within the lens and are also thought to be a consequence of aging.

Glaucoma

Glaucoma, which occurs commonly after the age of 60, is an increase of tension within the eyeball which arises if normal drainage of fluid from the eye is prevented by a blockage. Glaucoma gives rise to the same "red eye" as conjunctivitis and it can only be distinguished by a doctor. Any eye which suddenly goes red must be examined by a doctor very quickly. Glaucoma is a medical emergency because sight can be permanently damaged if the pressure gets too high for too long. Treatment includes eye drops to reduce the production of the aqueous humor, dehydrating agents, and possibly surgery to allow for efficient drainage and prevent further attacks. As the other eye may be susceptible before too long, you are advised to have both eyes done.

As you get older, the pupil is a tell-tale sign of your age. Gradually a pale ring, the arcus senilis, forms around the iris; this is a well-known medical sign for hardening of the arteries (see *Heart disease*).

Contact lenses, particularly the extended-wear soft lenses, are a popular alternative to glasses and can be used cosmetically to change the color of the iris. Not everyone can wear contact lenses, and some sight defects cannot be remedied with them.

Symptoms of medical conditions such as migraine, meningism and multiple sclerosis can first show up with eye symptoms. In migraine, before the headache begins, there are flashing lights. In meningism, the first sign of meningitis, the eyes become very sensitive to bright lights. In multiple sclerosis, the patient may first notice that there are black spaces in her vision. These are called scotomata.

Herpes infection of the eye is particularly serious (see *Cold sores*). This is most common with shingles. If vesicles form on the conjunctivae, they may ulcerate and heal by scarring, seriously affecting vision. Shingles or any herpetic infection which involves the face needs very careful treatment by a specialist.

Cosmetic surgery is employed around the eyes: to rid the upper eyelid of redundant puffy skin, to get rid of crow's feet and to remove bags underneath.

Mild exophthalmos or bulging of the eyes is a symptom of *hyperthyroidism*. Treatment of the thyroid disorder will not necessarily improve the exophthalmos; steroid drugs may be prescribed or the lids may be stitched together.

FACE LIFT

Face lift has come to mean any tightening, tucking and nipping of skin folds anywhere on the face, removal of bags under the eyes or removal of wrinkles around the mouth, eyes and chin. This can also take in tightening of the skin around the jaw line and neck. However, a total face lift is not usually a single operation; it can involve several operations. You can choose to have any or all of them done in any order you wish.

EYELID ALTERATION

This is also known as blepharo-plasty. The upper and lower eyelids are reshaped by taking out redundant skin and removing the fat pads. These fat pads cause the puffiness that commonly surrounds your eyes as you get older. Some people have noticeable bags under their eyes from an early age.

How is it done?
You will be admitted to hospital for about three days. The surgeon will discuss with you the extent and area you want removed and will mark the incision lines before the operation. Usually this operation is done under general anesthetic. The incisions are made along the natural crease when your eye is open. The lower incision is beneath the eyelashes and is usually slanted so that it looks like a laughter line. The skin and fat is trimmed away and stitched.

After the operation you will feel sore. Your eye will be covered with antibiotic ointment to prevent infection. The stitches are removed in 48 hours and the incisions smeared with the ointment once or twice a day.

What are the results?
There will be bruising around your eyes with swelling and you will probably want to wear dark glasses to cover this. Don't expect your appearance to return to normal too quickly. It usually takes three months for the swelling to settle down but the scars will by then be barely detectable and they will blend with your skin creases. If you are of a confident disposition, you can wear dark glasses and be back at work in three days.

Don't rub your face hard when cleansing or applying makeup.

DOUBLE CHIN REDUCTION

This can be achieved by the removal of excess fat and loose skin from under the chin. Most surgeons will not attempt this operation unless you are 40 years or over because the effects of the operation can be undone by aging. As the operation might have to be repeated in six to eight years, that would commit you to several operations within a normal life expectancy.

How is it done?
There are natural creases all over the body, known as Lange lines, and these are used by cosmetic surgeons when they decide where to make the incisions. Under a general anesthetic, the skin of your lower face is trimmed and the fat removed. The incision is then stitched. Your neck will be wrapped in a large dressing to maintain pressure on the wounds. You may even wear a neck collar for a day or two. Your chin and neck will be red and swollen. Half the stitches will be removed after about a week and the remainder within two weeks. The swelling should then subside in another week.

What are the results?
You will have a feeling of tightness around the chin and neck for about a month and the results are usually excellent.

FACE LIFT

This term is used specifically to describe the operation to lift the skin around the hairline. It does not touch the eyes, eyelids, mouth or chin. Most surgeons would be unwilling to perform this operation on someone under 40.

How is it done?
Small tucks of skin are taken in all around the hairline, generally tightening the skin of the face and pulling it upwards and outwards. The surgeon will have taken account of your expectations for your new face. The incisions will be traced on your face and, under general anesthetic, the first incision made on one side of your face. It usually starts at your temple, down the hairline to the front of your ear and then up and behind your ear. Excess skin and fat are removed and the skin reshaped and closed

EYELID ALTERATION
Blepharoplasty, to correct bags under the eyes, is a simple procedure with a short hospital stay.

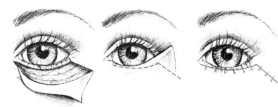

Excess sagging skin around the eyes is removed through an incision made along the fold of the eyelid or underneath the lashes which is subsequently stitched up.

FACE LIFT

with tiny stitches. The other side of your face is then done. You will be able to eat right away, though a large dressing will hold the wounds firm. You'll probably wear this for two days. Your face will be red and swollen, but the superficial swelling will subside within a month.

What are the results?
They are very good but don't usually become fully apparent until three months later. The effect may last for seven or eight years. This operation is particularly good for pulling out skin creases around the mouth. However, repeated operations of this kind can result in a perpetually smiling mouth and eyes which are stretched upwards, outwards and backwards.

TOTAL FACIAL REJUVENATION

This operation involves a face lift, a neck lift, eyelid repair and dermabrasion for mouth wrinkles. You should really be 45 years or over before you consider this as it involves a great investment of time, stoicism and money.

Because of the extensive tucking

and reshaping, you will need to have a number of operations. You will be red, swollen and stiff for some time afterwards. You'll wear bulky dressings but at the end of the surgery, the generalized swelling should subside in three weeks. You may experience numbness around the ears; it may take several months for feeling to return to normal. The results are good but may take six months to become fully apparent.

FACE LIFT

Pulling up loose facial skin and removing fatty tissue can eliminate wrinkles, jowls and sagging skin.

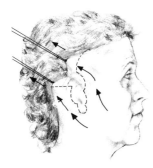

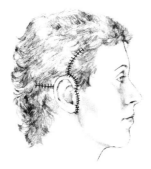

Skin is pulled back behind the ears. Loose chins and necks, drooping eyebrows and slack cheeks can all be corrected.

SEE ALSO:

COSMETIC SURGERY
DERMABRASION
EYE PROBLEMS
FACIAL TREATMENTS
OTOPLASTY
RHINOPLASTY

FACIAL TREATMENTS

Most women who seek facial treatments do so to stop the ravages of aging as they see it. Cosmetic surgery to lift bags under the eyes, re-align noses and do away with wrinkles is always popular. Vast amounts of money are spent each year on cosmetic creams and lotions to effect a transformation. However, gravity and the construction of the skin mean that these methods can only have transitory effects.

You inherit your skin type from your parents. As you approach middle age, the replacement of dead cells, which is going on all the time, is more erratic and with the loss of elasticity, your skin becomes drier and more wrinkled. When this happens depends on your inherited skin type and whether or not you have regularly exposed your skin to strong sunlight.

CARE OF THE SKIN

Handling, massage and gentle circular motions will keep your skin well nourished if done against the force of gravity and lines of natural wrinkling. So taking off and putting on makeup is beneficial as a massage and skin conditioner. If you have bad acne, don't worry about putting on makeup to hide unsightly break-outs. The skin can breathe and the pores aren't blocked.

Moisturizing

One of the greatest favors you can do for your skin is to moisturize it. The skin does not need oil, it needs water. You can either put moisture into your skin or prevent moisture loss from the skin. To put moisture into your skin is very difficult. Try a variety of moisturizing agents. None of them will have an effect lasting more than two or three hours. Some of them, the very light fluffy ones that disappear into the skin immediately, last no longer than 20 minutes.

Trying to prevent water loss is simpler. The skin is losing moisture as fast as you put it in and the drier the environment you live in, the faster it loses moisture. So before you apply makeup, use a very light, milky lotion and then on top put a heavier creamy variety which is formulated to mimic natural sebum. It is so efficient because it prevents water loss. This is a much better way of keeping the skin moisturized than by trying to put water into it.

Face masks

Whether you do it yourself at home or visit a beauty clinic, there are some fairly outlandish ingredients for face packs and masks. There is no evidence that oils of avocado or cucumber are more beneficial than moisturizing creams. Essentially the main benefit is the relaxation while they are on your face. Face masks can cleanse the skin and increase blood flow, leaving you looking healthy and pink, but they do no more than that.

FACIAL EXERCISES

To relax your facial muscles and prevent the lines and wrinkles that result from frowning, do these simple exercises. You should be

Massaging your face is pleasurable and a good way to help the blood circulation. Effleurage is one method you can do yourself to help drain fluid on your face. Place your fingertips on your jaw and, always working up and out, push a pad of flesh in front of your fingers. Use moisturizing cream to help you. Work along your jaw line, out from your nostrils and along your forehead. Don't massage the eye socket in this way as there is little supporting muscle or fat there.

BEAUTY TREATMENTS

For more serious marks on the face, such as deep acne scars and accidental injury, there are effective treatments that should only be undertaken by trained technicians. These include dermabrasion and chemical skin peeling.

A less drastic skin peeling or content with the laughter lines, but you might as well try to avoid those associated with worry and tension.

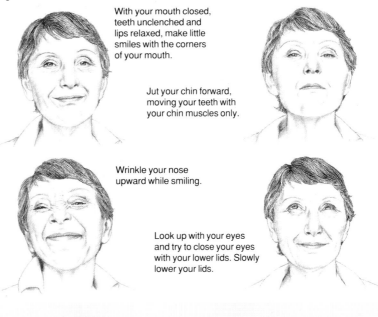

With your mouth closed, teeth unclenched and lips relaxed, make little smiles with the corners of your mouth.

Jut your chin forward, moving your teeth with your chin muscles only.

Wrinkle your nose upward while smiling.

Look up with your eyes and try to close your eyes with your lower lids. Slowly lower your lids.

exfoliation with a face mask or abrasive pad removes the top layer of dead cells that tend to give the skin a gray appearance. Some body scrubs containing ingredients such as oatmeal may make your skin feel tingling and fresh. However, the skin naturally loses dead cells in a process called desquammation. This occurs at a rate of millions of cells shed each day. If you seek to increase this shedding of cells, you will irritate your skin and the over-production will leave scaly patches, which is the reverse of what you want. In fact, dermatologists usually seek to prevent rapid cell replacement and so reduce the skin's sensitivity.

There really is nothing you can apply to your skin to prevent wrinkles and aging. Exercising facial muscles may limit the tension lines. Anti-wrinkle creams, injections with animal extracts, collagen implants and the application of electrical currents to your face may cause your skin to feel smooth and well moist-urized, and you to feel pampered and refreshed, but there is no reason to suppose that these expensive treatments are any more effective than a basic lanolin product.

CHEMICAL PEELING

This is a method for making skin blemishes less obvious. Fine lines, wrinkles, small pit marks and slightly discolored areas of skin and freckles can be removed in this way. How-ever, this method does not stop the aging process; the first effect wears off within months, certainly a year. Another comparable treatment is dermabrasion where the blemishes are "sanded" away with a high-speed abrasive tool.

How is it done?
One of the three chemicals is applied to the area, normally under local anesthetic. As the three main agents for chemical peeling are very strong – phenol, resorcinol and trichlorocetic acid – they should only be used by a medically qualified person.

Phenol when painted on the face causes coagulation, inflammation, swelling and peeling. It can be absorbed rapidly through the skin and can cause damage to the kidneys. It must therefore be used with caution and only on a limited area. It tends to be confined in use to treating small pitted scars of acne and superficial complaints such as small spots.

Resorcinol is used to deal with itchy skin or to remove scales and sometimes to treat acne. It acts by breaking the chemical bonds that hold the scales of keratin on the surface of the skin. Once broken they peel away. It must never be used on broken skin because it can cause serious side effects if absorbed into the bloodstream. Many derma-tologists are, therefore, of the opinion that the dangers of resorcinol out-weigh the advantages and it should be used very rarely indeed.

Trichlorocetic acid has the initial effect of producing a second-degree burn in the skin which turns whitish-gray in color. A brown crust then forms within three to five days and when this drops off the skin beneath looks pink, tight and with fewer wrinkles.

What are the risks?
The end result in the hands of an unqualified person could be a severely scarred face. Chemical peeling, therefore, should only be used where there is a clear and accurate diagnosis of the blemishes and how they will respond to such treatment.

As a general rule, chemical peeling is used as a treatment by beauticians and cosmetologists for mild conditions, and any serious scarring or pitting is reserved for doctors and dermatologists. I feel that there should be no distinction, and it should always be done by medical personnel. The best results are on fair skins as the bleaching effect is less noticeable.

SEE ALSO:

ACNE
BIRTHMARKS
COSMETIC SURGERY
DERMABRASION
FACE LIFT
WRINKLES

FAINTING AND DIZZINESS

A feeling of weakness and unsteadiness on your feet is usually the result of a sudden drop in blood pressure. You may also feel cold and clammy all over. Faintness is not usually cause for concern; perhaps you haven't eaten for some time and your blood sugar levels are low. If you do feel faint, lie down and raise your feet above your head so the blood flows back to your brain. If this isn't possible, sit with your head between your knees to achieve the same result. If you do lose consciousness momentarily, this is not usually cause for concern.

If you feel that you are spinning around or everything is spinning around you, this spell of dizziness is known as vertigo. Vertigo does not mean a fear of heights; that is acrophobia. Vertigo is a symptom of a disorder in the brain or the inner ear which affects your balance. You may even feel sick and faint. Your eyes may move sideways and then come swiftly back to their normal position. Although these sensations are frightening, they are usually only temporary. Lie down with your eyes closed.

If you have heavy periods, or you are taking certain drugs, particularly sedatives and antihistamines, they may make you feel weak and dizzy.

If you are unable to make a diagnosis from this information, consult your doctor. (*continued overleaf*)

NATURE OF THE PROBLEM	PROBABLE CAUSE
You feel dizzy when you jump out of a hot bath	The blood flow to your heart and brain is temporarily reduced because the blood supply to your skin has increased in the hot water, causing a drop in blood pressure. Get out of hot baths or sauna slowly and carefully.
You feel faint when you exercise strenuously	If you are panting, the rapid breathing caused by this exertion can cause temporary faintness.
You suffer from *anxiety* attacks	These can cause feelings of faintness. You may also feel faint after receiving an emotional shock because the nerves that control blood pressure may have been affected by the incident.
You feel faint during pregnancy	Blood supply to the uterus is increased, and if blood pools in the lower parts of the body because your system is more sluggish at this time, your brain can be temporarily deprived of blood. Sit down immediately to avoid falling. Put your feet up and allow the blood flow to return to normal. Avoid standing for long periods.
Unexpectedly upon standing up you feel faint	Standing up suddenly can cause your blood pressure to temporarily drop. Stand up more slowly.
You have high blood pressure (see *Hypertension*) and are taking drugs to combat it	Your blood pressure may fall too low because of the medication, causing faintness. See your doctor to check the dosage level.
You feel dizzy in the morning or late afternoon, or you don't eat regularly, or it has been some time since you ate	Low blood sugar levels can cause faintness and loss of energy. If you haven't eaten for some time, eat something sweet and starchy to make you feel better. Carry glucose tablets if you have these attacks often and eat frequent snacks of nutritional food instead of two main meals a day.
You suffer from a form of *heart disease*	A sudden alteration in heart rhythm can cause fainting. Consult your doctor right away.
You have been out in the sun, or in a hot and stuffy room	You may feel faint because of the heat. Lie down in a cool darkened room and have a refreshing drink.

FAINTING AND DIZZINESS

NATURE OF THE PROBLEM	PROBABLE CAUSE
You suffer from *diabetes*	You should recognize that faintness is a sign of hypoglycemia. See your doctor if your medication isn't preventing the attacks.
You feel that you are spinning, and there are other symptoms such as difficulty speaking, blurred vision, numbness and/or tingling in your hands or in any part of your body	Consult your doctor without delay as this could be because there has been a temporary interruption in blood supply to your brain. You may have suffered a stroke.
You feel dizzy and you have noticed some loss of hearing or noises in your ear	This could be Ménières disease, a rare disorder of middle age when fluid accumulates in your inner ear causing difficulty with balance. Consult your doctor.
You are vomiting and finding it hard to keep your balance	This may be caused by inflammation of the inner ear. The virus attacks the labyrinth which is the part of the inner ear responsible for maintaining balance. Consult your doctor.
You feel dizzy when you turn your head or look upwards	This could be *osteoarthritis* of the spine, especially if you are over 50.
You are anxious and your breathing is rapid	Hyperventilation leads to dizziness and numbness in your hands. Breathe deep and slowly.
You are taking medication for some other problem	Certain drugs may cause dizziness. Consult your doctor.
You suffer from *menorrhagia*	Chronic blood loss at menstruation can lead to *anemia* and a feeling of faintness.

FATIGUE

This can describe anything from tiredness to exhaustion. It can also describe the lack of energy that might occur during pregnancy or the days before menstruation, or with an illness such as anemia or the apathy experienced during a depressive illness.

An almost constant feeling of fatigue is something many women understand as they go about their lives combining the roles of mother, wife, worker and good neighbor. This could be described as a "busy" life but if it leads to lack of energy, inability to concentrate and neglect of yourself, and disinterest in sex and social life, there may be physical and emotional repercussions.

What causes it?

Fatigue can be a symptom of a physical disorder. Hypothyroidism, where the thyroid gland secretes only a small amount of a hormone called thyroxine, causes the body to slow down noticeably. Diabetes mellitus also produces this symptom, as does anemia. However, other more dramatic symptoms will probably be more apparent in these cases. Certain viral illnesses, particularly mononucleosis and hepatitis, can leave an aftermath of tiredness and depression for several months.

Recently, a new disease, myalgic encephalomyelitis, also commonly known as the post-viral fatigue syndrome, has been identified. Sufferers often report long bouts of exhaustion with no apparent cause, and almost constant fatigue. There is no known cure and symptoms are usually treated as they occur.

Excessive consumption of alcohol or social drugs can also bring on feelings of intense fatigue.

Should I see the doctor?

If you think your extreme tiredness may be a symptom of some medical condition, and if you are unable to make a diagnosis from this information, consult your doctor.
(continued overleaf)

NATURE OF PROBLEM	PROBABLE CAUSE
You are worried and consequently unable to sleep	This *insomnia* can cause you to feel fatigued during the day.
You have felt under the weather and short of energy for some time	Examine your diet and eat more sensibly. You could be skipping meals and missing valuable nutrients. Too little food leads to hypoglycemia and low energy levels.
You are pale, short of breath, have palpitations and feel faint	You could have *anemia*.
You are or could be pregnant	This is an early sign of pregnancy. If all your prenatal checks are okay, this is normal.
You feel extremely fatigued, with aching limbs so that you can't walk far, and your exhaustion seems constant	This could be a post viral syndrome - myalgic encephalomyelitis. See your doctor.
You are unhappy, anxious, uninterested in sex and unable to make decisions	*Depression* could be the cause.
You are passing a lot of urine, and your weight is going down	You could have *diabetes mellitus*.
You are middle aged and feel the cold more than before, and your skin and hair are coarse and dry and you are inexplicably gaining weight	You could have an underactive thyroid gland (see *Hyperthyroidism*).
You find yourself short of breath on exertion and you feel your heart racing	This could be a heart condition. Consult your doctor.
You regularly drink alcohol	Cut out for a week and see if you feel better. Regular consumption of alcohol in relatively moderate quantities has a depressant effect and can make you feel tired.
You are taking medication, for example, for hayfever	Many antihistamine drugs can cause drowsiness. See your doctor about changing the medication.
You have been ill for some time or had major surgery	Don't expect to feel your old self right away. Take it easy and rest as much as you can and build your strength up gradually.

FATIGUE

What will the doctor do?

Your doctor will treat the underlying cause of the fatigue. If you are depressed and fatigue is preventing you lifting yourself out of your sadness, your doctor will probably prescribe anti-depressive drugs to treat the depression. Take the full prescription; follow your doctor's regime carefully. You should not suddenly stop taking these drugs.

What can I do?

If your work is taking too much of your energy and you have family or other commitments, don't be afraid to admit them or the spiral of self deception about your inability to cope will lead to illness. Timetable your day or reschedule your program and remember you don't have to sleep to conserve your strength. All your vital organs will benefit from simply resting.

Look at your diet. Are you eating enough of the right energy-giving foods? Are you too busy, or feeding your family and forgetting yourself or trying to take off weight in a drastic way. Often skipping breakfast can lead to a feeling of irritability and mental tiredness so try to eat a balanced breakfast and take sensible snacks during the day.

You may need to get your priorities straight. Overwork and tiredness could lead to the relationships with your family and your sex life suffering. You must decide what you want to come first and this may require a rearrangement of your priorities for a more realistic life style.

Sometimes if you are very tired or rushing around, you may have trouble resting or finding a minute to revitalize yourself. By transferring the site of your breathing to your diaphragm, you will take deep breaths which have a relaxing quality.

SEE ALSO:

ALCOHOLISM
DEPRESSION
DRUG DEPENDENCY
PREMENSTRUAL SYNDROME

FETOSCOPY

This is a method of viewing the fetus directly with a fiberoptic lens to check for any abnormalities and to remove a sample for analysis. It is usually done in the 15th week of pregnancy.

Why is it done?

Investigations involving this level of risk are only undertaken at the instigation of a physician who thinks there may be something wrong.

Fetoscopy is now used principally to check the fetal blood for blood disorders that are genetically carried, such as thalassemia. Visible defects, such as cleft palate, may also be confirmed in this way.

A medical intervention of this kind is always taken seriously, and most doctors will make a determined effort to avoid it unless absolutely necessary. However, in obstetric units where high technology births are the norm, this test is more likely to be carried out.

How is it done?

A fetoscope is a needle, about 2mm in diameter, into which a light and a powerful lens is placed. Under a local anesthetic, a small incision is made in the woman's abdomen, either just above the pubic bone or below the navel. With constant monitoring with ultrasound to keep a watch on the fetus' movements, the needle is passed through the abdominal wall and the uterine wall into the amniotic cavity. The doctor can then look at the fetus and obtain a sample of blood, or sometimes skin.

What are the risks?

This test will not be done merely because you ask for it. There would need to be very good reasons as the risk of miscarriage is high. Ultrasound and amniocentesis have superseded fetoscopy as a check for congenital abnormalities.

WHAT THE FETOSCOPE SEES

Fetoscopic investigation entails a risk to the pregnancy and your doctor will have a very good reason for carrying it out.

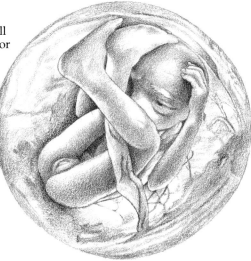

The powerful lens allows the doctor to look at the baby in the uterus. Any visible defects can be clearly seen. This healthy baby is 15 weeks old and her limbs are properly formed and the joints moving. Toe and fingernails are present.

SEE ALSO:

AMNIOCENTESIS
CHROMOSOMAL
   PROBLEMS
GENETIC COUNSELING
MISCARRIAGE
PREGNANCY PROBLEMS
ULTRASOUND

FEVER

If you feel very hot and sweaty, or shivery and unwell, you probably have a fever. This is a sign that your body is fighting infection. A temperature of 38°C (100°F) or over is a fever. If your temperature rises to 40°C (104°F), you should call your doctor immediately. Relieve a fever with aspirin, plenty of cool non-alcoholic drinks, and lie down in a cool, dark room.

Another means of reducing your temperature, if you don't feel too ill to move, is to take a tepid bath. This is good if you don't want to take drugs to reduce the fever. Rest will help your body combat the infection.

If you are pregnant, don't take any drugs, including aspirin, without your doctor's approval.

If you are unable to make a diagnosis from this information, consult your doctor.

NATURE OF THE PROBLEM	PROBABLE CAUSE
You have recently returned from abroad	This could be a symptom of a tropical disease. Call your doctor.
You have a headache and stiff neck, light hurts your eyes, you are drowsy and you have been vomiting	This could be meningitis, inflammation of the brain. Call your doctor immediately.
The fever is accompanied by a rash	You could have an infectious disease such as measles or chickenpox. If you are pregnant and you have a rash with swelling of the glands in your neck, this could be *rubella* (german measles) which can seriously affect your unborn child. If the rash is purple and remains on pressure, this could be an allergic reaction (see *Rashes*).
You also have a runny nose, aching limbs or sore throat	You probably have influenza. Relieve the symptoms with painkillers and bed rest. If you develop pain in your chest, breathlessness or yellow/brown sputum, this could mean the infection has spread to your lungs. It could be bronchitis or pneumonia. Call your doctor right away.
You have frequent or painful urination, pain in your back radiating to your groin or cloudy urine	This could be a kidney infection or *cystitis*.
You are breastfeeding and there is a painful red patch on your breast	This could be a breast abcess (see *Breastfeeding problems*).
You have pain in your lower abdomen and/or heavy, unpleasant smelling discharge	This could be *pelvic inflammatory disease*.
Your temperature fluctuates for no apparent reason, and you feel generally unwell	This could be a blood disorder and it is wise to see your doctor as soon as possible.

FIBROIDS

These are benign tumors of the endometrium, which is the muscle lining the uterine wall. They vary in size and number; they can be anything from the size of a pea to as large as a tennis ball. In neglected cases they may even grow larger. They increase the bleeding surface of the uterus.

About one woman in five develops fibroids by the time she is 45 years old.

There is often no reason for concern because the fibroids may never grow large enough to distort the uterus and present symptoms to alarm you. However, if you are trying to conceive, they may be the cause of your infertility because they are blocking the fallopian tubes. Large fibroids cause the muscular coating of the uterus to feel lumpy and bumpy to the doctor when palpating your abdomen during routine pelvic examinations. They can also be detected by a Pap smear.

· S y m p t o m s ·

- ▲ May be none
- ▲ Infertility
- ▲ Heavy menstrual bleeding
- ▲ Discomfort during intercourse
- ▲ Swelling of the abdomen
- ▲ Feeling of heaviness in the abdomen
- ▲ Pressure on the bladder and bowel causing frequency of urination, constipation and backache

Should I see the doctor?

If you are having difficulty conceiving, if you have increasing pain or bleeding with your periods or any other change in your normal menstrual cycle, see your doctor.

What will the doctor do?

Your doctor will do a routine pelvic examination and question you about the symptoms. You will then be referred to a gynecologist for further investigation which will

probably include ultrasound scanning of your uterus.

What is the treatment?

Fibroids are treated according to the seriousness of the symptoms and whether you wish to conceive. Once you are past childbearing days, the fibroids usually shrink and disappear anyway.

You may be referred for a hysteroscopy. This requires a local

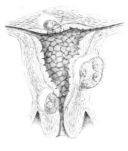

Location of fibroids
These non-cancerous lumps of tissue form on the uterus and increase its bleeding surface.

anesthetic. A fiberoptic tube is passed into your uterus through the vagina so the doctor can directly view the fibroids and assess their number and size. If you want children and they are numerous, your doctor will suggest a myomectomy. This removes the fibroids from the uterine lining and leaves the uterus intact and back to its usual shape. If the symptoms are very difficult and you have finished your family, a hysterectomy might be advised. You should consider this as a last resort and only after two opinions and full discussion with your doctors.

In November 1986, some Swedish scientists discovered that an anti-estrogen hormone preparation made fibroids shrink and wither, thereby relieving symptoms. This research is still in its infancy but may hold promise for the future.

What can I do?

Fibroids are the commonest reason for hysterectomy operations in the United States so be on your guard against an unnecessary operation of such a radical nature. If you are suffering from profound anemia or have unbearable symptoms, obviously you should consider it, otherwise look for alternatives. As there is a high incidence of uterine cancer in women who have benign fibroids, any bleeding or irregularity in your menstrual pattern should be investigated immediately.

SEE ALSO:

DYSMENORRHEA
HYSTERECTOMY
PAINFUL INTERCOURSE
PELVIC EXAMINATION
ULTRASOUND
UTERINE CANCER

FITNESS TESTING

Physical fitness and good health usually go hand in hand. The benefits of physical exercise are not disputed and you'll sleep better, feel better and look better as a result of it. You are likely to suffer fewer illnesses as well.

To become physically fit you can either devise your own exercise program or join a club or group. However, before you set goals, it is sensible to aim for the right fitness level for your age. Before you can do that, you have to know how unfit you are. This can be assessed in a simple way by examining the response of your heart to exercise. Strenuous exercise is enough to increase the oxygen requirements of your body above normal. This is termed aerobic exercise and the heart and lungs are only challenged when this kind of exercise is performed.

Oxygen requirements of the body

increase when exercise involves large muscle groups such as those of the legs, the hips, pelvis, the arms and shoulders. Good exercise therefore would be jogging, swimming, cycling, and rowing, though a brisk walk is also excellent.

You can measure the response of your heart to taking exercise by assessing the pulse rate. If you are unfit, your heart will start to beat very fast when you exercise strenuously because this is the only way it can pump more blood around your body to keep up with the increased demands for oxygen. On the other hand, a fit heart will not beat as fast because it can pump more blood with each beat than an unfit heart.

How do I know if I am fit?
The normal, average resting pulse is 80-90 beats per minutes until the age of 40 or so. The pulse rate varies with

age. A young baby's heart beats at 160 beats a minute reducing to 100-120 by the time a child is eight or nine. During mild or moderate exertion, your pulse rate should rise to between 120 and 130.

Until you are sure you are fit, you shouldn't exceed this figure during exercise. As you get older, the maximum allowable pulse rate diminishes, for example:

age	pulse rate
50-54	117
55-59	113
60-64	109

Should I see the doctor?
If you have heart trouble, high blood pressure or chest pain, or a family history of heart disease, or you are overweight, or over 35 and you have not exercised regularly before, you shouldn't undertake any strenuous exercise without consulting your doctor first.

Your doctor may give you some form of cardiovascular stress test which is designed to assess your overall fitness and the health of your heart (see opposite).

Some doctors may recommend a cholesterol blood test to check the levels of cholesterol in your blood. High levels may be inherited, but in most cases they are due to a diet high in saturated fats. To make your exercise program a thorough one, you will need to watch your diet, cut down on alcohol and stop smoking.

FINDING YOUR PULSE

The pulse is the wave of pressure that passes along each artery every time your heart beats. You can feel it wherever an artery lies close to your skin. The most common site is the radial pulse, on the underside of your wrist in line with your thumb. You can also feel your pulse under your jaw, just outside the midline on your neck, (this is the carotid pulse), up the arch of the

foot in line with the big toe and in the center of your groin.

Feel for the pulse with the tips of the first three fingers. Count the number of beats you can feel in 15 seconds and multiply by 4 to get the rate per minute.

A normal pulse is regular and strong; any abnormality such as a slow pulse or a fast, weak pulse is cause for concern.

What can I do?
Fitness testing aims to measure how long it takes a person to recover her normal pulse rate after mild to moderate exercise. A simple way of assessing the efficiency of your heart, lungs and muscles is to do the step test. However, if you can't walk up three flights of stairs (each of 15–20 steps) steadily without pausing for breath or are breathless when finishing – do not try the following.

Choose a bottom stair or any fixed platform about 8 inches high. Step onto it with one foot, bring up the

Pulse (heartbeat) counted in 15 seconds		
under 45 years	over 45 years	fitness rating
below 20	below 21	excellent
20-22	21-23	good
23-28	24-29	average
above 28	above 29	poor

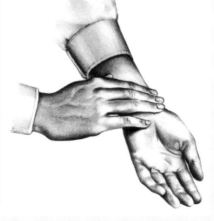

other, and then step back down onto the floor. Repeat at the rate of 24 times a minute for 3 minutes. Stop and wait for exactly one minute, then check your pulse rate (see opposite) to determine your fitness rating.

Stop the exercise at any time if you feel unpleasantly out of breath, dizzy, nauseated or uncomfortable.

Another simple test is to run on the spot for 30 seconds, take your pulse for 15 seconds and multiply by 4.

Testing during exercise

When you exercise, your pulse rate should not go higher than the rate achieved during mild to moderate exercise. The aim of aerobic exercise is to keep this pulse rate for 15-20 minutes; 30-40 is better. While you are exercising, continue to take your pulse every few minutes. If the rate goes over that which you have calculated, slow down and wait until you drop below 100 again before you start back on the exercise program. By stopping and starting, you will prevent excessive strain on your heart. As you continue to exercise day by day and week by week, the length of time you exercise without stopping will increase as your fitness increases.

Safety notes

◆ No exercise should be undertaken without warming up first. This consists of movements simply to get the joints and muscles working. Arm circling done with your feet wide apart and your arms loose, or side bends with feet wide apart and your hands on your hips, are all good and promote agility and good posture.

◆ Never exercise on a full stomach; always wait an hour at least and then spend a few minutes loosening up before beginning any strenuous exercise.

◆ Don't be over-zealous about increasing the length of time you exercise; slowly and surely is the best way.

CARDIAC STRESS TEST

This test is to determine whether people suffering from chest pain, breathlessness or palpitations during exercise have some form of heart disease.

The person is attached to an ECG machine which records the electrical activity of the heart. She then performs some exercise such as walking on a treadmill. The ECG recording is then examined for changes outside of normal. The patient also breathes into a face mask. The air is analyzed, usually by a computer, to ascertain how the lungs respond to exercise.

◆ Always check your pulse rate so that you are reaching the level of fitness for your age over a period of weeks; this should never be less than six weeks.

◆ Try to exercise at least three or four times a week once you have achieved your level of fitness in order to maintain it.

If you are jogging.

◆ Start by jogging at a comfortable rate for about 50 yards.

◆ Slow down and walk 100 yards.

◆ Keep repeating this cycle until you've been going about 20 minutes.

◆ Stop if you start to feel dizzy or sick or so out of breath you can't speak.

◆ Don't extend the time limit over 20 minutes until you can jog for the whole 20 minutes without stopping.

SEE ALSO:

HEART DISEASE
HYPERTENSION
SPORTS INJURIES

FLUID RETENTION

Fluid retention is the accumulation of fluid in the body tissues. It is also known as edema and is noticeable as puffiness or swelling, most commonly in the ankles and fingers when poor circulation or gravity causes stagnation in these extremities.

It is often a common problem during pregnancy and also premenstrually. For example, the tingling and tenderness in the breasts prior to menstruation is a form of fluid retention.

This condition is not usually a symptom of a serious disease unless you have a heart, kidney or liver problem. It is treated with diuretic drugs which cause you to pass more urine and thereby reduce the amount of fluid in the body. Salt in the diet may need to be reduced as this encourages fluid to be retained in the body tissues. Fluid retention may not be accompanied by pain, but it should be investigated.

If you are unable to make a diagnosis from this information, consult your doctor.

NATURE AND SITE OF PROBLEM	PROBABLE CAUSE
You are pregnant and your rings are tight, your face bloated and your shoes feel too small, especially in the last three months of your pregnancy	This could be a serious condition known as *toxemia of pregnancy* or pre-eclampsia, especially if your weight has also increased. You will be checked for puffiness at every prenatal visit.
If you stand for any length of time, you may notice that your ankles swell and your legs ache.	You may have *varicose veins*
You are a chronic drinker	Any obvious fluid retention may be a symptom of cirrhosis of the liver (see *Alcoholism*). Consult your doctor without delay.
The swelling is accompanied by pain, localized in one ankle and lower leg	This could be *phlebitis* or a *deep-vein thrombosis*.
You are gaining weight and your breasts increase in size	This may be a side effect of your contraceptive pill. Ask your doctor for an opinion, and perhaps change your form of *contraception*.
You are stung on the face or mouth, and your face starts to swell	This could be an allergic reaction known as angioedema (see *Skin problems*). Consult your doctor immediately.
Your breasts feel tender and swollen and you are in the week before your period	This could be part of the *premenstrual syndrome*.
Your ankles swell during a journey when you are seated for long periods	This is quite normal and should subside within 12 hours. The circulation in your legs has been reduced.
Your ankles are persistently swollen and additional symptoms include breathlessness, extreme tiredness and swelling in other parts of your body.	Consult your doctor in case this is a symptom of a heart or kidney condition.

FOOT PROBLEMS

Throughout our lives our feet, which ultimately bear the weight of the body, are worked really hard. They are the greatest distance from the heart so tend to be poorly nourished. By the time the blood reaches the extremities, its flow is rather sluggish, so nutrients are slowly dispersed.

Given the stresses and strains of everyday life, we should all take care of our feet, but most of us are neglectful. We put our feet to increased stress by the kind of shoes we wear. Feet are happiest and healthiest going bare. Worst of all are very high-heeled shoes with pointed toes. The heel tips the body forward so that the whole weight is directed downwards to the single joint of the big toe with the foot, hence the development of *bunions*.

The damaging effects of high heels are compounded if the shoes are narrowly pointed. This crowds the toes together, puts a strain on joints and causes friction in any part of the toe which is raised above the rest. If the friction continues for any length of time, a callus or corn will appear as a pad of thick and dead skin. This presses on nerve endings in the skin and the joint and can cause excruciating pain.

Even with the greatest care, areas of hard skin will appear in those parts of the feet that take a lot of wear and tear, around the edges of the soles and heels, for instance. This can be kept at bay by using a pumice stone or hard skin remover when it has softened up after a bath or shower. If you cream your feet too, they will remain smooth and soft and corns, calluses and bunions will be less trouble. If you use a silicone-based preparation on your feet, you will find that your feet slip more easily into shoes and blisters become a rarity.

Most of us think a podiatrist is a luxury until we reach middle age, but it's worth taking care of your feet from your early 20s onwards. A podiatrist can maintain young feet in a healthy condition, attend to problems before they become serious, and obviate pain and discomfort.

The feet are subject to a variety of infections, one of the commonest being a fungal infection, athlete's foot. This is contagious, and if left untreated can affect the toenails as well. Good hygiene and anti-fungal medication should clear it up quickly. If the *wart* virus attacks the foot, this is known as a verruca and can be painful, requiring removal. If you have sweaty feet, this is a common form of *body odor*. You can reduce odors by adopting proper hygiene.

Most women have swollen feet and ankles occasionally from the time they have their first child. This is partly because fluid is forced out of the blood vessels into the tissues. During and after a pregnancy swelling of the ankles (edema) is more likely. Swelling of the ankles is particularly bad in the week prior to menstruation. This is caused by general *fluid retention* due to swinging levels of hormones. You may notice other symptoms of *premenstrual syndrome* – your rings may feel tighter due to fluid in the fingers and your face may look puffy. *Varicose veins*, those that are swollen and twisted, can develop if there is interference with the bloodflow to the legs.

Ingrown toenails
When the toenail fails to grow straight out from the nail bed and instead curves over into the side of the toe, this is an ingrown toenail. It can be a problem, particularly if the nail is small and the big toe is fleshy. The nail seems to bite into the skin producing severe pain and, on occasion, nasty infections. A self-help measure involves cutting a small V shape in the top edge of the nail to relieve pressure on the side of the nail.

Chilblains
In the winter, many of us suffer from chilblains. These are small, red/blue itchy lumps usually on the backs of the legs, hands and feet. They are a reaction to cold. The chilblain itself is a group of blood vessels which dilate and swell when the legs are warm and then constrict down when cooling takes place. The chilblain becomes most itchy if you go from a cold environment into a warm one because the blood vessels suddenly fill and swell causing a stretching of the pain receptors in the skin resulting in exquisite itching. The way to treat chilblains is to avoid extremes of temperature. Few proprietary creams make any difference.

FORCEPS DELIVERY

This is a delivery when the birth of the baby is speeded up and assisted by the application of forceps around the sides of the baby's head. The forceps allow medical staff to pull the baby out gently in tune with the mother's contractions. They are rather like a cage protecting the baby's head from any pressure in the birth canal. Their use is confined to deliveries when the cervix is fully dilated and the baby's head has already descended into the mother's pelvis. Your doctor will decide when they should be used.

Forceps were used centuries ago as the first artificial aid to delivery. However, their use today in problem births has largely been overtaken by Caesarean section. Vacuum extraction is the other form of assisted delivery. This is a gentler method, favored in Europe, when the cervix need not be fully dilated. Most medical authorities agree, however, that premature babies should be delivered by forceps so that their heads are not compressed in the birth canal.

Why is it done?
A forceps delivery can be done in the following situations:
- Fetal distress
- Maternal distress
- Epidural anesthetic prevents you pushing the baby out yourself
- The umbilical cord is wrapped around your baby's neck
  Less usual presentation, for example if the baby's face is towards your front or when the face and not the crown is the presenting part
  Very long second stage of labor
- Premature birth

How is it done?
Your legs will be put in stirrups and local anesthetic injected into the perineum, unless you have had an epidural anesthetic when the area will be numb anyway.

You will be given an episiotomy

HAVING A FORCEPS DELIVERY

The two wide, blunt blades are shaped so that they cannot press too far in on the baby's head. They are used to protect the head in a breech presentation or in premature labor, or they can be used to turn the baby's head to a more favorable delivery position.

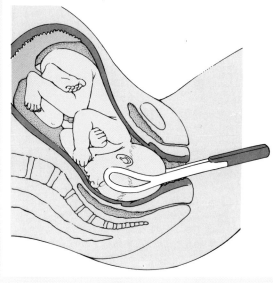

Depending on the use, different shapes of forceps are employed. These pictured here are used simply for lifting the baby's head out of the birth canal. For rotating the head, curved Kiellands forceps are used.

to allow room for the forceps. The two blades are then inserted into your vagina, one at a time. The doctor will have already determined where your baby's head lies and will fit the forceps around either side. The two blades are then clamped together outside your vagina. By pulling for 30–40 seconds at a time, your baby will gradually be brought down to the perineum.

You should feel no pain. When the head is delivered, the forceps will be removed and the delivery completed as normal.

The type of the forceps will depend on how far up your birth canal the baby's head lies. You may have a pudendal nerve block which is an injection to anesthetize your vaginal wall.

Are there any complications?
There are few problems with a forceps delivery, though you will be rather sore for a day or two. Your

baby will have slight markings on the head where the forceps have been. If you prefer to have your baby as naturally as possible, you should be explicit about this during your prenatal visits. A forceps delivery is, however, more likely if you opt for a high-tech birth in a large hospital with all the latest equipment where the administration of drugs and anesthesia can interfere with your own efforts to push the baby out.

SEE ALSO:

CAESAREAN SECTION
EPIDURAL ANESTHETIC
EPISIOTOMY
INDUCTION
LABOR
VACUUM EXTRACTION

GALACTORRHEA

This condition literally translated means too much milk, and relates specifically to the production of milk by a woman who is not pregnant or lactating. The condition occurs very rarely in men, too. The discharge from the nipple may not look like milk; it is simply a watery discharge of white, clear or greenish color which appears for no apparent reason.

Lactation is the result of secretion by the pituitary gland of the hormone prolactin, and excessive secretion of this hormone is usually the reason for galactorrhea. The pituitary gland may have a small tumor growing on it, or some medications such as certain tranquilizers or types of oral contraceptive could be disrupting the normal secretion of hormones. In about 50% of cases, no cause for the galactorrhea can be found.

The major problem with galactorrhea is if it is associated with amenorrhea; in this case, the hormonal balance will need to be corrected if you want to conceive. Very rarely, galactorrhea is a symptom of hormonal imbalance which has nothing to do with the sex hormones, such as Cushing's disease.

· S y m p t o m s ·

▲ Secretion of a watery, white or greenish discharge from both nipples

---

Should I see the doctor?
Consult your doctor if the secretions persist for more than a couple of weeks, if your periods have ceased, or if the secretion is brownish.

What will the doctor do?
Your doctor will examine you and take a detailed account of your gynecological history. If after specialist investigation, a tumor is found on your pituitary gland, drugs or an operation will correct the hormonal imbalance. Bromocriptine, which suppresses prolactin production, is the drug given to dry up the milk.

Treatment for any amenorrhea will be given to regulate periods if you wish to conceive.

What can I do?
Try not to stimulate milk production by handling your breast too much.

SEE ALSO:

AMENORRHEA
BREASTFEEDING PROBLEMS
INFERTILITY

GALLBLADDER DISEASE

This is a group of diseases that includes indigestion, gallstones and cholecystitis. The gallbladder is a pear-shaped sac about 80mm long which lies within the liver and stores bile. The presence of fat in the stomach stimulates the gallbladder to produce bile and pump it into the intestine to help digest the fat. Fat cannot properly be digested without bile. If the gallbladder contains stones or is distended or inflamed, then the formation of bile and the action of emptying the gallbladder causes discomfort and even severe pain.

Women are far more likely than men to have gallstones. They occur in 20% of post mortems on women (8% on men), though they may be symptomless in life. They are very rare in young people and increase with age. Women with many children are more often affected than women with none. Certain groups, including American Indian women, for unknown reasons, are extremely susceptible.

What causes gallstones?

Nobody is quite sure how gallstones form but usually they're due to the solidification of cholesterol from the bile fluid. There is, however, no direct connection between diet and the formation of gallstones so this doesn't mean they can be prevented by a diet low in cholesterol.

Early gallbladder disease is nearly always associated with indigestion. It may then progress to gallstones. If the gallstones are trapped at the entrance to the bile duct, the stagnating bile in the gallbladder can cause inflammation and swelling – this is known as cholecystitis. The severe pain experienced with cholecystitis, known as biliary colic, when a stone becomes caught in the bile duct that leads from the gallbladder into the intestine, resembles a heart attack and is a medical emergency. The pain is usually felt under the

margin of the right rib, near to where the liver is situated. It can be more central and may even grip the general chest area as though in a vise.

Should I see the doctor?

If you have troublesome indigestion, and you notice it occurs after a fatty meal or it is becoming more severe, see your doctor. If you have an attack of severe pain on the right side and when you press under your rib, the area is very tender, see your doctor immediately and if the attack is very severe with fever and vomiting, call an ambulance.

What will the doctor do?

Your doctor will question you about your diet and when the indigestion occurs. If, after examination, your symptoms aren't those of a more serious disorder, your doctor will advise you to avoid fatty foods, such as butter, cheese and cream. Attacks of gallbladder pain without fever require very little treatment other than the avoidance of fatty foods, and in most cases loss of some weight. Your doctor will warn you of the danger of jaundice developing and describe the symptoms in case you should notice them occurring.

· Symptoms ·

▲ Indigestion – this may go unnoticed if you are normally prone to heartburn or flatulence after a meal. The symptoms may be belching, a bad taste in your mouth, excessive wind or an uncomfortable feeling in the abdomen. If the indigestion becomes worse and follows a meal high in fat, this could indicate gallbladder problems

▲ Pain in degrees of severity just under the right rib, sometimes radiating to the left or around the body, with a fever and vomiting

▲ Jaundice with symptoms of yellowing skin and the whites of the eyes – chronic gallbladder disease may lead to blockage of the bile duct, thus damming up bile which spills over into the blood causing the jaundice

▲ Fever

stones trapped at entrance to bile duct

stone trapped in bile duct

gallbladder

duodenum

GALLBLADDER DISEASE

If you have cholecystitis, you will be given something to kill the pain, though attacks of this kind usually pass off suddenly. You may be admitted to hospital for ultrasound scans or an X-ray to confirm the diagnosis. You may be treated with antibiotics to overcome any infection of the gallbladder, advised to eat a bland, fatfree diet and take bedrest. Depending on your symptoms, especially if there are episodes of jaundice, and the acuteness of the attacks, you may be advised to have your gallbladder surgically removed. This operation is called a cholecystectomy.

What does a cholecystectomy involve?

For a thin person this is a simple operation. The gallbladder is removed under general anesthetic. The incision is usually on the diagonal on the right side. During the operation, the surgeon will check that no stones have passed into the bile duct. Post-operative management sometimes involves the setting up of an epidural block to numb the abdominal area for 48 hours. There will also be an intravenous drip to provide fluids and nutrients, a catheter if you have lost the sensation in your bladder because of the epidural and a drain to get rid of bile.

Often cholecystectomy patients are overweight and this can lead to a greater risk of post-operative infection, so your doctor may advise you to take off weight before the operation.

Recovery after the operation is usually straightforward and the cure permanent. It appears that we don't need our gallbladders.

What can I do?

If you have gallstones, eat sensibly and avoid the fatty, rich foods that bring on the attacks of biliary colic. You could try proprietary brands of antacid to combat the indigestion. If you have an attack of biliary colic, your doctor will probably have given you painkillers in case of an attack. Take one immediately and rest in bed. If the pain hasn't subsided in two hours, call your doctor.

SEE ALSO

DIGESTIVE PROBLEMS
EPIDURAL ANESTHETIC
OBESITY
ULTRASOUND

GENETIC COUNSELING

This is a procedure for couples who have had an abnormal child or who wish to have children but who have a history of a disease that tends to run in families. Any familial conditions such as sickle cell disease or spina bifida, for example, may be inherited genetically. Other conditions which can be inherited include cleft lip and palate, congenital heart disease, physical deformities such as extra fingers or toes or fusion of fingers and toes. The genetic counselor will attempt to predict the chances of the trait affecting your children. This will depend on the disorder and the frequency with which it has occurred in your families.

A large number of diseases have a genetic cause when the inherited genetic material, the genes, carry some defect or fault. This gene is normally recessive and so can't be detected in the carrier – that is one of the parents – so the risks have to be summed up by means of a careful look at family history. If you have already conceived, there are tests to find out if any abnormality has been passed on to your child.

Why is it done?
It is wise to seek genetic counseling before you become pregnant. There is a lot of information for you to absorb and it can be quite an emotional shock to realize that you and your partner may pass on a disease to your children. For most people it is difficult to come to terms with this. You also need to realize that if a test on your unborn baby is positive, you will have to make the agonizing decision whether or not to terminate your pregnancy. If this is not an option for you, then the counselor can help by setting out the possible effects, physically and emotionally, of living with an abnormal child in the family.

Genetic counseling is also given to couples who have had an abnormal child to help them under-stand how it happened and how to learn to cope with the child's disabilities.

How is it done?
Genetic counselors are usually either a pediatrician, your family doctor, or a trained geneticist. Their job is to help you understand and make an educated decision for yourselves. As a result of information about your family history, sometimes gained from post-mortem certificates, the counselor will tell you about the disease or condition you may be, or are, carrying which might be conveyed to your child.

You will be told how the condition is transmitted from one generation to another, what the chances are that your children will be affected with it and how serious an impediment to healthy life it will be for your unborn child.

The aim is to give you and your partner all the information you require to make up your minds about whether you want to risk having children, and if you do, what the chances are of them inheriting the unwanted disease.

As part of the genetic counseling, you will be told about the various tests which can determine if your baby is affected while still in utero. Not all the tests are done at the same time and certain tests cannot be done very early in your pregnancy. Some tests can't be done until you are at least 14–16 weeks pregnant before they give answers that can be relied upon. All this will be explained to you whether you are already pregnant or are seeking advice first.

Who should seek counseling?
All couples should seek to make sure they are in good health before conceiving. All of us take a risk, albeit a small one, when we decide to have a child. It is important to understand the risks and so if there is any family history of a disease or condition, you should seek genetic counseling.

Any woman who is over 35, or who has already had a child with a birth defect, or a woman on continuous medication, for example for epilepsy, or women who have had recurrent miscarriages should seek genetic counseling. Your family doctor will be able to put you in touch with a genetic counselor. The first line of action therefore is to go to your own doctor.

What are the most common tests?
If you already have an affected child, the child will be examined and have a chromosome analysis done.

Chromosome counts of the parents may give some idea as to what risk you run of having an abnormal child. This is a simple, painless procedure in which cells are scraped from inside your mouth and investigated under a microscope. Your count will be normal but it may show up an abnormal chromosome.

Other analysis of the parents' chromosomes, known as genetic probes, are becoming more widely available. Although the actual defective genes can't be identified, DNA markers have been identified, and these will be looked for on the parents' chromosomes. They are the pieces of genetic material which are known to be close to the defective gene on a chromosome.

If you are already pregnant, cells from the fetus can be taken during amniocentesis or a chorion biopsy. These are cultured and just before they divide, they are fixed with a special chemical and photographed. This shows the chromosomes in their pairs, numbered and sorted out. This is known as a karyotype (see over). Each cell in the body contains 46 chromosomes in 23 pairs. If, for example, the baby has Down's syndrome, there will be three number 21 chromosomes, making 47 in all.

GENETIC COUNSELING

CHROMOSOME ANALYSIS

Amniocentesis, chorion biopsy and certain blood tests are all able to provide fetal cells. By studying the chromosomes in such cells, certain abnormalities can be deduced and informed decisions on the continuation or termination of a particular pregnancy made.

Karyotype
The individual chromosomes are cut out from the photographic print and arranged into their correct pairs.

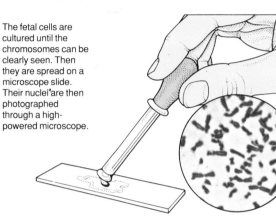

The fetal cells are cultured until the chromosomes can be clearly seen. Then they are spread on a microscope slide. Their nuclei are then photographed through a high-powered microscope.

Down's syndrome
The grouping reveals any abnormalities. For instance, an extra chromosome in pair 21 would indicate this genetic disorder.

Certain genetic disorders mainly affect male children but are usually carried by the female. Hemophilia and Duchenne muscular dystrophy are two such disorders.

Amniocentesis and chorion biopsy will show the sex of the child and a decision to terminate can be taken if the fetus is a boy. There will be a 50% chance of a boy inheriting the disease and a 50% chance of a girl being a carrier. Ultrasonic scans can pick up certain visible abnormalities such as brain or kidney conditions. Maternal blood testing such as alpha fetoprotein screening can detect a neural tube defect like spina bifida.

Rhesus incompatibility can be anticipated if the mother's blood group is Rh negative and the father's Rh positive. Amniocentesis will then determine if bilirubin levels are high and whether the baby needs an intrauterine transfusion.

A more invasive test that may be used if hereditary disease is possible is fetoscopy when a fiberoptic tube is inserted into the uterus to view the fetus directly. This will show any physical abnormalities and is a means of taking blood directly from the fetus to check for disorders such as thalassemia.

Many genetic disorders are apparent at birth and are therefore also congenital. On the sixth day after birth all babies have their heels pricked and a drop of blood taken for testing. This is called the Guthrie test. This checks for a serious digestive disorder, which is carried by the mother, called phenylketonuria (PKU). An excess of a certain enzyme in the body can lead to damage of the nervous system. Detected early enough, this disorder can be treated with diet during the child's early years.

SEE ALSO:
AMNIOCENTESIS
ANEMIA
CHORION BIOPSY
CHROMOSOMAL PROBLEMS
DOWN'S SYNDROME
FETOSCOPY
RHESUS INCOMPATIBILITY
TERMINATION OF
   PREGNANCY
ULTRASOUND

GENITAL HERPES

This is a common viral disease transmitted during sexual intercourse when the virus is active in the surface layers of the skin around the genital region. Millions of people are infected with the virus but probably only a quarter of those infected experience symptoms. In recent years it has increased alarmingly among women.

The disease is caused by the herpes virus. Another type of the same virus causes cold sores around the mouth and face but this is herpes simplex I; herpes simplex II causes the genital infection, although some doctors consider the distinction between the two to be less clear than previously thought.

The virus is transmitted through exposed raw areas of skin and is more common in women because their genital areas are warmer and moister than the males. The disease can also be spread by contact with other parts of your body, especially to the fingers and eyes. Herpes is highly contagious; there is a 90% chance of catching it if either partner has an active blister. However, new research indicates that the virus can also be transmitted by people who don't have symptoms.

Today, it is considered incurable; once in the body the virus stays there although treatment can help clear the symptoms or suppress active bouts. This waxing and waning course can cause much psychological misery as well as physical pain. In addition to severe physical problems, a sufferer is often depressed and anxious about her loss of control over her body and whether she has transmitted the disease to another.

The symptoms appear between three and twenty days after sexual contact with an infected partner.

Should I see the doctor?

See your doctor immediately if you feel numb and sensitive in the genital area or if you have had

---

· S y m p t o m s ·

▲ The skin on the vulva feels sensitive to the touch, ticklish, even numb – the infection can spread to the anus and even to the upper thighs

▲ Blisters appear within a few hours; enlarge, burst and become painful ulcers within two or three days

▲ Pain on urination

▲ The ulcers form scabs and take 14–21 days to disappear

▲ There may be a raised temperature and swollen glands in the groin

---

sexual relations with anyone with the herpes virus.

What will the doctor do?

Your doctor will probably diagnose genital herpes by examining a sore and asking you about your symptoms. A sample of the blister may be taken for analysis. A Pap smear or blood tests may also be performed.

What is the treatment?

There is no cure for genital herpes but new hope has been given to herpes sufferers by the latest anti-viral agents. One of these, Zovirax, is very potent and often effective in limiting the blisters and shortening the attack if applied early enough. However, it is very expensive.

There are few anti-viral agents that can be guaranteed to treat any virus with success.

Location of herpes virus
Once in the body, the virus can retreat to nerve cells near the base of the spine. If the virus is reactivated, it can return to where it entered the body and cause a recurrence.

Unfortunately, none of these medications helps to prevent a recurrence of the virus (see below).

Other remedies include daily douches with providone iodine solution, or painting the blisters with gentian violet.

Your doctor may prescribe a painkilling cream or antibiotic to prevent infection.

Are there any self-help measures?

When ruptured blisters are causing extreme pain, there are a number of things you can try to get relief. A long soak in a tepid bath can help as can cold packs applied directly to the labia and vulva. Make certain the water comes from the tap; do not use ice cubes.

Can I prevent it recurring?

Not all people have recurrences; some have a few and for some it recurs regularly. Normally the initial attack is the most severe. Recurrences don't necessarily depend on having intercourse with an infected partner. Irritation of vaginal tissues from other causes is known to trigger attacks. It's important to clear up any vaginal discharge from a coexisting infection. During intercourse adequate lubrication can help protect you from too much friction. The use of a condom can protect your partner from excessive rubbing. Other causative factors include emotional stress, fever, cold, menstrual periods, and tight fitting clothes.

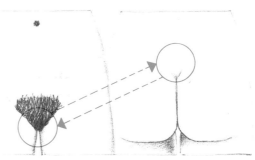

GENITAL HERPES

What can I do?

All you can hope for if you contract genital herpes is that the treatment prescribed for you means that the attack is shortened and the pain reduced. About 50% of herpes sufferers have another attack so you should be prepared to recognize the early warning symptoms and use the medication that works for you as soon as possible or go to the nearest clinic for sexually transmitted diseases. If you take note of the early symptoms before the blisters appear and treat them, the attack may even be avoided.

The way to avoid the virus is not to have sexual intercourse with someone who is infected and don't have sexual intercourse with anyone yourself if you have the disease and it is active. You should always avoid oral-genital sex if a cold sore is present. It is absolutely necessary to have a responsible attitude towards sex and to the disease.

You can do a lot to prevent genital herpes recurring. Get plenty of rest and eat a balanced diet with nutritional foodstuffs – fresh fruit and vegetables, wholefoods and plenty of liquids. If your life is stressful, manage your stress by learning relaxation exercises or taking up yoga.

You also need to come to terms with the disease itself. Many sufferers feel unclean, unwanted and stigmatized. You must try to overcome this feeling through counseling or joining a herpes sufferers group. If you feel in control of your body, you may find the attacks are less frequent.

Remember the virus can lie dormant for a number of years and can arise in even a steady, long-standing relationship. So try not to feel resentful or angry and let it threaten your relationship. You should seek sex therapy or counseling.

GENITAL HERPES AND PREGNANCY

If you or your partner have had an attack of genital herpes, this should be recorded in your notes. You will be checked for an active infection during the third trimester of your pregnancy. Your doctor will take a smear of the secretions in your vagina. If the virus is present, you will need to be delivered by Caesarean section because the baby may contract the virus during the birth and this can cause severe damage such as blindness and brain damage.

What are the long-term effects?

There is a greater risk of cervical cancer occurring in women who have had herpes infections. It's extremely important, therefore, that you continue to have regular Pap smears.

SEE ALSO:

CAESAREAN SECTION
CERVICAL CANCER
COLD SORES
DEPRESSION
GENITAL PROBLEMS
SEX THERAPY
SEXUALLY TRANSMITTED
  DISEASES

GENITAL PROBLEMS

Problems that occur around the genital area can usually be traced to the vagina or to a skin irritation. The lining to the vagina is glandular and the glands secrete mucus which keeps the vagina soft and well lubricated. At the menopause when the level of female hormones gradually diminishes, several changes occur in the vagina – somewhat less mucus is secreted so it may become dry, sore, even cracked. This results in tenderness and itching and *vaginitis* can be a problem. Any unexplained irritation is known as *pruritis vulvae*.

Because of the proximity of the anus, there is always the possibility of cross-infection from the feces, the most common being *yeast infection*. If yeast infection takes hold in the vagina, and is re-infected from the anus, a red, scaly and itchy rash may spread onto the inner sides of the thighs. In undiagnosed *diabetes mellitus*, where there is a lot of sugar in the urine there may be a rash on the thighs, the vulva and lower abdomen which exactly mimics that of yeast infection.

Genital warts are caused by the same virus as *warts* on the hands and fingers. They are associated with a high incidence of *cervical cancer*. *Genital herpes* is not as yet curable, but newer methods of treatment can reduce the number of attacks.

Bartholin's cysts
There are two glands, the Bartholin's glands, on either side of the vagina which secrete a mucus to keep the vulva moist, lubricated and healthy. Occasionally the exit from one of these glands may become blocked and a cyst forms with a large swelling. This condition can be treated simply under a local anesthetic when the cyst is drained. If the gland becomes infected, this will form a painful lump known as a Bartholin's abcess which may need lancing and draining, and a course of antibiotics.

Urethral caruncle
This is a small, bright-red polyp-like growth at the exit from the urethra found in post-menopausal women. It can be painful when touched or during urination and can cause bleeding into the urine. It is treated painlessly with electrocautery.

GONORRHEA

This is the commonest venereal disease and it is caused by a bacterium *Neisseria gonorrhoeae*. It affects both men and women though in five out of six women affected, there are no symptoms which makes it more dangerous. The most serious aspect of the disease is the chronic form which sets up inflammation in the pelvis; if the ovaries and fallopian tubes are affected, they may become blocked, and the scarring may cause sterility.

The risk of contracting gonorrhea seems to be higher if you are using the contraceptive pill – the infection seems to spread more quickly. The most common way women suspect they may have the disease is if they notice the recognizable symptoms in their male partners.

· S y m p t o m s ·

▲ There may be a discharge from the urethra, but more often vaginal discharge with pain and burning when passing urine

▲ The entire perineum may be sore and inflammation of the rectum causes pain when passing a stool

▲ A sore throat if the bacterium has been passed there during oral sex.

▲ Back or abdominal pain and/or fever.

▲ Blindness can be a rare result of advanced gonorrhea as the infection can be passed by hand to the eyes.

▲ Babies born to infected mothers may be born with serious eye infections.

Should I see the doctor?
If you suspect that you have gonorrhea or you have had sexual intercourse with someone who has it, if your sexual partner has any discharge from his penis, or any sores around his genitals, or if you have any sore around your genital area that doesn't heal within a day or two, go immediately to your doctor or your nearest clinic specializing in sexually transmitted diseases and don't have any sexual contact with anyone until you are clear.

What will the doctor do?
Diagnosis of gonorrhea is difficult and relies on the correct swabs being taken. Samples of the secretions from your urethra, cervix, rectum and possibly throat will be taken for laboratory examination. There is no reliable blood test. Special clinics should give the best results so even if you have a negative test and you know or think you may have had intercourse with someone with gonorrhea, insist on more tests or treatment.

What is the treatment?
Penicillin is the mainstay of treatment and may be given in a slow-release injectable form which requires only the one injection, making treatment quick and convenient for you. If the organism is resistant, other courses of medication may be used. You should then have a full gynecological examination to make sure that the disease has not caused pelvic inflammatory disease and affected your internal organs. And you should obtain a repeat gonorrhea culture to ascertain that the infection is gone.

Because gonorrhea can mask the symptoms of other sexually transmitted diseases, you should be tested for syphilis, too.

What can I do?
If you discover you have gonorrhea, make sure you tell the doctor or clinic the names of your sexual contacts so that they can get treatment before they infect others. You and your partner(s) should limit all sexual activity until you have been treated.

If your treatment is taking some time and you have an IUD, you would be wise to have it removed. You can have a new one fitted when you are clear of infection.

Gonorrhea is most common in young people under 25 who have many sexual partners. If you fit into this category, you would be wise to have a check-up every six months or so. Using condoms will decrease the probability of you getting an infection or being reinfected.

What is the outlook?
Reinfection is common even after successful treatment. If symptoms persist or if you have a positive culture after treatment, make certain your partner seeks medical attention or confirmation of whether or not he is a carrier as he may be reinfecting you.

SEE ALSO:

PAINFUL URINATION
PELVIC INFLAMMATORY
  DISEASE
SEXUALLY TRANSMITTED
  DISEASES
SYPHILIS
VAGINAL DISCHARGE

GUM DISEASE

By the time a woman reaches adulthood, the majority of problems she may have with her teeth will not be due to cavities from eating sweets but will result from gum disease, most often as a result of plaque. Even if you brush your teeth regularly, you can still have dental problems because of gum disease.

What is plaque?

Plaque is a thin film, made up of bacteria and saliva, that forms over the teeth. If this sticky deposit isn't removed frequently, it is trapped in a hard scale known as calculus within which bacteria can flourish, leading to soft, soggy gums and erosion of the alveolar margins around the teeth. This calculus can only be removed by a dentist.

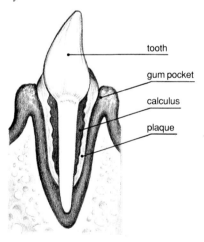

tooth

gum pocket

calculus

plaque

Results of gum disease
At an advanced stage of gum disease, the bacteria eats into the bone and tissue that supports the tooth and causes it to loosen in its socket. The loosened tooth will have to be taken out.

If plaque is allowed to build up at the gum margins, the gums will become irritated and swollen. The large amounts of sugary foods in our diets mean that the build-up of plaque is more likely unless dental hygiene is given a high priority.

During pregnancy, the gum margins are softened because of the influence of progesterone, predisposing

them to infection. This necessitates very careful tooth cleaning. There is no truth in the saying that you lose a tooth for every child, but pregnancy is a time when you are more susceptible to gum disease.

BLEEDING GUMS

Inflamed or swollen gums bleed easily – during tooth cleaning routines or while eating hard foods, for example. The commonest cause of bleeding gums is plaque. Treatment is therefore aimed mainly at keeping plaque at bay with frequent tooth-brushing and the use of dental floss. Regular visits to the oral hygienist for cleaning twice a year are also essential.

Your dentist may take a bacterial swab to check for infection and will give you instruction on the correct way to brush your teeth.

MOUTH ULCERS

Aphthous mouth ulcers are commonly seen on the tongue, cheeks and gums. They may be linked with psychological stress. They start out as a sore patch on the inside of the mouth, enlarging to form a painful yellow crater which slowly heals. The whole process may take 10 – 14 days and no proprietary medicines will speed things up. An injury caused by a jagged tooth or some other sharp object can also produce an ulcer if it becomes infected – and it generally

does – since the mouth is such a bacteriologically dirty place. If you get crops of ulcers, consult a doctor and avoid acid foods until your mouth is healed.

ABSCESSED TOOTH

The root of a molar can be infected if chronic tooth decay penetrates the living pulp at the center of the tooth. Infection travels along the hollow root to its tip where it is halted by the jaw bone. The condition is acutely painful because the collecting pus cannot expand into the rigid bone. Instead, it normally spreads under the gum giving rise to a soft, exquisitely painful swelling.

Treatment is in two stages: first the pus is released, either by puncturing the gum or by opening up the tooth; then the tooth is treated and filled. Despite the agony, there is no need to have the tooth removed; with modern dentistry a completely dead tooth can serve you well for 30 years.

GINGIVITIS

Sore, red, swollen, inflamed gums which bleed easily on brushing, and even if touched, indicate gingivitis. The condition needs specific treatment from a dentist or doctor because your gums are infected; proprietary mouth washes are not usually effective. Plaque is nearly always the underlying cause.

GUM DISEASE

If the condition becomes chronic, it is very difficult to eradicate. Chronic infection of the gums is known as pyorrhea and this puts the teeth in jeopardy. Treatment consists of antibiotics. In severe cases, gingivectomy (cutting away the inflamed gum margin) is sometimes the only way to rid the mouth of pockets of infection. After gingivectomy the use of dental floss or dental sticks to harden the gum margin is important.

If the gums become secondarily infected, the extreme condition could be trench mouth when small abcesses form around the gum margins with pockets of pus. This condition is so named because it was prevalent in the trenches in the First and Second World Wars, largely because of the habit of sharing drinking utensils which quickly became contaminated and spread the infection from one drinker to another. If the condition is left untreated, the teeth may eventually become loose in the gums and bone, and have to be extracted.

The treatment for trench mouth depends on antibiotics and regular washing of the mouth with an astringent mouth wash. Not all infections heal with this treatment and it may be necessary to perform gingivectomy to eradicate the infection completely .

The health of the gums should be maintained with careful and regular toothbrushing, if possible after every meal but certainly late at night and first thing in the morning. A waterpick used after each meal to get rid of food particles from between the teeth may be useful.

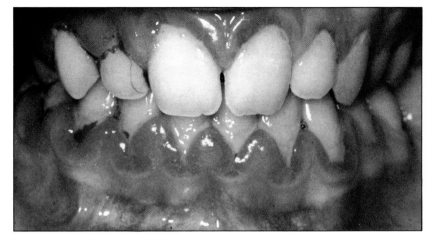

Swelling of the gum margins can be clearly seen as they appear to ride up the teeth. The pockets of bacteria make the gums soft and they bleed easily.

Disclosing tablets are available over the counter. They contain a dye which stains plaque. If you chew one of these tablets after toothbrushing and spit out the residue, you will be able to see from your teeth whether your toothbrushing technique is adequate to remove all the plaque from the surface of your teeth. Any stains left can be removed with a further brushing and dental floss.

EFFECTS OF DRUGS ON GUMS

In susceptible people, anti-convulsive drugs such as Dilantin may cause swelling of the alveolar margins of the gums. This causes the edges of the gums to grow up the teeth, and become thick, puffy and red. If the drug is stopped, the gums normally recede. If lead is ingested, this shows as a grayish-blue line along the edge of the gum margins. This is a diagnostic sign of lead poisoning, which is usually seen only in those who are exposed to high concentrations.

SEE ALSO:

COSMETIC DENTISTRY
DENTAL PROBLEMS
MOUTH PROBLEMS
PREGNANCY PROBLEMS

HAIR LOSS

Hair loss or alopecia may consist of only a tiny patch on the scalp or the hair over the entire body may be shed (alopecia universalis).

For reasons unknown, certain parts of the scalp lose hair more readily than others giving rise to the standard type of male baldness which, though usually found in men, can be found in women – especially after menopause. Thinning of the hair at the crown and the frontal area is common after menopause but never progresses to complete baldness.

What is it caused by?

Alopecia has many causes. Ionizing radiation, such as is found in X-rays, may produce permanent baldness even after a single dose. Chemical agents, like perms, may cause complete destruction of hair follicles and baldness can occur with severe shingles, ringworm and some scarring skin diseases.

General thinning of the hair is common after pregnancy. The pregnancy hormones throw most of the scalp hair into a growing phase. Under normal circumstances, hairs are at different stages of resting and growing phases and therefore hair loss is gradual and imperceptible. The dramatic hair loss associated with pregnancy is because great numbers of hairs come out of the resting phase at the same time and are lost simultaneously. This kind of hair loss may go on for anything up to eighteen months to two years. Though very frightening when it occurs, this is no cause for alarm because it is self-limiting and always recovers – though it may take a long time to do so.

Chronic scratching of the scalp, particularly at the back near the nape of the neck, is quite common in women and can give rise to hair loss. However, this is rarely complete and always recovers if you stop scratching.

Hair pulling, or trichotillomania, can occasionally be bad enough to cause bald patches but it can always be diagnosed because hair loss is never complete and there are quite often broken hairs of different lengths present in the bald patches. Like chronic scratching, trichotillomania nearly always has a psychological cause.

Certain drugs cause hair loss, the commonest being anti-cancer ones. But as treatment is warranted in malignant disease, therapy cannot be discontinued and hair loss must be suffered.

Should I see the doctor?

See your doctor right away if you think you have ringworm as this is infectious and may spread to the rest of your family. If you are otherwise unsure about the hair loss, see your doctor for a diagnosis.

What will the doctor do?

There have been a great many methods of treatment for alopecia but there is no proof that any of them has a significant effect, with the exception of steroid therapy.

Steroids, particularly triamcinolone, may be effective in re-growing hair. As the side effects of triamcinolone are considerable, it should never be given for long periods by mouth. In special hair clinics, this steroid treatment can be given by injection into the scalp itself to help stimulate hair growth, but results are unpredictable.

Other causes of alopecia, such as

ALOPECIA AREATA

This is the commonest form of hair loss and quite often there is a family history. The onset is sudden with complete loss of hair in round or oval patches. There may be only two or three of these or the whole scalp may be affected. Sometimes hair of the eyelashes, eyebrows, the armpits and the pubic area may be lost at the same time.

No one knows the cause, and there are no signs of inflammation or damage to the scalp. The course of the disease is capricious and unpredictable – new patches appearing while hair is returning to older ones. In about two-thirds of all these areas there is re-growth of hair and return to normality. In about 20% there may be no re-growth at all. Quite often finger nails may become pitted and ridged; the severity of nail changes being parallel to that of the alopecia.

ringworm, should be treated promptly by a dermatologist.

What can I do?

▲ Try not to worry – anxiety can make alopecia worse. Very often it is worth considering wearing a wig so that the psychological effect of the hair loss doesn't take too great a toll.
▲ Be very gentle with combing and brushing your hair.
▲ Be careful washing your hair and comb very carefully after washing as the scalp is soft and hair can be pulled out.
▲ Always use a conditioner after hair washing to prevent tangling.

SEE ALSO:

NAIL PROBLEMS
PREGNANCY PROBLEMS
RADIATION THERAPY

HAIRINESS

The commonest form of excess hair or hirsuteness of women is not a disease but a normal variation. A few dark and slightly coarse hairs can be a great source of distress yet it is commonly seen among Latins and people from Eastern Mediterranean countries as a racial characteristic. This trait is often inherited through families and women are nearly always perfectly healthy with no hormonal imbalance. Some races, such as the Chinese, have very little body hair.

Hirsuteness, nonetheless, can give rise at the very least to disquiet and in severe cases to psychological trauma in women who have the ill-luck to live in a society which finds hairiness in women offensive.

Hirsuteness due to endocrine abnormality, though often discussed and quoted, is rare. So rare in fact that unless accompanied by other signs of virilism, such as an enlarged clitoris, a deep voice and amenhor-rea, investigations are largely wasteful.

During pregnancy or menopause, the drop in estrogen levels may cause an increase in hair growth. Many pregnant women notice, for example, that their hair seems thick and healthy. This is due to the high levels of progesterone, which stimulate the sebaceous glands on the scalp (also sometimes causing acne). Women with dark skins may find that their body and facial hair darkens. In some cases this does not return to its former color.

Should I see the doctor?
For increased hairiness during pregnancy and at the menopause, the best treatment is no treatment. This is normal as is the appearance of hair at puberty.

The most important clue regarding hormonal status is your menstrual history. If this is completely normal, the possibility of an hormonal imbal-ance or a virilizing syndrome is completely ruled out. Only if your menstrual history is abnormal

should you see your doctor for referral to an endocrinological clinic. Virilizing syndromes are extremely rare; they nearly always involve chromosomal abnormalities and endocrine dysfunction.

If the extent of your hairiness worries you, then see your doctor or go to a clinic that specializes in removing unwanted body hair.

What will the doctor do?
Your doctor will probably take a blood sample to test for levels of the male hormone testosterone. If they are high, you may be prescribed a drug to reduce the secretion of the hormone by the hair follicles, or a contraceptive pill, if this is suitable for you, because estrogen in the pill balances the male hormone.

Even if a precise diagnosis is reached, treatment of hirsuteness may never be completely successful, even with hormone treatment. There-fore your doctor may advise you to seek cosmetic methods.

If your periods are infrequent, your doctor may refer you to a gyne-cologist in case this is a symptom of polycystic ovaries or a tumor on your ovaries.

What can I do?
You can either use the cosmetic aids yourself or attend a special clinic. If the hairs are few in numbers, plucking gives temporary relief and is not harmful unless performed over-zealously.

Shaving is obviously the safest temporary method but is unsatis-factory for most women. The fallacy

that shaving increases the growth and coarseness of hairs will not die but it has no basis in fact.

When hirsuteness is mild and the hairs are not too coarse, bleaching with a peroxide solution provides some concealment.

Modern depilatories are effective and do not cause irritation. They rely on strong agents.

Hot and warm waxing can remove hair from deep in the skin and one treatment should last six weeks. Even hair from the upper lip can be suc-cessfully removed.

Electrolysis is the only method that will remove hair permanently. A galvanic current is used and if the hairs are not too numerous or close together only a few treatments may be necessary. If the hairs are numer-ous and closely packed together, as is sometimes the case on the upper lip and on the chin, many painful sessions may be required and tiny pitted scars remain. This treatment should only be carried out by a trained technician.

SEE ALSO:

AMENORRHEA
CHROMOSOMAL PROBLEMS
MENOPAUSAL PROBLEMS
PREGNANCY PROBLEMS
OVARIAN PROBLEMS
SEX DIFFERENTIATION

HEADACHES

Headaches are an occurrence in all our lives, and are usually the result of tension or lifestyle. They are brought on by sitting in a stuffy room, skipping meals, drinking too much alcohol or going out in the hot sun without a hat. Take the recommended dose of a painkiller, lie down in a darkened room with a cool compress on your head and rest until the headache goes. If a headache is severe and longlasting or recurs, this is a symptom you should not accept as normal.

If you are unable to make a diagnosis from this information, or if you cannot relieve the headache with the self-help measures outlined above, consult your doctor.

SITE AND NATURE OF PAIN	PROBABLE CAUSE
The headache is on one side, and it is preceded by flashing lights and/or nausea	This could be a migraine. See your doctor for a diagnosis and suitable medication as these headaches can interfere with your normal life.
You feel nauseous and you have a severe pain around your eye, and your vision is blurred	This could be acute glaucoma, particularly if you are over 40 (see *Eye problems*).
The headache starts at the back of your head and/or feels like a tight band around your head	This is probably a tension or vascular headache. These headaches are usually caused by poor posture, intense concentration or emotional stress resulting in neck muscle strain or tension in the blood vessels in your head (see *Anxiety*).
You have a fever and sore throat and aches and pains	This could be sinusitis, influenza or other common infectious illness of which a headache is often a symptom.
You have a stomach upset and have been vomiting frequently over a period	A headache is a common after effect.
Pain is felt in the cheeks, especially when you are exposed to cold winds	A decaying tooth can be the cause of these facial headaches. See your dentist.
You have regular headaches which increase in severity and are accompanied by nausea or vomiting	This may be a brain tumor. See your doctor immediately.
The pain in your face is severe and you may have a shooting pain, like a knife, which is hard to bear	This could be the result of a damaged nerve, when it is referred to as facial neuralgia. Consult your doctor.
You have been drinking alcohol	This is a common aftermath. Cut down on your alcohol intake and drink water at the same time to reduce the concentration of alcohol in your blood stream (see *Alcoholism*).
You have recently started medication for some other condition or have started the contraceptive pill	This could be a side effect. Discuss this with your doctor.
The headache is very severe and you can't tolerate bright light and your neck is stiff	This could be meningitis, inflammation in the brain. See your doctor immediately.

HEART DISEASE

There are many types of heart disease including defects present at birth as well as various infections. Here, however, I'm concerned specifically with coronary artery disease. While women are presently less at risk from coronary artery disease, its incidence is rising rapidly. Moreover, women who take the contraceptive pill after the age of 35, and all women who smoke or are overweight, are at greater risk.

Younger women are fortunate in that they are protected from greater risk of this disease by their hormones. Our female hormones protect us throughout our fertile lives until the menopause. After the menopause, when the ovaries become inactive, and there is no more monthly cycle with rising and falling levels of estrogen and progesterone, the frequency and risk of heart disease in women is equal to that of men. In general, too, women are more concerned about their diets – poor diet is a central cause of heart disease (see below).

What is coronary artery disease?

Coronary artery disease, or atherosclerosis, is a narrowing and hardening of the arteries anywhere in the body by deposits of fatty tissue known as plaques. (Arteriosclerosis is something different; it is the name given to the diseases that cause the arteries to become thick.) When it is the arteries leading to the heart that are affected, this can cause heart disease.

Postmortems show that athero-sclerosis is widespread; it has even been noted in children. Often there are no symptoms; in other cases there may be a heart attack or angina. These fatty deposits are almost certainly related to the amount of fat and cholesterol taken in the diet, and a lack of exercise which would expend the fat for energy. Not every fat causes atherosclerosis. The worst offenders are saturated fats – animal fats and some plant fats such as those found in nuts. On the other hand, polyunsaturated fats, found in corn oil and sunflower oil, do not encourage high levels of cholesterol in the blood.

What happens?

The commonest result of heart disease is coronary thrombosis or heart attack. This occurs when one of the already hardened and narrow coronary arteries is blocked by a blood clot, cutting off the blood supply to part of the heart. Angina is another common complaint; it is the name given to the pain felt when, because of atherosclerosis or high blood pressure, the heart has a reduced supply of oxygen. Angina sounds a warning of the possibility of more serious disease. If you are rushing about, the pain is felt when oxygen is most needed by the heart; when the angina sufferer slows down, the pain reduces. In women, obesity and heavy smoking cause damage to the coronary arteries because the heart pumps with more pressure than is necessary for the usual flow. The arterial walls become damaged as a result and fatty tissues appear on the damaged site.

· Symptoms ·

- ▲ May be none
- ▲ Pain in the chest, spreading down the left arm and sometimes into the jaw, usually felt on exertion – this is angina
- ▲ Severe crushing pain tightening and squeezing the chest in a grip and spreading down the arms – this is a heart attack
- ▲ Dizziness, sweating, nausea, difficulty breathing, fainting, chills
- ▲ Bluish skin color
- ▲ Pupils dilated
- ▲ Faint pulse

Should I see the doctor?

There is no doubt that you can inherit a tendency to heart disease. If close members of your family suffer from heart disease, or died prematurely of a heart attack, then you are a person at risk, particularly if you are over 35 and smoke. You should have regular check-ups and consult your doctor if you have any cardiac symptoms.

What will the doctor do?

If you do experience the symptoms of angina, your doctor may refer you for tests to find out the cause of the pain. Your blood pressure will be taken to exclude this as a cause. You may be given a blood cholesterol test to check for high levels in the blood. A chest X-ray helps the doctor to see the size of your heart – enlargement of the heart occurs with heart strain. An electrocardiogram (ECG) measures the efficiency of your heart function and an arteriogram involves a dye being pumped into your artery so that it can be seen on an X-ray. The catheter containing the dye is usually passed through from the groin under local anesthetic. On X-ray, the arteries can be seen as blocked or narrowed.

A quick check on the health of your circulatory system can be done by your doctor if he examines your eyes with an ophthalmoscope. If the vessels in your retina appear damaged, this is an indication of the condition of blood vessels elsewhere in your body.

What is the medical treatment?

Whether you have angina or have had a heart attack, medical treatment after diagnosis relies on supporting the heart with a variety of drugs and a regime of healthy diet and exercise. Drugs to combat angina brought on by effort can be placed under the tongue for quick relief. You may be able to anticipate the pain and use the drugs before you exert yourself. Other drugs help

Effect of hypertension
Abnormally high blood pressure can affect all the arteries in the body. Here, a normal retina with clearly healthy and intact retinal veins and arteries (right) is contrasted with a retina of a person suffering from hypertension (far right). The latter has areas of fluid – to the right of the optic disc in the center – which have oozed from the blood vessels.

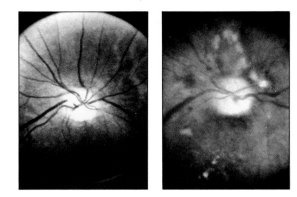

BALLOON ANGIOPLASTY

A modern technique for unblocking coronary arteries involves the use of a balloon catheter. This is inserted via a major artery in the thigh, and once it reaches the blockage, the balloon is inflated in order to clear the obstruction.

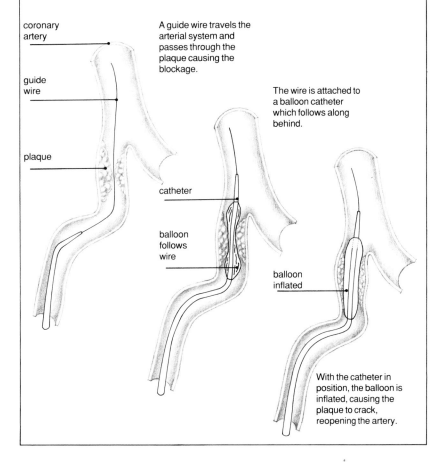

coronary artery

guide wire

plaque

A guide wire travels the arterial system and passes through the plaque causing the blockage.

The wire is attached to a balloon catheter which follows along behind.

catheter

balloon follows wire

balloon inflated

With the catheter in position, the balloon is inflated, causing the plaque to crack, reopening the artery.

HEART DISEASE

to keep the heart beating regularly and strongly by reducing the heart rate and thus the oxygen needed. These are known as beta blockers. Anti-diuretic drugs cause the body to lose water and this can relieve the strain on heart muscle by lowering blood volume.

If your problem is hypertension, your doctor will give you drugs to lower it, thereby lowering the risk of a heart attack.

What is the surgical treatment?
Surgery is used in suitable cases with good results. Cardiac artery bypass operations are done for patients who are found to have atherosclerosis. Less commonly the operation is performed in an emergency. This surgical procedure takes pieces of healthy vein from the leg. These are sewn into the coronary arteries and literally bypass the narrowed segments. This operation relieves the pain but does not cure the underlying cause of heart disease.

In balloon angioplasty, a fine catheter with an inflatable segment is carefully passed along a narrowed coronary artery, and then inflated to stretch the constriction. The results are excellent and many lives have been saved. Angioplasty is also being used to open up narrowed heart valves in elderly patients. Experimental work, using lasers, is also being carried out.

In a few, rare cases, heart transplant may be performed. You will be connected to a heart-lung machine which will take over the work of your heart and lungs, and your diseased heart will be removed. A donor heart will then be put into place, connected up to existing blood vessels. You will then be given immunosuppressant drugs to try to prevent rejection of the new heart by your body. Over 80 percent of patients survive the first critical year, followed by a death rate of around five percent a year after that.

PACEMAKERS
For patients who suffer from irregularities of the heartbeat due to a breakdown in their electrical conducting system there are pacemakers which pass electrodes to the heart muscle to keep it beating regularly. A pacemaker consists of a battery driven, electronic impulse which can be strapped to the body or, in a micro model, slipped underneath the skin in a simple operation done under local anesthetic. The impulse is conducted to the heart wall via a thin tube which is pushed through a vein. The only problem pacemakers present is that you can't pass through security screens.

What can I do?
We are all, to a certain extent, born with a blueprint which determines whether we will have a heart attack or not and when it will occur. But even if your blueprint predisposes you to a heart attack in your middle sixties, that is not a death knell. You can give up smoking now and eat the right food and exercise.

If you are still of childbearing age, to have a healthy heart in later life, you must plan fairly early in life. Pay attention to diet, make sure you don't become overweight, don't smoke and exercise as much as you possibly can. For women, the best exercise is taken upright – jogging, horseriding, tennis, skiing, and cycling. To prevent your children suffering from heart disease in later life, you need to start them on the right track when they are very young by providing them with a good diet and making sure they maintain healthy eating habits.

Some sufferers from heart disease say that their pain becomes worse when they are stressed, worried or anxious. Stress may be involved with heart disease, either as a direct effect on the coronary arteries by causing them to go into spasm, or by raising blood pressure – both lead to heart attacks. So try to manage the stress in your life and take as much stress out of your life as you can.

Cut down severely on fats, particularly animal fats. They are contained in egg yolks, shellfish, and creamy, dairy products. Blood fat levels do rise after a fatty meal. High blood fats and high blood cholesterol are certainly connected with the deposition of fat in the arteries. So although it isn't a guarantee, it seems wise to cut down on the amount of animal fats and cholesterol in your diet. Cholesterol is made by the body and the amount made depends on the foods we eat. Saturated fats encourage the body to make cholesterol and polyunsaturated fats discourage high levels. Cut back on the sodium in your diet too. Salt in the diet is believed to encourage high blood pressure.

If you are over 35 and still on the pill, have a check-up and ask your doctor's advice about an alternative form of birth control.

SEE ALSO:

HEMORRHOIDS

These are varicose veins of the rectum. Mostly they occur inside the anus, but occasionally, particularly if you strain to pass stools, or during childbirth, they prolapse outside the rectum and feel rather like a soft, spongy bunch of grapes.

How are they formed?
Healthy veins have a valve system to prevent blood falling back with the force of gravity. This helps to keep blood pumping around the body. If the valves become damaged or weak, the blood will be constantly forced back down the veins. This prevents the valves working and results in pooling of blood in the veins. The walls of the vein weaken and balloon out to produce venous swellings which are clearly visible as varicose veins on the legs. In the anus they mostly occur because of the pressure exerted during attempts to pass stools when constipated.

Once they develop, the thin membrane is easily ruptured by the passage of stools and often the only indication of the disorder is blood with the stools.

· S y m p t o m s ·

▲ Soreness, irritation and itching around the anus
▲ Clear mucus if the hemorrhoids have irritated the anal canal
▲ Small amount of red blood when you defecate
▲ Severe pain if the varicosity gets nipped in the anal muscles. Very severe pain if the varicosity becomes twisted outside the anus (strangulation of the hemorrhoid)

Should I see the doctor?
There is no medical treatment to improve hemorrhoids other than to stop exerting pressure when coughing or straining to defecate. If you have bleeding from the anus, you should see your doctor in case this is a symptom of a more serious disorder such as cancer of the colon.

THE EFFECT OF PREGNANCY AND CHILDBIRTH

The pressure of the uterus in late pregnancy may restrict the return of blood from the rectum, causing hemorrhoids. Straining during childbirth can cause the hemorrhoids to prolapse. If you suffer from hemorrhoids after childbirth, your doctor may prescribe a soothing cream and advise you to keep up the fiber content in your diet to ensure your stools are soft and easy to pass. The hemorrhoids usually get better after delivery. Cold ice packs reduce irritation and pain. Don't have very hot baths as these cause the hemorrhoids to worsen.

What will the doctor do?
Your doctor will examine you and advise you to improve your diet to make the passage of stools softer and easier. Any prolapsed hemorrhoids will be replaced manually. Your doctor may prescribe soothing creams or suppositories so the area is less painful while the constipation is improved with dietary measures. Injections can be given which cause the varicosities to wither and shrink.

What is the surgical treatment?
For a permanent cure in severe cases, surgical hemorrhoidectomy is performed under a general anesthetic. This involves stripping out the venous varicosities so that the rectum and anus return to normal. This in no way impairs the natural function of the rectum and anus. We have millions of veins to do the job of those removed.

What can I do?
The use of proprietary medicines does no good, so resist over-the-counter local anesthetics and suppositories. It is essential to keep your stools soft so eat a diet rich in vegetables, fruit and high-fiber cereals. Drink at least $1^1/2$ liters (3 pints) of liquid per day and take regular exercise.

Try not to strain when you defecate. Don't lift heavy weights or cough – you should give up smoking if this causes coughing.

SEE ALSO:

COLORECTAL CANCER
CONSTIPATION
VARICOSE VEINS

HIP REPLACEMENT

A hip replacement operation is when a damaged hip joint is surgically removed and replaced with an artificial hip joint. Women are more likely to have this operation because fractures of the neck of the femur are common in older women due to the effects of osteoporosis and osteoarthritis.

Why is it done?

Osteoarthritis, an exaggerated aging of the joints, tends to produce extra outgrowths of bone around joints which cause limitation of movement, stiffness and pain. These changes are speeded up in any joint which is strained and over-stressed such as through any type of trauma including twists, sprains or fractures. The hip joint, one of the main weightbearing joints, is constantly over stressed but particularly if the individual is overweight.

Osteoarthritis of the hip joint can make walking without a limp impossible and restrict movement so that the normal gait becomes a waddle. The pain of osteoarthritis of the hip can be excruciating, and hip replacement is done more often to bring pain relief than for any other reason. Without this operation, all that is possible is symptomatic relief with painkillers. Occasionally anti-inflammatory drugs are used but do not bring any special benefit because there is very little inflammation in an osteoarthritic joint as opposed to a joint affected by rheumatoid arthritis.

Nonetheless, by the time a patient gets to surgery, the ball and socket joint of the hip may be grossly deformed, even partly destroyed. The smooth ball at the upper end of the femur may be pitted, eroded and rough. The normally smooth arc of the hip bone, which forms the socket of this ball-and-socket joint, can be flattened and scarred with craters.

How is it done?

During the operation, the whole of the head of the femur is removed at the level of the neck and is replaced

ARTHROPLASTY

Hip replacement was the earliest and is still the most successful "spare parts" surgical procedure. The muscles and tendons that overlie the joint keep it stable. These are pushed to one side or cut during the operation and replaced and repaired afterwards.

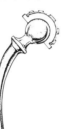

The artificial ball-and-socket joint is fixed in place to the femur and pelvic bones with a plastic cement.

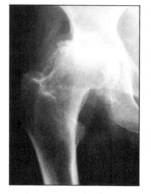

before the operation

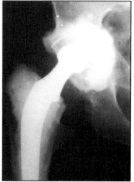

after the operation

by an artificial head of femur on a shaft which is driven into the hollow femur bone. Much engineering and technical research has gone into fashioning replacement hips, concentrating on the strength of the material, its non-allergic, non-irritating nature and its durability.

The present standard is exceptionally high; artificial joints can now be made to measure. Patients with unusually shaped bones can have artificial joints made to an individual fit now that doctors have teamed up with engineers using computer-aided design systems. X-rays of patients with small or unusually shaped joints can be sent to a designer who draws up a near perfect match from the X-ray directly onto a computer screen. An exact fit can be made by placing a steel ball from one of the standard sizes of implant in the plane of the X-ray so that the outline of the ball can be computerized along with the patient's joint. Using the dimensions of the standard model as a reference point, a custom-made implant can be fashioned for an accurate fit.

About 5–10% of patients in need of hip replacements have unusually shaped skeletons because of abnormal bone growth, injury or previously failed joint operations.

What are the risks?

Hip replacement is one of the most successful operations undertaken. The success rate is between 90 and 100%. Many patients feel that they are given a new lease of life, not only because they can return to near normal activity but also because of the relief from pain.

Very few of the operations go wrong, but even if they do the outlook is good. The femur is one of the strongest bones in the body and hip replacement can be repeated. With new techniques being developed, this is needed less and less often.

SEE ALSO:

ARTHRITIS
OBESITY
OSTEOARTHRITIS
OSTEOPOROSIS
RHEUMATOID ARTHRITIS

HORMONE REPLACEMENT THERAPY

Hormone replacement therapy, or HRT, also referred to as Estrogen Replacement Therapy (ERT), is a means of treating troublesome symptoms which arise during the menopause. A similar treatment is prescribed for women who have undergone a premature menopause as a result of surgical removal of the ovaries or following radiation treatment for ovarian cancer or premature ovarian failure for unknown reasons. Hormone replacement therapy does not, in fact, bring hormones back to their pre-menopausal levels; the smallest appropriate dosage is given.

Why is it prescribed?
A fall in estrogen and progesterone levels occurs naturally after the menopause when the menstrual cycle ceases. The sudden reduction of estrogen often causes distressing symptoms such as hot flashes, night sweats, and vaginitis which can lead to loss of libido. Either because of the lack of sleep or the negative feelings about the menopause, insomnia, depression and irritability may be other symptoms. Many doctors advocate the use of hormone supplements following menopause. They help to reduce the symptoms and also delay some of the long-term consequences of reduced estrogen levels in old age including osteoporosis, and atherosclerosis (fat deposits in the arteries).

Is it always necessary?
About 20% of women have no noticeable symptoms at all, and others require little treatment. However, if your symptoms are having a significant effect on your daily life and making you miserable, consult your doctor.

What will the doctor do?
Your doctor should talk to you in great detail to establish the extent of the symptoms and whether they are true menopausal symptoms and whether they are due to estrogen lack. You will also be examined externally and internally to reveal any changes in your vagina which can become dry and sore, making intercourse painful.

What is the treatment?
There are many different ways that your doctor may prescribe hormone therapy. The most common form is a course of estrogen and progesterone pills. These pills are prescribed in a three-stage cycle that is repeated each month: estrogen will normally be taken for 25 days of each month; for 10 to 14 days, progesterone will be taken along with the estrogen; a period of approximately five days is completely drug free after which the course begins again for the next month. There is no real need to coincide your treatment with the first of each month but this can make calculations easier.

Previously, doctors merely prescribed a course of estrogen (hence the name "Estrogen Replacement Therapy"), but now are much more likely to indicate an estrogen *and* progesterone course. Intake of estrogen alone has been linked to the build up of the uterine lining thus leading to possible uterine cancer. However, it has not been conclusively proved that adding progesterone is a completely satisfactory safeguard against this possibility. You should, of course, fully discuss the procedure and its potential risks with your physician.

How will it affect me?
The number of hot flashes can lessen dramatically within a week.

However, you will start to menstruate again during the days when you are not taking the tablets. Also, it may cause fluid retention, nausea and vomiting, breast tenderness, headache, dizziness, and depression although taking account of the relatively low doses of the medication, side effects are unlikely.

Once you start the regime, you will have routine six-monthly check ups of your blood pressure, your breasts and possibly an internal examination. A urine test and a Pap smear should be done every year. You may need menstrual extraction if you have a lot of breakthrough bleeding. In this way, the endometrial lining can be checked for other problems which may arise because of the therapy. Hormone therapy should never be given for prolonged periods without regular full medical checks and without breaks between courses. Signs that your dosage is too high include

WOMEN AT RISK
Hormone replacement therapy is not advised for women

With existing circulatory disease
Because estrogen is implicated in circulatory problems, there are some risk factors that your doctor will have to consider. You will probably not be prescribed any hormone therapy if you: suffer from high blood pressure, have a history of thrombosis, are diabetic, or suffer from chronic liver disease

With a cancerous condition
A history of breast, vaginal, cervical or endometrial cancer, particularly hormone-dependent cancers, are a non-indication

Overweight women
Especially those who cannot take weight off

Smokers
This automatically puts you into a higher risk group than women who don't

HORMONE REPLACEMENT THERAPY

breast tenderness, nausea and a feeling of bloatedness.

What is the alternative?

Some doctors prefer not to prescribe hormone therapy. Other treatments such as an estrogen cream for itching of the perineum, jelly to lubricate the vagina prior to intercourse or tranquilizers and sleeping pills for depression and insomnia may be sufficient. Placebos have also been found to be effective. Sometimes symptoms can be relieved by hormone therapy for a year or two and then you can take a break to see if you can tolerate the symptoms without treatment.

If you want to try hormone therapy and your own doctor won't supply it for you, ask to be referred to a gynecologist. The benefits of the treatment for you have to be weighed against the possible side effects.

What are the risks?

There has been a great deal of publicity about the risks of hormone therapy. There is still a lot of uncertainty and the safety of hormone therapy is not yet clear.

There is concern that uterine cancer increases with hormone therapy, particularly if estrogens are prescribed unopposed by progesterone. Care should be taken with breakthrough bleeding. Even though this is normal with hormone therapy, it can mask the symptoms of serious disorders such as uterine cancer and fibroids. Always alert your physician if the bleeding is heavy or if it lasts more than seven days.

There is no clear evidence that estrogen used in hormone therapy increases the risk of heart disease or circulatory problems. Your doctor would not prescribe the treatment if you were known to be at risk.

There is no evidence that breast cancer is more common. The risk increases in women over 50 anyway, and these women should perform

regular self-examination of their breasts and undergo yearly mammography.

There is an increased risk of gallbladder disease.

Is hormone therapy effective?

For the common symptoms of the menopause, this treatment is almost 90% effective. It is particularly recommended for women who have a premature menopause. Within two to three weeks of starting the therapy, most women find the sweats, flashes and vaginal dryness are relieved. As a direct result, libido tends to return and any depression and insomnia lifts. Another advantage is that hormone therapy is thought to arrest the natural bone softening that occurs in post-menopausal women (osteoporosis), although a calcium-rich diet combined with exercise throughout life has been shown to be important in preventing this, too. There is also some evidence to suggest that hormone therapy may protect women against developing heart disease.

However, the problems of the menopause and aging cannot be completely eradicated with hormonal treatment. The treatment only helps with the symptoms, it does not prevent the menopause from occurring. Some doctors use tranquilizers and counseling to steer their patients through the worst symptoms and help them to manage this time in their lives.

SEE ALSO:

CANCER
HEART DISEASE
MENOPAUSAL PROBLEMS
MENSTRUAL EXTRACTION
OSTEOPOROSIS
PAINFUL INTERCOURSE
UTERINE CANCER
VAGINITIS

HYPERTENSION

Doctors measure two types of blood pressure: the systolic and the diastolic. The systolic pressure is the head of pressure which results from the pumping action of the heart. The diastolic pressure is a "holding" pressure which is mainly dependent on the back pressure from the veins and keeps up the blood pressure between heart beats. Both are measured in millimeters of mercury.

When written down the systolic pressure is always put on top of the diastolic pressure, so, a reading of 120 over 80 (120/80) means that the systolic pressure is 120 millimeters of mercury (mmHg) and the diastolic pressure is 80 millimeters of mercury.

120/80 and any reading lower than that is considered normal although most doctors base their judgments upon each individual case. In most countries blood pressure is rarely considered to be too low; low blood pressure is considered healthy. If either reading is higher than that, however, then a degree of hypertension is present though no one would be concerned unless three consecutive resting readings were raised. A rise of 20 for the systolic and 10 for the diastolic blood pressure is abnormal.

The systolic blood pressure increases physiologically under certain circumstances, for example when you get excited, tense or emotional. If you do anything which raises your heartbeat, the systolic pressure will rise but such a high reading is not considered abnormal because it will come down to normal levels when activity ceases. Doctors only get worried if blood pressure stays up for long periods of time, hence the necessity to take three separate recordings of the blood pressure after you have been lying down for 15 minutes and after an interval of at least a week. High blood pressure can never be diagnosed on one single test unless the readings are extraordinarily high.

· **S y m p t o m s** ·

▲ Headaches
▲ Palpitations
▲ Shortness of breath
▲ Angina
▲ Swelling of the ankles

How is it lowered?

The diastolic pressure has the most significance. This is because a raised diastolic pressure produces damage to the heart and the blood vessels much more easily than does a high systolic pressure. In addition, once a diastolic pressure is increased it is much more difficult to bring down than a systolic pressure. For instance, simply cutting salt out of your diet and not adding it to cooking can bring down your systolic pressure by 10 millimeters of mercury; it has a somewhat lesser effect on the diastolic pressure. In a similar way, losing weight can bring down the blood pressure.

The reasons why doctors want to lower the blood pressure is that people with a high blood pressure run the risk of heart attacks, strokes and chronic disease of the arteries.

Should I see the doctor?

Left untreated, hypertension can be dangerous; it can continue to rise thereby presenting a hazard to your heart and circulatory system. If blood pressure is brought down, the long-term outlook is good if you risk a heart attack due to coronary thrombosis. This is particularly so for patients in middle age who have no previous history of heart disease. Many people with high blood pressure don't know they have it. Therefore see your doctor annually for a blood pressure reading. This is not painful and takes only a minute.

Make sure your blood pressure is monitored during pregnancy. High blood pressure in pregnancy can lead to complications such as toxemia.

Your doctor will advise on dietary measures if these are appropriate

and, depending on your symptoms, prescribe anti-hypertensive drugs. High blood pressure is a disorder that the medical profession can treat really efficiently. Anti-hypertensive drugs are at the forefront of medical research; their sophistication is much greater than almost any other class of drugs. We know how to find the exact dose for each individual so that the effectiveness is optimum and side effects are kept to a minimum.

Your doctor will assess your blood pressure at regular intervals. You may also be given a diuretic to remove fluid from your body thereby lessening the burden on the heart.

The kidneys are one of the first organs to be damaged by high blood pressure. Your doctor will therefore keep an eye on their function by testing your urine.

If your heart is affected you will be given cardiac drugs as appropriate for the heart condition.

What can I do?

Restricting salt in your diet and losing weight are two of the main ways by which it's possible to lower blood pressure.

◆ Cut salt from your diet and don't add salt to food.
◆ Check labels for sodium.
◆ Bring your weight down to the normal range and keep it down.
◆ Exercise as much as you can; this naturally brings the blood pressure down, although if you are over 35 you might consider checking on your fitness first.
◆ Reduce stress in your life by practicing relaxation therapy or yoga.
◆ Stop taking the contraceptive pill.

SEE ALSO:

FITNESS TESTING
FLUID RETENTION
HEART DISEASE
OBESITY
PRENATAL CARE
TOXEMIA OF PREGNANCY

HYPERTHYROIDISM

The thyroid is a gland in the lower neck. It manufactures the hormone thyroxine which controls our basal metabolic rate (BMR), the rate at which chemical reactions occur in our bodies. For no apparent reason, the whole gland or part of it (sometimes called a "hot" nodule) may become overactive and secrete too much thyroxine. In this case the BMR is raised with many accompanying symptoms. This condition is known as hyperthyroidism, thyrotoxicosis, toxic goiter or Grave's disease, depending on the cause of the problem.

Thyrotoxicosis is a severe state of hyperthyroidism; the symptoms are extreme and your heart may be affected. Quite often there are symptoms concerning your eyes.

· S y m p t o m s ·

Hyperthyroidism
- ▲ Person is very active, quick and mercurial
- ▲ Sweaty and/or trembling hands
- ▲ Intolerance of heat, need to wear light clothing all the time
- ▲ Increased appetite but weight loss
- ▲ Diarrhea
- ▲ Amenorrhea

Thyrotoxicosis
- ▲ Protruding eyes
- ▲ Swelling in the neck where the gland is enlarged – a goiter
- ▲ Atrial fibrillation (flutters of the heart)

Should I see the doctor?
Although these are fairly rare disorders, they are most common in women, so if you notice any combination of these symptoms, see your doctor for tests and a diagnosis.

What will the doctor do?
You will be given a blood test. Circulating levels of l-thyroxine, the active form of thyroid hormone, is a good indication of the gland's activity. High levels of l-thyroxine suggest an overactive gland and vice versa.

A radioactive iodine uptake test

HYPOTHYROIDISM

If the thyroid gland fails to produce sufficient thyroxine and the BMR is lowered, this can quite often result in a condition known as hypothyroidism.

The symptoms of hypothyroidism are the reverse of those for hyperthyroidism: lethargy and fatigue, dry, puffy skin, sensitivity to cold all the time, weight gain despite little appetite, constipation, heavy periods and loss of interest in sex.

Thyroid hormone deficiency can be treated with thyroid hormone supplements in the form of l-thyroxine tablets. Each individual is

will be performed. Iodine is an essential part of thyroxine; most of us get enough in our diets. Overactivity shows as a more rapid than normal uptake of iodine by the gland to manufacture the hormone thyroxine. The gland will be scanned for radioactivity to see whether or not a hot nodule is present. If the gland is underactive, iodine uptake is lower than normal.

Other thyroid function tests involving thyroid stimulating hormone (TSH) may be performed to assess the activity of the gland and as a basis for treatment.

Very high levels of thyroid hormone as in thyrotoxicosis may affect the heart causing flutters or palpitations. Cardiac function tests including an ECG may be performed.

What is the medical treatment?
If you have an overactive gland, you will be prescribed anti-thyroid drugs. Radiation therapy is occasionally used with a carefully measured dose of radioactive iodine. This therapy is most often given in the form of an isotope of iodine (I.131). Its action depends on uptake by the thyroid cells which are destroyed by the effect of radiation on the nucleus of the cell. The advantage of I.131 is that it can be given to out-patients and it

different and the dosage may have to be changed once or twice before a suitable dose is found. Tests of thyroid function check that dosage is adequate.

Another form of hypothyroidism, Hashimoto's disease, starts as an autoimmune disease when the thyroid gland becomes allergic to itself and produces antibodies which attack and damage the gland making it less able to secrete thyroxine. Hashimoto's disease may run in families. Quite often the early phase of Hashimoto's disease is hyperthyroidism.

causes no discomfort. The recurrence of hyperthyroidism with this form of treatment is rare. However, there may be a four to 12 week delay before the full effect is seen and overactivity is completely controlled.

Surgical treatment
A hot nodule on the gland can be removed surgically. Part of the thyroid gland itself may be removed surgically to treat hyperthyroidism.

SEE ALSO:

AMENORRHEA
AUTOIMMUNE DISEASES
FATIGUE
NUMBNESS AND TINGLING
PALPITATIONS
SEXUAL PROBLEMS

HYSTERECTOMY

This is a uniquely female operation involving major abdominal surgery for removal of a woman's most important reproductive organ, the uterus. A more radical form of the operation may include the removal of the fallopian tubes, cervix and the ovaries. If the ovaries are removed, you will go through a premature menopause and will need to take hormone supplements, probably until you reach the age of the natural menopause, around 50.

How common is it?
In the United States, 25% of all women over 50 have had simple or radical hysterectomies. Often the operation is performed for no good reason, such as the removal of small fibroids. In countries where surgery is more often used to treat gynecological disorders, the rate of hysterectomies is alarmingly high. Some doctors even advocate it once child-bearing is over to forestall the risk of cancer.

The decision to have a hysterectomy should never be taken lightly and it should only be performed when absolutely necessary.

Why is it done?
The operation, whether simple, or radical, will be advised for the following reasons:
◆ To remove cancer in the pelvic organs
◆ To treat severe and uncontrollable pelvic infection
◆ To stop severe hemorrhage
◆ In certain conditions affecting the intestines and bladder, which threaten the woman's life, when it is impossible to deal with the primary problem without removal of the uterus
◆ Excessive fibroids which are causing bleeding and pain
◆ The operation is sometimes done, depending on the circumstances, to treat prolapse, as a method of sterilization (though this should not be necessary), to treat severe endometriosis, because of some injury to the pelvic muscular structure at childbirth, severe enough to interfere with bowel and bladder function, and when vaginal bleeding results in anemia and is unchecked by hormone treatment.

What should I do?
Question your doctor carefully about the reasons for your hysterectomy and be satisfied in your mind that it is absolutely necessary. Explore all the possible alternatives and involve your partner and family.

Check whether your ovaries need to be removed as well, and find out about the hormone treatment for premature menopause. If you are prepared, any trauma will be less severe.

How is it done?
Under general anesthetic, an incision is made in the lower abdomen, though sometimes the uterus is removed through an incision in the vagina. The latter is more difficult but leaves less post-operative discomfort and no scar. It is performed, for example, for treatment of a prolapse or cervical

TYPES OF PROCEDURE

Hysterectomy is a major operation which should only be undertaken for certain life-threatening conditions. It should never be done as a matter of routine after child-bearing has ceased or when other, more minor, treatment is available.

Total abdominal hysterectomy involves removal of the uterus and cervix through a horizontal incision in the lower abdomen. The ovaries and fallopian tubes are left behind, so hormone treatment is not necessary.

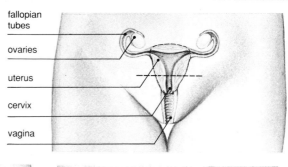

fallopian tubes
ovaries
uterus
cervix
vagina

Less and more extensive operations can be done. In sub-total hysterectomy (far right) only the uterus is removed. In total abdominal hysterectomy and bi-lateral salpingo-oophorectomy (right), the uterus, cervix, fallopian tubes and ovaries are all removed.

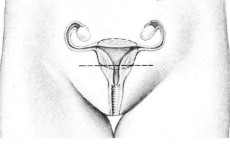

cancer. The vagina will be slightly shortened.

After the operation you will have an intravenous drip for fluids or blood, and perhaps a catheter to drain urine. There will be some discharge from the vagina for a day or two. If your ovaries were removed, hormone replacement will be planned.

You will be encouraged to get out of bed after a couple of days. If you suffer discomfort with gas or you find urination difficult, tell the medical staff.

What can I do?

When you go home, maintain a moderate level of activity, but stop the minute you feel pain. You need to build up your strength and energy again. Gentle activities can be started by the fourth week; moderate activity like light shopping or housework, can be done by the fifth week. By the sixth week you should feel nearly back to normal, though tiredness will probably still be a problem.

By the eighth week you can resume sexual intercourse, as the top of the vagina will have healed. There is no reason why sex should be any different for you and many women report increased satisfaction. Any problems with sex can probably be attributed to a premature menopause, with symptoms such as insufficient vaginal lubrication and loss of libido. Talk to your doctor and ask about hormone therapy. After a hysterectomy you have no periods and are sterile, so birth control methods are no longer necessary.

Are there psychological changes?

Nearly half of all women having hysterectomies are satisfied with the operation. Because the internal organs move to fill the space left by the uterus, there is no sensation of emptiness and the vagina will be the same size as it was before,

unless the operation was a radical total hysterectomy because of some disease of the cervix.

Dissatisfaction is related to whether the operation was done for a very good reason and after full consideration by the woman of the options available. Women who find it the most difficult are those of child-bearing age and inclination, and those whose ovaries are removed pre-menopausally. The majority of women who suffer depression after hysterectomy are those for whom the operation was for a non-life-threatening condition. It seems easier to bear if you know that the operation saved your life or has made a great improvement as for women who become pain-free after the removal of multiple fibroids or free from the pain of endometriosis.

HYSTERICAL BEHAVIOR

In the medical sense, hysteria means exhibiting an abnormality which has no anatomical foundation. The symptoms are therefore imaginary but to the hysterical person there is no difference between what is apparent and what is real. For example, amnesia is a rare form of hysterical behavior when loss of memory is the over-reaction to something the sufferer wants to forget.

Hysteria, now more commonly known medically as a somatization disorder, usually begins before the age of 30 and leads to numerous investigations by many different physicians. Sometimes, unnecessary surgery and other treatments are performed.

The problem of hysterical behavior is much more common among women than men; the prevalence is said to be 1 in 100 women, many of whom have a family history of antisocial personality disorders in their male relatives.

Hysterical behavior is not a psychosomatic illness which has real physical symptoms that originate because of emotional factors, such as stress-induced skin rashes and migraine headaches. Even friends and relatives of the hysterical person will probably assume the symptoms are real.

Why does this happen?

An hysterical illness can be a response to an unpleasant situation which can't be managed so the illness is used as leverage or as a show of helplessness. The hysterical symptoms may be simply attention seeking, such as an asthmatic attack. Hysterical behavior can also be seen as a woman's attempt to express her needs and feelings. The individual becomes manipulative and deceiving in an attempt to gain attention and be understood. So often this has the reverse effect and she is grossly misunderstood and even more unhappy. A woman who suspects her husband of an affair may develop symptoms that prevent her leaving the house, thus confining him too.

· S y m p t o m s ·

Depending on the hysterical illness – can be
▲ Neurological and include headaches, paralysis, loss of memory, double vision, seizures and weakness
▲ Gynecological and include painful menstruation and pain on intercourse
▲ Gastrointestinal and include abdominal pain and nausea

What should I do ?

Hysteria is very difficult to diagnose and if you suspect someone of faking symptoms, diagnostic tests should be done first to ensure that hysteria is the cause of the problem, so encourage her to go to the doctor. Hysterical behavior and related symptoms can recur so you will need to be alert to symptoms and seek professional help as soon as possible.

What will the doctor do?

Because there are no physical symptoms to treat, the treatment of hysteria is always through psychotherapy and counseling. The individual will probably be very sensitive to being called a faker and so care should be taken in approaching psychotherapy. A frank talk with the family doctor, therapist or counselor might be enough to solve a minor problem.

In severe cases, formal psychiatric help with counseling, hospitalization and analysis will be necessary to discover the underlying problem. The doctor may prescribe tranquilizers to calm the patient during the therapy. Hypnosis is also used to bring the suppressed trouble to the surface.

SEE ALSO

ANXIETY
DEPRESSION
PHOBIA

HYSTEROSALPINGOGRAM

This is an X-ray picture of the womb and fallopian tubes, including the ovaries. In the simplest form, the outline of the organs is achieved by pumping the abdominal cavity up with air or carbon dioxide, known as tubal insufflation. This gives a sufficiently clear picture to determine whether the cavity of the uterus is clear and that the fallopian tubes are not blocked.

If a more accurate and detailed picture is required, such as precisely where the blockage is, a radio-opaque dye can be injected directly into the uterus and tubes so that their cavities show up on X-ray. If there is no blockage, the air or the dye passes into the cavity and is harmlessly reabsorbed into the body. A blockage of either the uterus or the fallopian tubes can be easily seen because the dye does not flow beyond it.

Why is it done?

An hysterosalpingogram (HSG) is most commonly performed as part of investigations for infertility. It is also performed after an ectopic pregnancy and to establish the site and extent of scarring or deformity or a total blockage of the fallopian tubes.

The X-ray pictures will show whether there is any distortion in the uterine cavity such as that caused by a fibroid or cyst. It will also show if the fallopian tubes are blocked and pinpoint where the blockage occurs. What it can't do with any accuracy is show the state of the organs, and if there is any doubt remaining after the hysterosalpingogram, the doctor will probably arrange for you to have a laparoscopy so the organs can be viewed directly.

How is it done?

This procedure can be done under a local anesthetic or without anesthetic. It is normally performed in the X-ray department of a hospital or in a radiologist's office on an out-patient basis, which is quite safe, need not be painful, and allows you to go home on the same day. It takes about ten minutes to perform. If you find you have to have a hysterosalpingogram, ask your doctor what is available at the local hospital and make your choice.

Firstly the cervix is exposed by the insertion of a speculum into the vagina. A hollow metal tube is then inserted and a water-based dye (radio-opaque fluid) injected into the uterus. X-rays are taken while the dye is injected and these can be seen on a television monitor situated nearby. The doctor will watch as the liquid fills the uterine cavity and flows into the fallopian tubes. If there are no blockages, the dye disperses into the abdominal cavity.

What are the risks?

This is not a difficult or painful procedure although as the dye is injected into the uterus there may be some cramping sensations.

FERTILITY TESTING

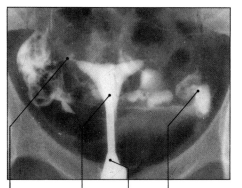

fallopian tube | uterus | nozzle | dye dispersing

This X-ray of the pelvic organs shows the pelvic bones, uterus and fallopian tubes of a fertile woman. There is no sign of any blockage in the fallopian tubes or distortion of the uterine cavity. The cervix and vagina is visible at the base of the picture.

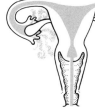

Right-hand tube is open but the left tube is blocked near the uterus

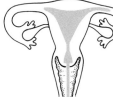

Both tubes are blocked at different distances along their length

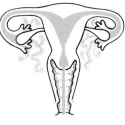

Both tubes are open but the uterus is divided within its cavity

---

SEE ALSO :

ECTOPIC PREGNANCY
FIBROIDS
INFERTILITY
LAPAROSCOPY
OVARIAN CYSTS

INCONTINENCE

This is the involuntary leakage of urine when you are unable to control your bladder; some degree of incontinence is very common, especially in older women. Incontinence used to be an unmentionable subject, kept secret by most of its victims, but today we recognize that many women may suffer from a degree of incontinence for transient periods from their middle twenties onwards, particularly if they have borne children.

· S y m p t o m s ·

▲ Inability to control your bladder, particularly when you exert pressure on the abdominal muscles
▲ Frequency of urination, even when your bladder is not full
▲ Urgency, even when your bladder isn't full

What causes it?
There are three important factors that produce incontinence. It is an aftermath of pregnancy if the pelvic and perineal tissues become so stretched that a prolapse of the vaginal wall, urethra or bladder occurs. If a small part of the urethra (a urethrocele) or the bladder (a cystocele) accompanies the prolapse, this nearly always leads to urinary symptoms of some kind be it urgency, hesitancy, frequency and/or pain.

If the exit valve from the bladder is slightly weakened, usually as a woman gets older, stress incontinence can result. This is not uncommon during pregnancy but goes away after the birth. Urine may leak away if pressure inside the abdominal cavity is increased when we cough, strain to open our bowels or lift a heavy weight.

If the muscles of the bladder wall become over-sensitive to the presence of urine in the bladder, they respond by contracting uncontrollably and trying to empty the bladder even when there are only small quantities of urine present.

This is sometimes called irritable bladder.

Should I consult the doctor?
It is very important that women seek help for the treatment of incontinence as soon as their symptoms appear. The earlier incontinence is treated, the less likely it is that weaknesses will persist and the condition become chronic.

What will the doctor do?
The good news is that both stress incontinence and irritable bladder can be treated. Your doctor will take a mid-stream urine sample to check whether there is any urinary-tract infection, such as cystitis, present. You may also be referred for a special X-ray of your bladder. This takes place while you are passing urine. It is called a voiding cystourethrogram.

You will be advised to strengthen your pelvic floor muscles (see index). As obesity weakens the pelvic floor, so you may be advised to consult a dietitian or exercise to take off weight if that is a contributory cause.

Treatment for prolapse involves wearing a special ring or sponge in your vagina in the daytime.

If treatment for stress incontinence fails to work, you can have a surgical operation to tighten up your pelvic floor muscles.

If you are suffering from an irritable bladder, your doctor may encourage you to hold onto urine for as long as possible to strengthen the bladder muscles. There are also drugs to relax the muscles. If this doesn't work, there is a surgical operation to stretch the urethra.

What can I do?
Pelvic floor exercises are an excellent way of combating the symptom of incontinence. Research has shown that even in a woman as old as 80, a regime of pelvic floor exercises carried out regularly over as short a time as three months, can allow her to regain bladder control and vastly

improve any incontinence.

Various forms of prolapse are implicated in urinary problems but the important thing to remember is that every prolapse is preventable as long as you are aware of situations in which you become vulnerable and maintain the health of the pelvic floor muscles throughout your sexually active life and beyond.

SEE ALSO:

CYSTITIS
LABOR
OBESITY
POSTNATAL CARE
PROLAPSE
URINARY PROBLEMS

INDUCTION OF LABOR

This is when the onset of labor is triggered artificially because labor has failed to begin spontaneously, or the doctor decides that delivery should not be delayed for important reasons. Induction is nearly always planned in advance so you will be admitted to hospital the night before you are to be induced.

The methods used for induction are sometimes employed to speed up a spontaneous labor if it is not progressing quickly enough for the health of the mother and baby.

Why is it done?
All induction of labor is an intervention, therefore you need to be sure that the reasons for inducing you are acceptable to you. Make sure that your medical advisers know how you feel. However, it would be wrong for you to oppose the induction of labor if your doctor provides you with very good reasons why it should be done. (Electing to have the induction on a certain day or time of day used to be fashionable but is now questioned as unnecessary intervention.)

Medically advisable reasons include:
◆ The baby is late for dates or postmature. It is often difficult for the mother and doctor to be absolutely sure of the expected delivery date. There are diagnostic methods of checking such as ultrasound scanning and measuring the height of the fundus (the top of the uterus). However, 80% of babies who are born with a spontaneous labor arrive after the due date. Only 5% actually come on the due date.
◆ If your baby is 14 days overdue, and particularly if you stop gaining weight, the doctor may recommend induction mainly because the placenta may be inadequate to support the baby who is outgrowing its food supply (placental insufficiency).

AMNIOTOMY
The bag of waters has to be removed in order to allow the baby to pass down the birth canal. Usually it ruptures naturally towards the end of the first stage of labor but sometimes it must be artificially ruptured.

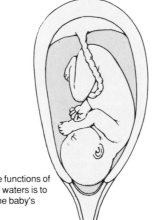

One of the functions of the bag of waters is to cushion the baby's head

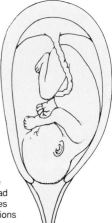

Once ruptured, the pressure of the head on the cervix causes increased contractions

◆ You are over 35 and particularly if this is your first baby when you may be unflatteringly referred to as an elderly primigravida. Obstetricians are sensitive to the possibility that the placenta is more likely to fail in a woman over 35. As long as you are closely monitored, you should not be unnecessarily induced just because of your age.
◆ If the fetus is suffering from retarded fetal growth because of some condition of the mother such as high blood pressure, antepartum hemorrhage, diabetes or Rhesus incompatibility. The baby will be induced as it has a better chance of developing normally outside the womb than inside.

Labor will be speeded up by artificial means if:
◆ The cervix fails to dilate, or labor fails to progress smoothly, but stops and starts and the mother and fetus are becoming distressed.

How is it done?
There are many methods, both natural and medical, to induce labor. One or more methods may be used depending on the condition of the cervix and the reasons for induction. Before any induction, the doctor will examine your cervix to determine whether it is "ripe" - soft and perhaps partly dilated. This is a sign that labor is imminent. If the cervix is not ripe, then artificial hormones will need to be used to induce labor.

AMNIOTOMY

Amniotomy is only performed at term because the risk of infection once the waters have broken means the baby must be delivered inside 24 hours.

Membranes are ruptured with a small pair of forceps or a tool not unlike a crochet hook. This is inserted into the uterus and an opening made in the bag of waters. It is usually painless and the waters escape in a rush.

The bag of waters provides a cushion for the baby's head as it presses against the cervix. Once the membranes have been ruptured, the head presses directly onto the cervix, and if labor was indeed imminent, this could be enough to start the contractions and speed up labor.

If you are already in labor, rupturing the membranes causes the contractions to increase in intensity because the baby's head is lowered. This should bring the first stage of labor to completion much more quickly.

In a normal labor, the membranes don't usually break until late in the first stage. The disadvantage of rupturing the membranes when labor has started spontaneously is that everything speeds up alarmingly and if the baby has the cord around its neck, the release of the cushioning bag of waters can increase the pressure and affect the flow of blood to the baby through the cord.

If your doctor plans to monitor the fetal heartbeat with an electrode, the waters will need to be broken to attach the electrode to the baby's head. Inspecting the waters is also a way of checking whether the baby is distressed or not. If she is, there will be traces of the first bowel movements – meconium – in the waters.

OXYTOCIN

Oxytocin is a natural hormone which is secreted by the pituitary gland in the brain. It stimulates labor and if given in a synthetic form, via the drug Pitocin, it can start labor and keep it going. It can be administered in several ways:

The most common and preferable way that Pitocin may be given is through a drip directly into a vein. The speed of the drip can be slowed down if you go into labor too quickly and the cervix is well dilated.

The disadvantage of a Pitocin drip is that labor may be so quick and strong that the need for pain-killing drugs may be greater. Also the contractions are usually close together and this can affect the fetus as the blood supply to the fetus is shut off during every contraction.

The drip won't be removed until after the baby is born because the uterus needs to continue contracting to prevent postpartum bleeding.

What are the risks of induction?

Many women are delighted to be induced, particularly if they have had a long, unpleasant labor in childbirth before. The speeding up of a prolonged labor is greeted enthusiastically by some mothers. No one would argue that a planned induction should not be contemplated if the fetus is in danger but this would seem to be the case in only a small percentage of pregnancies and in some centers about half the births use some form of artificial induction.

The intensity of contractions in an induced labor means that painkilling drugs, fetal monitoring and other methods of intervention such as forceps and episiotomy may be much more common. The baby is more likely to be jaundiced. This makes childbirth a very different experience if you had hoped for a natural one.

SEE ALSO:

DIABETES MELLITUS
EPISIOTOMY
FORCEPS DELIVERY
LABOR
RHESUS INCOMPATIBILITY

INFERTILITY

Infertility means the inability to bear a child. Very few women and couples are infertile; a much higher number are sub-fertile – in other words they have difficulty in conceiving.

Infertility is not a matter of either partner exclusively but of the couple as a unit. Your fertility is indivisible from the fertility of you and your partner. It must therefore be investigated with the co-operation of both of you. It is unrealistic to expect difficulty in conceiving to involve only one partner.

About 10 percent of all couples have some period of sub-fertility in their lives.

Should I see the doctor?
If you've been having unprotected intercourse for at least a year, twice a week, and you haven't become pregnant, consult your doctor. If you are over 30, however, consult your doctor after six months.

What will the doctor do?
At whatever stage you consult a doctor if you are having difficulty conceiving, your doctor will still question you closely about your menstrual history, how long you have been trying to have a baby, when you stopped contraception, and your family's medical history. You will also be asked about your medical history: any surgical operations such as an appendectomy; illnesses such as anorexia nervosa; specific gynecological problems such as terminations or sexually transmitted diseases.

You and your partner must be honest and thorough in your answers. Investigation of fertility can take a long time and be very frustrating and embarrassing at times. If you are prepared for this, the strain will be easier to bear. While these investigations can cause irreparable damage to a relationship, other couples find that they are brought closer together.

Your doctor will then give you a physical examination to check the condition of your reproductive

WHAT CAUSES INFERTILITY?

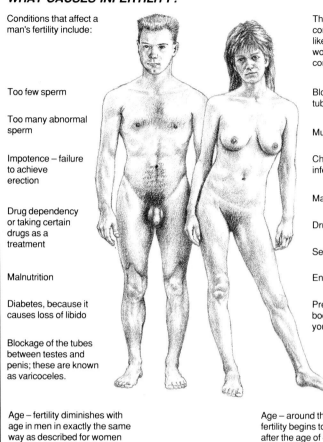

Conditions that affect a man's fertility include:

Too few sperm

Too many abnormal sperm

Impotence – failure to achieve erection

Drug dependency or taking certain drugs as a treatment

Malnutrition

Diabetes, because it causes loss of libido

Blockage of the tubes between testes and penis; these are known as varicoceles.

Age – fertility diminishes with age in men in exactly the same way as described for women

There are certain conditions which are likely to prevent a woman from conceiving:

Blocked fallopian tubes

Multiple fibroids

Chronic pelvic infection

Malnutrition

Drug dependency

Severe heart disease

Endometriosis

Presence of antibodies immobilizing your partner's sperm

Age – around the age of 25 fertility begins to diminish and after the age of 45 only half a woman's cycles are ovulatory. A woman over 45, therefore, has only half as many fertile periods annually as a younger woman.

organs and your general health. The precise examination will depend on your medical history. This may involve your doctor looking into your eyes to check the retina or feeling your neck for any differences in your thyroid gland.

You may have a Pap smear and the doctor, if necessary, will take a small piece of the lining of your uterus – the endometrium. This indicates whether ovulation has taken place and is always done in the second half of the cycle. This examination will also show whether there

are growths such as fibroids in the uterus or any cysts on the ovaries.

This initial examination will help the doctor to determine the first line of action. The tests and investigations then begin. If you are an older woman wanting a first baby, ask for the program to be speeded up as it takes time and you should expect priority treatment.

Your partner will also be asked about his medical and family history. For example, if his testes did not descend naturally, and about his work environment; environmental

MAJOR SYMPTOMS

These can alert your doctor to common causes of infertility.

Failure to ovulate

Amenorrhea usually shows that a woman is not ovulating, unless of course she is already pregnant or breastfeeding. Failure to ovulate can be the result of some problem in your pelvic organs or in the release of hormones from your brain. Surgical exploration, usually laparoscopy, is a method whereby the surgeon can clearly view your pelvic organs and spot any reasons for failure to ovulate. You will have a general anesthetic and the laparoscope is passed through the abdominal wall to view your uterus, fallopian tubes and ovaries.

If your menstrual history has already shown scanty or irregular periods, then hormone levels will be implicated and tests done to determine what is wrong. For example, if certain hormones are being over produced, levels will be measured with a blood test and if they are abnormal, an X-ray of your skull will show if there is a tumor on the pituitary gland, the gland that secretes the sex hormones. Drugs are used to lower hormonal levels and surgery can remove the tumor on the pituitary.

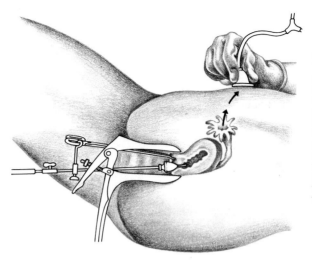

Insufflation
This is a safe procedure to check for blockages in the fallopian tubes. Carbon dioxide gas is passed from the vagina into the tubes. The doctor listens through a stethoscope to the escaping gas. The site of the blockage can even be determined, though the test cannot indicate the damage done.

Other reasons for a failure to ovulate include severe weight loss (anorexia nervosa), emotional problems, (even jet travel can cause temporary amenorrhea) and diseases such as diabetes. Some women may experience menopause as early as 35. This results in permanent infertility.

Fallopian tube disorders

Any interference with the fallopian tubes, such as an ectopic pregnancy, adhesions after abdominal surgery or pelvic inflammatory disease, can block the tubes,

preventing fertilization of the egg by the sperm.

Insufflation is a test where gas, usually carbon dioxide, is passed through the vagina into the tubes. The doctor listens at your abdomen to the sound of the gas in the tubes and can determine whether they are releasing the gas into your abdominal cavity or not. If they aren't, then the assumption is that the tubes are blocked.

Another test to see whether there are blockages or other problems is a hysterosalpingogram where dye is passed through the vagina.

---

factors can result in a low sperm count (see overleaf). Childhood illnesses such as mumps, and sexually transmitted diseases are also relevant.

What tests are done?

If your doctor suspects some anatomical obstruction, basic tests will be carried out right away. If, however, there seems no immediate and obvious reason for your inability to conceive, your doctor will first ask your partner to produce a sample of semen. There wouldn't be much point in going on with the female

tests if your partner was infertile. This is known as semen analysis. Your partner will also be examined to see if there is any obvious physical reason for infertility.

You will need to keep a menstrual chart for a couple of months. This involves recording your temperature every day with a special thermometer. If you ovulate, there should be a temperature rise around day 14.

Another basic test is a postcoital test, which should be arranged around the time when you ovulate. You will be asked to arrange an appointment and have sexual inter-

course within three hours of this visit to your doctor's office. You will be advised not to wash or douche until after the doctor has examined you. You will be given an internal examination to remove a sample of cervical mucus to see if the sperm have reached the cervix, and if the sperm are still moving about. If they are immobilized, this could indicate the presence of antibodies in the cervical mucus. The antibodies in your body see your partner's sperm as a foreign body and fight them off.

Routine blood and urine tests help your doctor to estimate hormone

INFERTILITY

levels and this can pinpoint a failure to ovulate. Ultrasound will show up any ovarian cysts.

Once the semen analysis and preliminary tests have been completed, it should be clear whether it is you or your partner who needs treatment.

What is the treatment?

This of course depends on the results of your tests and what the problem is thought to be. Treatment may be with fertility drugs (see box) or different surgical procedures. Both types of treatment have proved successful.

If endometriosis is the cause of your infertility, hormone treatment is usually the most common method of clearing up this painful condition. Depending on the severity of your case, after about a year of the treatment, you should try to conceive. Pregnancy clears up endometriosis completely in some cases.

SURGICAL TREATMENT

Laparotomy is an exploratory abdominal operation to locate the source of the problem and carry out the appropriate treatment. Blocked fallopian tubes, for example, can be opened up again, although not without some risk, either by forcing fluid through them or with microsurgical techniques (salpingostomy).

Once opened, the chances of an ectopic pregnancy are higher, and even with microsurgery, the tiny, delicate tubes can easily be damaged. If the tubes are irreparably damaged, then in vitro fertilization may be the only chance. A new method known as GIFT (Gamete intrafallopian transfer) introduces the sperm and ovum directly into the fallopian tube to fertilize there.

Ovarian cysts and fibroids in the uterus can be removed surgically. Other surgical procedures may be necessary for a woman who ovulates, and may even have become pregnant, but miscarries every time for

ENVIRONMENTAL FACTORS

Check whether or not you or your partner work with certain chemicals, lead or radiation. Some industrial substances can damage sperm, lead to spontaneous abortion and make conception difficult. Spending a long time at high altitudes or exposure to high temperatures can affect the production of sperm.

It is also known that too much drinking and smoking can reduce a man's fertility.

some reason and is unable to carry the baby to full term. Abnormalities in the shape of the uterus and a cervix that does not remain tightly closed may be two reasons for this.

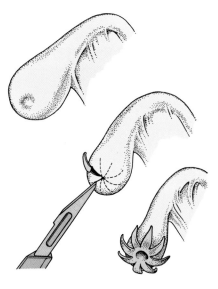

If fallopian tubes are blocked (top), they can be opened up (center) with microsurgery. This is known as salpingostomy.

ARTIFICIAL INSEMINATION

If you have developed antibodies to your partner's sperm, or some condition which prevents full intercourse makes you infertile as a couple even though both of you are fertile, then artificial insemination by husband (or partner) – AIH – may be the method used. If the man is infertile, artificial insemination by donor may be considered (AID).

What can I do?

Don't lose heart; be determined and ask for referrals to clinics where the most advanced research techniques are being investigated and used. If your medical advisers can give you no hope, you should consider adoption, though this is becoming more difficult.

Surrogacy is another method where a woman bears a child for another woman and has been used mainly by wealthy couples. This method has received much publicity which should serve to communicate to any intelligent person that it is a road with many pitfalls.

However, there are now numerous permutations as a result of in vitro fertilization. For instance, a woman can carry an ovum donated by another woman and fertilized by her husband or an embryo belonging to another couple entirely. The limits of this technique are only just being explored and, in future, may offer a variety of alternatives for the infertile.

FERTILITY DRUGS

These are used when a hormone defect has been diagnosed. The therapy will be adjusted according to the individual and often involves more than one drug. The risk of multiple pregnancy is great. Side effects include headache, hot flashes and abdominal pain because the ovaries are enlarged.

The basis for clomiphene treatment is to encourage the pituitary gland to increase hormone release so the ovaries produce an egg. Throughout this therapy, where the drugs are administered for short periods during the cycle, your doctor will monitor your temperature changes and cervical mucus to see if ovulation is occurring. The dose will be increased in subsequent months if there is no indication of ovulation. Blood tests in the second half of the cycle show if progesterone is being produced, another indication of success. You will then be advised when to have intercourse.

If this treatment fails to stimulate the ovaries, there is a more complicated treatment of hormone injections to encourage the ovary directly to release an egg. This involves gonadotrophins. This method can result in multiple pregnancies, and because of the monitoring of hormone levels with ultrasound and urine tests and therefore frequent visits to the doctor, it is expensive and time consuming.

The newest method is the wearing of a hormone pump. It is strapped around your waist and a catheter is introduced under your skin, usually in your arm. The syringe in the pump releases a small amount of luteinizing hormone on the days following your menstrual period. This method reduces the frequent visits to your doctor required for the direct stimulation treatment, and the risk of multiple pregnancy because only one follicle is stimulated. The pump replaces the natural release from the brain which occurs in normally ovulating women with little inconvenience and no discomfort.

TIMETABLE FOR DRUG TREATMENT

The graph shows normal hormone fluctuation during the menstrual cycle as well as the timing of the fertility drug therapy, which is administered according to the specific hormone defect.

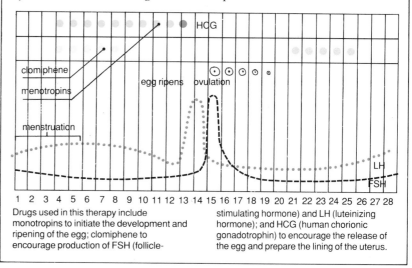

Drugs used in this therapy include monotropins to initiate the development and ripening of the egg; clomiphene to encourage production of FSH (follicle-stimulating hormone) and LH (luteinizing hormone); and HCG (human chorionic gonadotrophin) to encourage the release of the egg and prepare the lining of the uterus.

SEE ALSO:

ARTIFICAL INSEMINATION
DRUG DEPENDENCY
ENDOMETRIOSIS
FIBROIDS
HYSTEROSALPINGOGRAM
IN VITRO FERTILIZATION
LAPAROSCOPY
PELVIC INFLAMMATORY
  DISEASE

INSOMNIA

This is an inability to sleep and it can take two forms. You may have difficulty getting off to sleep no matter how tired you are, or you fall asleep quickly and wake a short time later or early in the morning.

What causes it?

Most people suffer from sleepless nights from time to time, usually because something has made them anxious or because they are uncomfortable, perhaps due to a minor illness. In the middle of the night, all unpleasant things seem exaggeratedly worrying and frightening. If you are feeling resentful, reliving injustices in the night can raise your blood pressure and make your brain race. Large quantities of alcohol may induce sleepiness but after a short time you wake and find it impossible to drop off again. Thinking about it only makes it worse.

Persistent sleeplessness can be caused by psychological problems including anxiety or depression, or by pain and discomfort arising from a physical disorder.

Should I see the doctor?

In the darkness, wakefulness seems interminable but studies have shown that our estimate of insomnia is greater than it actually is. If you are anxious about your inability to sleep, and you feel it is affecting your health and the self-help measures don't alleviate the problem, consult your doctor.

What will the doctor do?

If a lack of sleep is affecting your general health, your doctor will probably prescribe a short course of sleeping pills so that you can relearn new sleeping habits. The most commonly used class of sleeping drugs is the benzodiazepines, which have comparatively few adverse effects and are relatively safe in overdose. They include well known names such as Valium. Doctors don't usually prescribe them continuously. You should have a review of the drug

NATURE OF THE PROBLEM	PROBABLE CAUSE
You are overworked, anxious and your mind won't stop racing	*Anxiety* or stress of any sort can cause insomnia.
You have a new baby	This can result in ceaseless insomnia for the first 6-8 weeks. Work out a schedule with your partner for the diaper change and quiet night feeds.
You are unhappy, can't concentrate and have lost interest in sex	You may be suffering from *depression*.
You are pregnant	Insomnia can result if you need to get up frequently to urinate, or the baby's movements and discomfort with your enlarged uterus causes you to remain awake. Use pillows to get yourself back to sleep in a comfortable position.
Your partner snores, or there is a dripping tap or creaking pipe	This may be disturbing you. Do something about them.
You are in pain	Sleep won't come until you remove the pain. See your doctor about painkillers; don't just take sleeping pills. This is pointless unless you treat the cause of the pain.
You have been taking sleeping pills for some reason and have recently stopped	This can cause insomnia because it may take you a while to get back to normal. Don't be tempted to go back on the pills; this could lead to *drug dependency*.
You wake at around 2 a.m. with abdominal pain, and it is relieved with a drink and snack	This could be a gastric ulcer (see *Digestive problems*.).
You are going through *menopause*, and you experience symptoms such as night sweats	Waking soaking wet is bound to cause insomnia. This can be successfully treated with *hormone replacement therapy*. Our need for sleep does decline with age.
You wake feeling breathless	Consult your doctor. This could be a disorder affecting your heart or lungs.
You drink a lot of alcohol, coffee or tea before going to bed	You are not likely to sleep well as these are all stimulants.

treatment and the problem after one month.

Antihistamines can induce sleep in the elderly, and some antidepressant drugs may also be used to promote sleep in depressed people.

Barbiturates, the first drugs to be used widely to produce sleep, are now used rarely because there is a risk of abuse and dependency with them. Even non-barbiturate, non-benzodiazepine sleeping drugs, safer alternatives to barbiturates, have been less commonly used since the introduction of the benzodiazepines.

How long should the drugs be taken?
The effectiveness of sleeping drugs rapidly diminishes after the first few nights so they should only be used for limited periods. When taken they very quickly produce drow-siness and slowed reactions, so that they should always be taken shortly before you go to bed. The sleep induced by these drugs is not the same as natural sleep, and you may not feel as well rested as you might have thought. Some people even experience a "hangover" effect. Daytime drowsi-ness, dizziness and unsteadiness may also result.

Are there any risks from sleeping drugs?
If these drugs are taken regularly for more than a few weeks, especially if taken in larger than normal doses, they may produce psychological and physical addiction. If they are with-drawn abruptly, sleeplessness and a minor form of anxiety can arise. Nightmares and vivid dreams may occur because the amount of time spent in dream sleep increases.

There is always the temptation to take a larger dose of the drug once its effect has diminished. This is particu-larly dangerous if you are on a barbiturate drug.

What can I do?
If you've been unable to sleep because you are worried and can't stop your thoughts racing at night, talk to someone and try to get your feelings sorted out. The worries will become worse if you are tired and stressed.

If you have been prescribed a sleeping drug, try not to rely on it in the long term. If you become dependent, the withdrawal period will be characterized by the insomnia you are trying to cure. If you have been taking them regularly and you want to stop taking them, seek your doctor's advice on how to reduce the dosage gradually so as to avoid experiencing withdrawal symptoms.

If you are unable to make a diagnosis from the chart opposite, consult your doctor.

Self-help measures
Sometimes if you are emotionally upset your breathing is rapid and sharp. You should take two or three deep breaths and try to relax this way. There are other ways you can induce drowsiness and sleep.
◆ Limit your intake of stimulants such as alcohol, coffee, tea and cola drinks before going to bed.
◆ Have a warm bath and hot milk.
◆ Take advantage of temporary insomnia and do something constructive with it. Catch up on reading or do the household accounts. Don't lie there allowing the frustrations to build up.
◆ Sex is not a good hypnotic for women; there is usually the opposite effect.
◆ Fix things that may be diverting you – squeaking floor boards, creaking pipes and dripping taps.
◆ Keep the air temperature in your room equable. Leave a window open so the atmosphere isn't stuffy.
◆ If your insomnia is chronic, catnap during the day whenever you can. Indulge in catnaps, don't avoid them.
◆ Practice the deep breathing techniques used in childbirth.

INSOMNIA DURING PREGNANCY
During pregnancy, the baby's metabolism knows no day or night and turns over at top speed, keeping you awake with the kicks and nudges just when your metabolism has slowed down for the night. Other problems include the frequency you need to pass urine as the uterus presses on your bladder, and the increased blood supply which causes sweating and hot flashes. At night you wake dripping wet and uncomfortable, unable to get back to sleep again.

If you are pregnant and insomnia is a problem, don't take sleeping pills, find non-medical ways to deal with it. Wear cotton bedclothes to absorb the sweat. Don't lie flat on your back, lie on your side with pillows to support your abdomen and upper thigh or sleep partly propped up so that pressure of the uterus doesn't inhibit your breathing and press on the nerves in your back.

After the baby is born, you may have trouble sleeping when she wakes in the night for a feed or a cuddle and leaves you wakeful and alert. Getting through this phase is often a learning process for you too and you may find you acquire the ability to drop off to sleep after the night feed. The knowledge that you may be working or looking after small children the next day can make you even more irritated and anxious to get back to sleep.

IN VITRO FERTILIZATION

This is a method of treating infertility. It is still reserved for cases in which other methods have failed. The term "in vitro" literally means "in glass", because fertilization is usually accomplished in a test tube, hence the phrase "test tube baby".

In vitro fertilization (IVF) is particularly successful where there are blocked or damaged fallopian tubes or damage to the ovaries.

Why is it done?

In vitro fertilization, though very expensive and time consuming, is now established as a treatment for infertility since its first success in 1978. The couples who will be offered this method of conception are those where the woman has blocked or damaged fallopian tubes which means that the ova and sperm can never meet to achieve conception, where all investigation has found no obvious reason for the infertility after five years, where the male has a low sperm count and AIH was not considered because the chances of fertilization would be lessened.

How is it done?

IVF is not available at many centers and so you would need to approach your own doctor and hospital consultant first. Certain criteria such as the number of years of trying to conceive and the age of the woman will be taken into account. Women over 40 are not considered to have a good chance.

Before IVF can take place, there must be careful monitoring of the menstrual cycle to determine as near as possible the time of ovulation. All available means including ultrasound techniques are employed. Because the woman will already have undergone investigations for infertility, such as laparoscopy, the condition of her ovaries and fallopian tubes will be on record.

TUBAL SPERM-EGG TRANSFER

In vitro fertilization occurs in a glass tube with culture conditions as close as possible to those in the human fallopian tube. GIFT (Gamete intrafallopian transfer) is a variation on the standard in vitro fertilization. A laparoscope is used to introduce sperm and egg into the fallopian tube where fertilization can then take place in a more normal environment.

GIFT is suited to women for whom there is no reason why an egg cannot implant in the uterus and develop into a pregnancy. The main drawback is that the procedure must take place under a general anesthetic and this may have to be repeated a number of times.

Right: in in vitro fertilization, ovum and sperm are mixed in a petri dish and examined microscopically for successful fertilization.

Far right: in GIFT, ovum and sperm are introduced via a laparoscope into the fallopian tube so that fertilization can take place there.

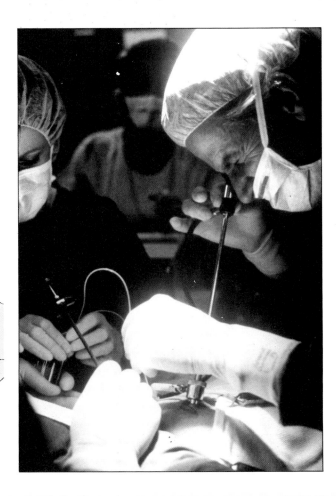

Fertility drugs are used to stimulate the follicles to produce several mature ova which can be retrieved from the ovary via laparoscopy at the time of ovulation. The ova are then sucked out through the abdominal wall by means of a hollow needle and transferred to a test tube. This is sometimes called the "egg harvest". Another technique uses ultrasound scanning to detect the follicle. This is easier for the woman as it can be performed, like amniocentesis, without a general anesthetic.

The ova are then mixed with a fresh sample of the partner's sperm which has been prepared to make it as close as possible to its condition as it passes up the fallopian tubes. If fertilization is successful, the embryos are grown to the two- or four-cell stage. This takes about three days when they are ready to be transferred via a fine tube through the cervix and high up into the uterus.

As many as three embryos are deposited in the uterus but it is very rare for all three to implant successfully. Three is thought to be the optimum number required to achieve implantation and pregnancy. Any unused embryos may be stored in case the first implantation is unsuccessful. This factor raises difficult ethical and moral issues.

There is then no more treatment until the time when a pregnancy test shows a positive result, although blood tests are used to give an earlier, accurate confirmation of the pregnancy.

What are the risks?

More than a quarter of IVF patients have a pregnancy, but as few as 15% have a successful birth. With the decrease in babies for adoption, there is an overwhelming demand for infertility treatment and the supply cannot meet the demand.

The major ethical question at present seems to center on the use of the excess embryos for research.

ALTERNATIVE METHODS

A new method, GIFT (Gamete Intra-fallopian Transfer), has been developed in Australia. Under general anesthetic, the ova are harvested and mixed with the sperm in the fallopian tube using laparoscopy to pinpoint the position. Fertilization then may take place in the fallopian tube as it does normally. This removes the religious objection to fertilization taking place outside the body. It doesn't seem to lead to ectopic pregnancy. It is an ideal method for couples where there is no impediment to pregnancy in the woman.

SEE ALSO:

ARTIFICIAL INSEMINATION
INFERTILITY
LAPAROSCOPY
ULTRASOUND
UTERINE PROBLEMS

ITCHING

If your skin feels itchy, and you can see no sign of a rash, you can often do more damage to the skin by scratching, so it is important to discover the cause of the irritation.

There are usually three root causes of itchiness; allergic reaction, dry skin and problems in the genital area. The allergic reaction may be food or drugs and even though children commonly suffer from food reactions such as hives, don't imagine that they can't arise in adults too, although there will nearly always be a history of allergic conditions, such as asthma or hayfever.

Itching in the genital area can be most distressing but it can arise for so many different reasons that you should look for a swift diagnosis; it could be a sexually transmitted disease, a contact dermatitis or a vaginal infection that shows itself on your vulva.

In pregnancy, the increased levels of estrogen can sometimes cause the skin, especially over the abdomen, to be very itchy.

If there is a rash, see *Rashes and skin changes*.

If you are unable to make a diagnosis from this information, consult your doctor.

NATURE AND SITE OF ITCHING	PROBABLE CAUSE
The itching is around your anus	This could be *hemorrhoids*, or if it is worse at night, it could be worms which you may have caught from your children. Check them for worms too and administer the treatment, which is available from pharmacists, to all the family as soon as possible.
You experience itching at night in your pubic hair	This could be a *sexually transmitted disease* – pubic lice.
The itching is confined to your genital area, and is accompanied by a vaginal discharge	This is probably a *yeast infection*.
The itching is confined to your scalp and bald patches appear	This is probably ringworm, a fungal infection. Consult your doctor.
The itchiness is between your toes and your toenails are yellow	This is athlete's foot, a fungal infection. (See *Foot problems*).
You have had a severe bout of diarrhea and your anus is itchy	This is a common after effect. Apply soothing cream or ice packs.
Your skin is dry	This can cause itching anywhere from your hands to your vulva.
Your skin and/or the whites of your eyes are yellowish	You could have jaundice, a liver disorder, which may be brought on by *gallbladder disease*. See your doctor.
You feel itchy around the genital area, and there seems no obvious reason for it	This could be *pruritis vulvae*.
Your scalp is itchy, and you notice white flakes on your shoulders	This is probably *dandruff*.
You feel very itchy around your genital area and this is followed by a crop of blisters	This is probably *genital herpes*. See your doctor

LABOR

Labor is the culmination of a pregnancy and should be an enjoyable experience for you and your partner. If you learn about what is going to happen to you, you should be prepared for most eventualities. Some decisions, such as whether to accept pain relief or be wired up for monitoring, can be written into your notes, but be prepared for a change of view should your medical advisers give you good reason.

POSITIONS FOR LABOR

A decade ago the traditional position for labor was lying on your back with your legs held up in stirrups. This is known as the lithotomy position and it was prescribed by doctors and midwives largely because it made their jobs easier. Little account was taken of a mother's wishes or of the strong natural forces, including the force of gravity, which were completely canceled out by this unnatural position. This position has several disadvantages:

◆ Labor becomes slower, longer and more painful.
◆ Blood pressure may drop so the amount of blood and oxygen reaching the baby is less.
◆ The perineal tissues are not stretched gradually by a baby pressing downwards, leading to a greater need for an episiotomy. One of the commonest reasons for prolapse is over-stretching of the pelvic tissues including the pelvic floor muscles during labor. This can occur if stage two is accomplished too quickly before the tissues are given a chance to stretch.
◆ A slow labor is more likely to lead to fetal distress and so the need for a forceps delivery is increased.
◆ Spontaneous delivery of the placenta is nearly always slow.
◆ There is more chance of getting low back strain in this position than if you are upright.

Natural positions

A woman left to her own devices and in the company of other women in the delivery room will nearly always adopt an upright position and there are very good reasons for this:

◆ Utilization of the tremendous pull downwards of the force of gravity to help the baby come out.
◆ When the uterus contracts, it contracts downwards vertically.
◆ The downward pressure of the baby gives a chance for the cervix and the perineal tissue to stretch over a period of time. This means that tears are infrequent and episiotomies are hardly ever needed and prolapse is less likely in the future.
◆ The birth canal is given the chance to expand gradually which means that forceps are rarely needed.
◆ The upright posture takes pressure off the diaphragm making all breathing easy and comfortable.
◆ Muscular tension and back pain is reduced and therefore less distracting during labor.
◆ The upright position is mechanically efficient, putting less strain on the spine and the joints of the pelvis. It's easier for a partner or friend to help during labor.

None of the positions for labor is right or wrong; you will need to find the most comfortable position for you and that is likely to change as your labor progresses.

You can minimize the possibility of damaging the pelvic floor muscles during labor by performing pelvic floor exercises all the way through pregnancy to keep the muscles and tissues firm. During labor, try and opt for an upright position and move about for at least part of the time. As soon as your baby is born try to start doing your pelvic floor exercises.

POSITIONS FOR LABOR

Lean on your partner so that the baby's weight is taken off your spine. He can massage your back.

Place a cushion over the back of a chair, and lean onto it with your knees bent. This is comfortable during the first stage of labor.

If your baby is in the posterior position, get down on all fours to relieve pressure on your spine.

LABOR

PAIN RELIEF

A big decision for women is whether or not to go for natural childbirth which relies on breathing exercises to counteract anxiety and pain without recourse to synthetic painkillers, or to take advantage of the array of analgesics which are available for childbirth.

This is not always an easy decision to take and you should talk over the subject with your partner, as many friends as possible who have had children and your doctors and midwives. Also gather as much information as you can on alternatives by reading about them.

In my experience, the decision not to have painkillers seems easier for women than the decision to accept pain relief. If you do accept pain-killing drugs in labor, remember that besides relieving pain they will make you feel calm and sleepy and some may send you to sleep. Others may make you feel light-headed and not quite in the normal world because you will lose some awareness of what is happening around you. As many women want to experience the full force of childbirth, this interference with their normal function is unacceptable.

You must also consider that most drugs will cross the placenta to the baby once you have taken them and will probably be in a higher concentration in your baby's blood than in your own. Some women cannot accept this.

Quite rightly, every woman enters labor believing that she is stoical and able to go without painkillers. However, it's impossible to know your own pain threshold in advance and any problems can't be predicted, so go into labor with an open mind and if you really feel in need of pain relief, consider it seriously when offered. If you accept it, don't feel guilty. On the other hand, don't be forced to take analgesics earlier than you want. A supportive word from your partner or friend may help you to get through a sticky patch. Don't feel victimized into going without painkilling drugs.

Tranquilizers

Given in small doses during the first stage of labor, these are designed to reduce anxiety and make you sleepy. The most common tranquilizer used in childbirth is Valium.

If you fall asleep or are too drowsy, you may wake confused and unable to get to grips with your labor. These drugs may depress the baby's respiration too.

Analgesics

These numb the pain center in the brain and are used to reduce anxiety and tension as well as dull the pain. They are used much as a surgeon uses premedication to relax a patient prior to surgery.

In many hospitals, meperidine (Demerol) is given routinely in the first stage of labor. The argument for analgesics such as meperidine is that if the first stage of labor is protracted, the mother will be exhausted, but with modern aids, protracted labors are less likely and meperidine doesn't work as a painkiller for all women anyway. It does have side effects, such as nausea and a sense of unreality. It is a narcotic after all. Added to that, it crosses the placenta making the baby drowsy at birth.

Inhalation analgesia or gas and air (often a mixture of oxygen and nitrous oxide) is self-administered just before the peak of the contraction and makes you feel light-headed. One of the main advantages of this form of pain relief, even if it doesn't work, is that it gives you something to do during difficult contractions.

Inhalation analgesia is best used during the first stage of labor. You need all your wits about you at the second stage when you push the baby out. The nitrous oxide does reach the baby but so does the oxygen, so there are benefits.

Anesthetics

These dull your conscious appreciation of pain and are the most successful means of having a "pain-free" labor.

Epidural anesthesia relieves the pain but leaves you consciously able to participate in the birth. The epidural is used even with Caesarean sections. It does greatly increase the technology surrounding your birth as you will need an intravenous drip to keep your fluid levels up should your blood pressure fall, a catheter because you may lose the sensations in your bladder, a fetal monitor and a monitor to record your contractions.

A general anesthetic is only necessary if you need an emergency Caesarean section.

Local anesthetics are used at delivery in case you need forceps or vacuum extraction, or when you have a tear or episiotomy stitched. These are administered into the perineum or the vaginal wall.

Other methods

Acupuncture is used successfully by women in labor. You will require thorough knowledge of how it works and be familiar with what is required of you.

Transcutaneous nerve stimulation (TENS) is a method from Sweden which uses the body's natural pain-killers, the endorphins. They are stimulated by means of an electrical current, administered through electrodes attached to your body, and you can regulate their intensity to suit your needs.

NATURAL CHILDBIRTH

The combination of relaxation techniques and breathing as a means of relieving pain during childbirth is an old idea. One method is known as psychoprophylaxis – using the mind to prevent fear and pain.

There are many different methods and they are taught at childbirth classes and through childbirth groups. You will be advised to attend

POSITIONS FOR DELIVERY

During labor you will have found comfortable positions you prefer and it could be one of these that you choose to deliver in.

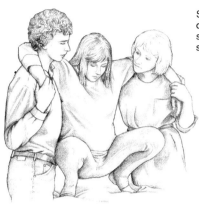

Squatting is an ideal delivery position. If you squat on a bed, you should be supported.

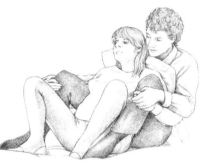

In this semi-upright position, you can lean back against your partner as support.

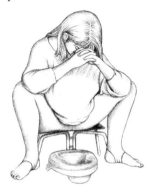

Forms of birthing stool have been used for centuries. Try one out to see what it's like.

the classes and practice regularly with your partner.

This method requires that you understand fully what is happening to you at any stage in your labor. You will need to learn how to relax both physically and mentally. You can be helped here by your partner through eye contact or massage, for example.

BREATHING TECHNIQUES

If you learn the different levels of breathing you can use them for different stages of labor to help you to relax, control your body and calm yourself down as the contractions become stronger.

Deep breathing
This is ideal at the beginning and end of contractions. To check that you are doing it properly, get someone to place their hands on your lower back. As you inhale, their hands should move. Deep breathing is calming.

Light breathing
At the height of a contraction, you should breathe fast and short. You only aerate the top part of your chest so that you move hands placed on

your shoulder blades. Keep your lips slightly apart and breathe in through your throat.

Featherlight breathing
During transition when the contractions are fast and difficult, yet you are trying not to bear down until the cervix has fully dilated, you should pant to stop yourself pushing. These breaths are short and rapid, limiting your ability to push downwards, but don't hyperventilate or you'll feel faint. Pant for 15 seconds and then hold your breath for 5 seconds. You can even think the rhythm of the "pant, pant, blow."

PHYSICAL RELAXATION

If you tense some part of your body, such as your fist, and then let go, you can notice the difference. This is the basis for one relaxation technique during childbirth. To learn this technique, you give orders in sequence to parts of your body to tense and then release the tension. You will then be able to appreciate the sensation of relaxation and you can achieve this during a contraction and let the uterus contract without the rest of your body tensing up too. Your

partner can help by recognizing whether you are tense, and indicating this with a gentle touch so you let go. You can practice this daily.

- ◆ Lie down in a comfortable position and close your eyes.
- ◆ With your hands by your side, palms upwards, think about your right hand.
- ◆ Tense it and let it go. Tell your hand to feel heavy and warm.
- ◆ Press your elbow into the bed or floor and let go.
- ◆ Concentrate on the right side of your body and tense and relax through your forearm, upper arm and shoulder. Raise your shoulder and let go.
- ◆ Repeat on the left side of your body.
- ◆ Relax your hips by rolling your knees outwards. Press your back into the floor or bed and let go.
- ◆ Your breathing should have slowed down by now. Check that it has.
- ◆ Shut your mouth and drop your jaw, with your tongue on the floor of your mouth. Think about your face and smooth it in your mind to get rid of any frowns.

LABOR

ELECTRONIC FETAL MONITORING

If you decide to accept the high-tech birth that your hospital offers, you will be wired up for electronic monitoring to check on your contractions and the baby's heart beat. What the equipment amounts to is a high-tech stethoscope and fetoscope.

How does it work?

You'll have belts strapped around your body and a tiny electrode will be clipped to the baby's head. Your contractions and the baby's heart beat are recorded on a paper print-out. There is also a video screen recording contractions and heart beats as visible waves, punctuated by flashing lights.

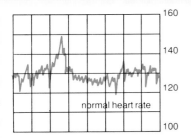

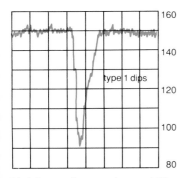

A baby's normal heart rate is around 130 beats per minute. The rate rises on contractions but any dip either during or between contractions can indicate fetal distress.

During a contraction, blood flow to the placenta is blocked for a second. If the baby is getting enough oxygen, the heartbeat should remain steady. The hospital staff will be watching the print out for signs of a dip in the line that traces the heart rate.

To have the electrode applied to your baby's head, the waters are broken when the cervix is at least two to three centimeters dilated. In addition to the baby's monitor, which picks up its heart beat, a second may be placed between the baby and the wall of the uterus to measure the pressure inside the uterus as it contracts and the rate of uterine contractions. An obvious disadvantage of this kind of electronic fetal monitoring (EFM) is that you are unable to move around during labor.

Another more subtle disadvantage to EFM has shown up. Because staff are more aware of small changes, they are more likely to intervene in the labor than let it take its natural course. In addition, three times as many babies who are electronically monitored are delivered by Caesarean section.

EFM greatly increases the amount of electronic equipment in the delivery room making it sterile and clinical in atmosphere, as are the staff who concentrate more on the machine than on you.

The latest type of EFM uses radio waves. This is known as telemetry. There are no wires or connections to the monitoring equipment, therefore you are free to walk about the room. The baby's monitor is attached to a transmitter strapped to your thigh.

When is it necessary?

You will always have electronic monitoring if you are being induced or your labor is being accelerated for any reason. High-risk pregnancies, such as if you are diabetic or have high blood pressure, or where you have an epidural, also need monitoring.

PROBLEMS IN LABOR

With vigilant prenatal care any possible problems during labor should be anticipated. These include conditions such as placenta previa when the placenta is low in the uterus and can impede the birth of the baby. Disproportion, when the pelvic cavity is too narrow to permit the baby's head to pass down the birth canal, should be picked up at your first prenatal visit. In these cases, a Caesarean section will probably be carried out, although your medical advisers may allow you to undergo a trial of labor to see if a normal vaginal delivery is possible.

The position of the baby in the uterus will be established by the 36th week. If the baby is breech, occipito posterior or transverse, this can lead to a prolonged labor.

Some factors that aren't always predicted are a prolonged labor because of a so-called "lazy" uterus when the uterus can't contract strongly or regularly enough. You may need an intravenous drip to induce stronger contractions, a Caesarean section or forceps.

About 5% of babies are born before 37 weeks when they are premature babies. A baby born at 39 weeks but weighing less than 2.5kg (5lb) may also be called premature.

The baby will probably need to go into the neonatal intensive care unit so that temperature, feeding and respiration can be monitored and controlled. You will have to be patient and stay near to your baby's incubator and involve yourself with your baby as much as is possible.

SEE ALSO:

CAESAREAN SECTION
EPIDURAL ANESTHETIC
INDUCTION
MULTIPLE PREGNANCY
PLACENTA PREVIA
PRENATAL CARE
PROLAPSE

LAPAROSCOPY

Certain conditions can be diagnosed accurately only if they are actually viewed. Laparoscopy is a procedure which enables a doctor to see the inside of the abdominal cavity, and organs such as the gallbladder, liver and uterus. Its most common use is in gynecology to view the pelvis and pelvic organs.

The instrument used is called a laparoscope. It is a long metal tube with a lens and a light source at one end and a telescope at the other. The lighting source allows the abdominal cavity to be seen through the telescopic eyepiece.

Why is it done?

Laparoscopy is most commonly used to examine the female reproductive organs to discover or diagnose:

◆ Reasons for infertility
◆ Reasons for abdominal pain
◆ Vaginal bleeding
◆ Fibroids or cysts
◆ Ectopic pregnancy
◆ Whether conception has occurred.
◆ Sometimes the laparoscope is used in minor surgical operations such as during the sterilization technique tubal ligation.

How is it done?

If laparoscopy is for a minor operation such as tubal ligation, you may be offered an epidural anesthetic, but generally laparoscopy is done under a general anesthetic.

First the abdomen is cut open, usually just below the navel so that no scar is visible afterwards. A needle is inserted into the abdomen and carbon dioxide gas is pumped into the abdominal cavity. This inflates the cavity and clears a space so the area is better seen. The needle is withdrawn and the laparoscope is passed in. The doctor angles it to get a clear view of the area as well as the suspect organs. If other instruments are being used, these are inserted through a second incision above the pubic line.

The procedure usually takes about 30–40 minutes and you will have one or two stitches. After about two hours, depending on the reason for the procedure, you should be allowed home. Any remaining gas and the site of the incision may give you a little discomfort for one or two days but there should be no other problems. This is a very safe procedure and it is now more commonly used than culdoscopy where an incision is made in the vaginal wall.

HAVING A LAPAROSCOPY

The procedure may involve an overnight hospital stay, or it may be an out-patient procedure in which you may leave, with assistance, after a few hours. A local or general anesthetic will be given. Exploration such as for endometriosis involves only one small incision. Any operative technique, such as tubal ligation, will require two incisions in order to permit the passage of instruments. Carbon dioxide gas is used to inflate the abdominal cavity so a good view can be obtained of the internal cavity.

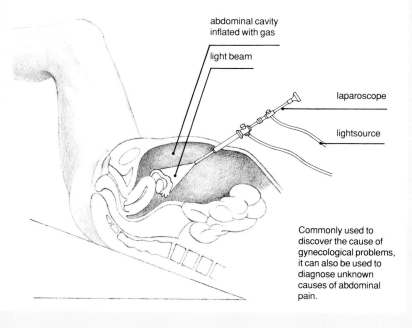

abdominal cavity
inflated with gas

light beam

laparoscope

lightsource

Commonly used to discover the cause of gynecological problems, it can also be used to diagnose unknown causes of abdominal pain.

SEE ALSO:

ENDOMETRIOSIS
FIBROIDS
INFERTILITY
OVARIAN CYSTS
**PELVIC INFLAMMATORY
  DISEASE**
TUBAL LIGATION

LUNG CANCER

There are two basic types of lung cancer. The most common is known as bronchogenic carcinoma. It is highly malignant and rapid growing. Bronchogenic carcinoma is associated with smoking, being triggered by certain chemicals including the tars in cigarettes. It does, however, take 10, 15 or even 20 years to develop.

A second type, oat cell carcinoma, is unrelated to smoking; it is much rarer than the first.

At one time bronchogenic carcinoma was extremely rare in women; it was predominantly a disease of men. (Oat cell carcinoma has always affected men and women equally.) The incidence of bronchogenic carcinoma mirrored our smoking habits. Very few women smoked until the last world war, but now they do increasingly. Smoking is declining among the male population, but not the female. Now the figures for lung cancer in women are a quarter those of men. It is expected that in the next few years lung cancer will become the number one cause of death from cancer in women – overtaking deaths from cancer of the breast.

· **S y m p t o m s** ·

▲ Lung cancers are nearly always "silent" until they are large enough to cause symptoms
▲ Troublesome chest symptoms that won't go away or keep recurring. Bronchitis is present in about half the people who eventually contract lung cancer
▲ Dry cough, not just the usual smoker's cough
▲ Yellow sputum
▲ Blood streaked sputum
▲ Loss of weight
▲ Lack of appetite
▲ Tightness in the chest, some difficulty breathing

Should I see the doctor?
If you are a smoker, you may develop symptoms of some of the other

SMOKING AND WOMEN

More women are smoking than ever before. Men seem to have responded to the anti-smoking campaigns of the last 20 years. In 1965, the proportion of men who smoked was 52%, whereas in 1987, it was only 33%. The proportion of women who smoked in 1965 was 34% and in 1987, that proportion had gone down only to 28%.

Smoking is still seen as a mark of independence in a woman, and many women have not got to the point of taking anti-smoking publicity seriously.

Women have also increased the number of cigarettes they smoke. Up until the 1940s it was considered not quite the thing for a woman to smoke; by 1950 the average woman was smoking about half as many cigarettes as a man, but now women have made up much of the difference.

Girls are starting to smoke earlier than they ever did and in some Western countries there is a greater proportion of young girls smoking than young boys. It is the first time that this has ever occurred in the history of smoking; smoking rates have doubled since 1964, but have remained stable for teenage boys.

Women find it harder to stop smoking than men. They have lower success rates in all the socio-economic classes, every kind of professional occupation and all age groups. Even when groups are highly motivated, men are twice as successful at stopping smoking than women, irrespective of the method they use. Another sad statistic is that women who give up smoking seem to return to cigarettes more rapidly than men. A Canadian study showed that after a year, one third of the men were true non-smokers whereas only one fifth of the women had been successful.

smoking-related health problems such as bronchitis, emphysema or heart disease. Any change in your cough or chronic chest symptoms should lead you to consult your doctor. However, in many cases it could be symptoms from the spread of the cancer to a secondary site that cause you to visit your doctor. Lung cancer most often affects the brain, bones, liver and skin.

If you ever see blood in your sputum, report it immediately to your doctor.

What will the doctor do?
Routine chest X-rays are the only hope of picking up an early lung cancer and are essential every year for women who smoke. Your doctor will refer you for a chest X-ray and possibly bronchoscopy when a fiber-optic tube is inserted into your lungs to look for cancerous growths. If the disease is present and suspected in

the early stages, surgical removal of the affected part of your lung offers the best chance of a recovery.

If the disease is advanced, radiation therapy treatment will be applied. This slows down the progress of the cancer and can relieve symptoms.

Another method of treatment is with cytotoxic drugs. These have been fairly successful although they have the disadvantage of unpleasant side effects. They are administered over a long period of time.

The treatment you are offered will depend on your general medical condition and the spread of the disease.

What is the prognosis?
The prognosis for cancer of the lung is never very good. This is because the blood supply to the lungs is so rich that the possibility of one or two cancer cells breaking off, getting into the blood and finding their way to a

HEALTH RISKS OF SMOKING

Women's adherence to smoking shows up in the health statistics. In 1985, 38,839 American women died from lung cancer. It has been worked out that one woman dies of lung cancer every hour of every day thoughout the whole year – almost all due to their smoking.

Cigarettes are a major cause of heart disease in women just as they are in men. This is the number one killer of both genders. In the United States, 398,175 men and 372,938 women died of heart diseases in 1985. This means that more women die of heart disease than all forms of cancer combined together.

Irrespective of other risk factors, a woman who smokes 20 cigarettes a day is twice as likely to die of a heart attack as a women who doesn't smoke at all. A woman who smokes and takes the oral contraceptive pill as well will multiply the risk. Thus a woman who smokes 20 cigarettes a day and takes the oral contraceptive pill is about 40 times as likely to have a heart attack as a woman who neither smokes nor takes the pill.

distant part of the body where they re-grow is extremely high. It is very difficult to treat distant spread effectively. Cancer of the lung characteristically spreads to the brain with an uncomfortable and unpleasant death.

What can I do?

There are a number of ways you can avoid or prevent lung cancer:

◆ Don't start smoking.
◆ If you do smoke, stop. If cancer hasn't started, you have a good chance of never contracting the disease.
◆ From the age of 40 onwards, have annual, routine chest X-rays as part of your general medical check-ups.
◆ Report all chronic chest complaints to your doctor.
◆ If your partner smokes, insist that he stops, and if you work in a smoke-filled environment, change jobs. You are at risk from "passive smoking."

What is passive smoking?

The first evidence on passive smoking came from Japan where it was suggested that non-smoking wives of smokers suffer a higher risk of developing lung cancer than the wives of non-smokers. Since then, further research has been done in several other countries and it is now estimated that the non-smoking spouse of a smoking partner has a 30% increased risk of developing lung cancer over two non-smoking partners.

Perhaps the worst effect of a smoker in the house is on children. The children of smokers not only become smokers more often than the children of non-smokers but they also suffer worse health. They are prone to coughs and colds in the winter, they have more chest disease and are admitted to hospital more often for serious chest infections.

SEE ALSO:

CANCER
COUGHING
HEART DISEASE
RADIATION THERAPY

MAMMOGRAPHY

This is a diagnostic tool for detecting breast cancer. It is a technique that uses X-rays in small doses to examine the breast and show up variations in consistency. A baseline mammogram should be done between the ages of 35 and 39.

Why is it done?

A tumor will appear as a white patch, denser than the rest of the breast and therefore impenetrable to certain X-rays even before it can be felt by manual examination. Mammography can sometimes even detect the difference between benign and malignant conditions.

Should mammography be used routinely?

It is recommended that women have a baseline mammogram between the ages of 35 and 39. From the ages of 40 to 49, women should have a mammogram every one to two years or as their physician advises. Screening for breast cancer is recommended annually only for women over 50 and those who fall into a high risk category. This is because the doses of radiation absorbed during the procedure may cause cancer to develop if the X-rays are taken too frequently. Mammography is also used during check-ups following mastectomy to check the health of the other breast.

SEE ALSO:

BREAST CANCER
BREAST OPERATIONS
BREAST SELF-EXAMINATION
MASTECTOMY

HOW A MAMMOGRAM IS DONE

This is a painless procedure for which you strip to the waist and sit in front of a small table. Your breast is placed in various positions under a cone-shaped device which takes the X-rays. This technique is particularly useful for the examination of large breasts because there is a greater contrast. However, a trained radiologist will detect any cysts or tumors in even the smallest breasts.

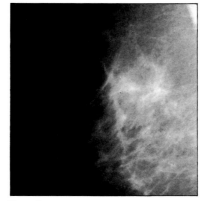

Normal

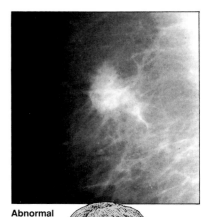

Abnormal

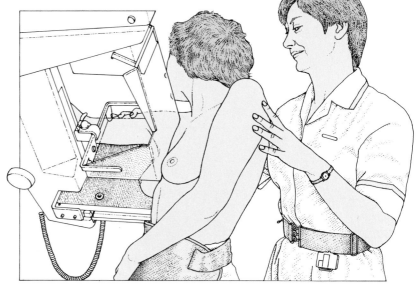

Each breast is placed on a small examination plate and up to 3 different pictures made for diagnostic purposes

MASTECTOMY

This is the partial or complete removal of the breast as a method of treatment for breast cancer. It is used in conjunction with drugs and X-ray therapy whenever there is danger of the cancer spreading. Some women who suffer from intractable benign breast disease where lumps and cysts keep developing may be offered mastectomy and reconstruction to give them peace of mind.

There are various kinds of mastectomy.

What choice have I got?

On the whole, the more destructive operations are no longer performed because the medical profession has accepted the huge psychological stress involved in any type of breast surgery. Physicians today seek to rebuild a woman's sense of self along with her breast. They also regard the avoidance of unpleasant side-effects as a high priority. The two-stage approach whereby only a biopsy is performed before the cancer is categorized according to its spread and potential, means that surgeon and patient can take a careful, considered approach to the treatment. Then, the least destructive surgical option and a combination of radiation therapy and drugs will mean less unpleasant side effects, and the least change to a woman's previous shape.

The ideal reconstruction is achieved with cosmetic surgery because the majority of women want to forget about their cancer and an external prothesis serves as a reminder, too.

What happens during the operation?

The procedure is carried out under general anesthesia in hospital, and takes from one to two hours depending on the type of mastectomy performed. In radical mastectomy, the skin incision extends from the armpit, sweeps across the breast to encompass the nipple and a quantity of skin overlying the cancerous lump, to end near the midline. The surgeon removes the whole of the breast including its axillary tail (that which extends into the armpit), the chest muscles, and any lymph glands with their surrounding fat from the armpit. The skin which has been undercut to remove as much tissue as possible is then stitched to cover the bare ribs. A suction drainage tube is used to prevent any collection of blood or tissue fluid in what is an extensive raw area under the skin. Sometimes a skin graft is needed to close the wound without undue tension. The skin scars are extensive, but fade within the year.

For a simple mastectomy, the whole breast, the nipple, some skin overlying the cancer and often part of the chest muscle, are removed using a shorter skin incision and not extending into the armpit.

In a lumpectomy only part of the breast containing the cancer with a fringe of normal tissue is removed through a small incision.

LUMPECTOMY

This is the first option for a very small tumor which has not yet spread to the lymph nodes in the armpit – the axillary nodes. It involves surgical removal of the lump, and at the same time, the lymph nodes are checked for the spread of the disease. Lymph nodes are capillaries which drain the breasts (and other organs). In this role, they may hold up the spread of the cancer cells. If no cancer cells are found in the lymph nodes, this is a sign that the disease is not yet spreading.

With the lump removed, spread of the disease is prevented with X-ray therapy or anti-cancer drugs or a combination of both. Anything more than a lumpectomy is clearly not justified if the cancer has already spread to various organs

How long will I be in hospital?

You will usually spend a week in hospital – less for removal of a lump, more for a radical procedure. The drainage tubes remain for 2-3 days, the bulky dressing is changed and reduced in volume as healing proceeds, and the stitches are removed alternately from the fifth to the tenth days.

Because the nerves will have been severed, your whole chest will feel numb for some time. Sensations in the chest and upper arm can take months to return. If you experience any restrictions in arm function, you will be given physical therapy to help you regain your physical fitness and to help blood circulation and healing. Return to normal activity may take up to six months; fatigue and tightness over the scar will be the major problems.

What happens after leaving hospital?

There are three stages of recovery after this operation. The immediate in the body.

Whether you have a lumpectomy, with or without radiation therapy, will depend very much on the stage of your disease. If you fall somewhere in the middle between a small tumor and established cancer, only your surgeon can advise you on the best course. If your breast cancer is diagnosed early, you should always discuss the possibility of a lumpectomy with your doctor.

After the operation, your breast will not look very different from the way it did before.

MASTECTOMY

MASTECTOMY OPERATIONS

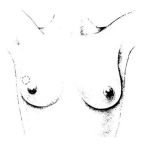

Lumpectomy or tylectomy
Only the lump is removed. This is done when lumps are small. It's the least invasive procedure and the breast will look almost completely normal.

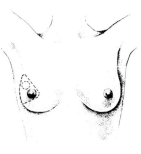

Partial mastectomy
The tumor and a sizeable amount of surrounding breast tissue plus the underlying skin and tissue are removed. The affected breast will be smaller after the operation.

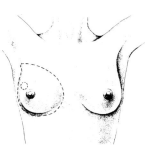

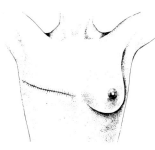

Modified radical mastectomy
This is based on the Halsted operation, but the pectoral muscles are not removed.

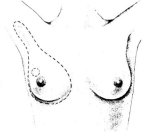

Simple (or total) mastectomy
The whole of the breast is removed, leaving the pectoral muscle and the axillary nodes. The last lymph node in the breast itself is taken out to check if the cancer has spread. This is the most common surgical treatment.

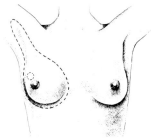

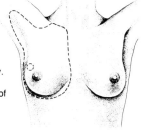

Extended radical mastectomy
This is rarely performed today. It is extremely mutilating and sometimes involves removal of ribs and the nodes above the collar bone.

Radical mastectomy
This operation was perfected by Dr. Halsted in 1894 and as it is so mutilating, it is rarely used today. It involves removal of all the tissues of the breast, axillary lymph nodes and pectoral muscles. As the pectoral or chest muscles help you move your arm, impairment of your arm function may be a permanent result of this operation.

Subcutaneous mastectomy
The internal breast tissue is shelled out, leaving the areola and nipple intact and enough skin to cover a silicone implant. The implant is usually done some months later. The axillary lymph nodes may be removed too. This is a highly skilled operation and is not universally available as it requires specialist cosmetic surgeons.

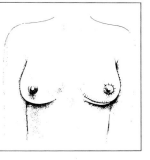

post-operative period will involve counseling and support to help you get over grief about the mutilation and perhaps some physical therapy. You will then need a post-operative course of drugs and/or X-ray treatment in which case you will be visiting the radiation therapy department regularly. There are often unpleasant side effects, such as hair loss, retching and sore throat or tongue. Tell your therapist about any symptoms you have and the doses will be readjusted accordingly.

You will have checkups at about three-monthly intervals when you will be thoroughly examined. This will include liver palpation, blood count and mammograms to screen the other breast. If there is any suggestion that your tumor is hormone-dependent, you may need hormonal therapy or be advised to consider surgical removal of your ovaries (ovariectomy), adrenal and pituitary glands.

After your operation you will be given a temporary breast form to fit inside your bra. This removes any embarrassment about your shape. It is very light and won't press against the scar tissue. When the tenderness around the scar fades, you can have a prothesis fitted. These are inserted in your bra to give you back your normal shape. It moves like a breast and is the weight of a normal breast so you don't feel lopsided. It can fit into a pocket in your bra or be held in place by ribbons or velcro.

The final stage is reconstructing the breast by mammoplasty. This can be done three months after mastectomy and for many women is a vital component before a return to normal life after breast surgery.

Because most mastectomy patients are now prepared for the removal of the breast before it happens, the adjustment is not so difficult for those with the close support of partner, family and

Breast prostheses
There is a variety available which can be simply fitted into a bra, or you can have a bra made which incorporates one. Materials used simulate the look, texture and feel of a normal breast. Most breast cancer units have special departments where prostheses are individually designed and made.

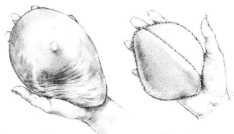

For general wear   For swimwear

specialists. Women whose relationships were rocky before or who are menopausal and perhaps already had psychological problems may have a harder time and should seek all the help therapists and psychiatrists can provide.

What can I do to help myself?
After the amputation of a breast you not only have to recover from the physical discomfort but also from a heavy mental strain. It is therefore quite understandable that you will sometimes suffer from depression. In your own interest and in your family's interest, you should, however, attempt to regain your joy of living as soon as possible and try to continue your normal every-day life as usual.

Be confident! You will see that your optimism will inspire the same in the people around you. Your partner, children, friends and relations will stand by you; trust in them. Don't hide your feelings. To cut yourself off would be fundamentally wrong. Socialize, and make certain you continue to see people even when you feel you don't want to.

Try to make contact with women in the same situation as yourself. There are self-help groups associated with mastectomies and with breast cancer. If you exchange ideas and experiences with others in the same situation you will feel less alone and isolated and they may have practical solutions to

problems that are worrying you.

Pay attention to your posture. After a mastectomy some women have a tendency to walk slightly bent forward. This will neither improve your back nor your figure.

Exercise can be especially important as the arm and shoulder on the side of the missing breast are often stiff after a mastectomy. Special exercises will be shown you in the hospital. Make certain you practice them regularly.

Points to bear in mind
◆ Make certain you see your doctor regularly
◆ Immediately report the following symptoms: swelling of the arm changes in the area of the operation changes in the remaining breast

---

SEE ALSO:

BREAST CANCER
BREAST OPERATIONS
COSMETIC SURGERY
MAMMOGRAPHY
OVARIAN PROBLEMS
RADIATION THERAPY

MENOPAUSAL PROBLEMS

Menopause or "climacteric" means the cessation of monthly periods. It is the transition between the child-bearing and non-reproductive years. Many women experience the symptoms, which signal menopause, during the time that menstruation begins to decline. Periods become less and less frequent or heavy and then menstruation finally stops. Old-fashioned phrases like the "change of life" imply that menopause means an unavoidable decline in life. This is not so. In fact, most women find that life improves.

What causes them?

The decline in monthly periods is only a symptom of a parallel decline in the production of female hormones by your body. What started at puberty with your first periods and the change in your physical shape, now wanes as ovarian activity falls off and you fail to ovulate. Nearly all the symptoms of menopause are referrable to decreasing levels of estrogen and progesterone in your blood.

How does it happen?

During your late forties or early fifties, raised levels of stimulating hormones cause an imbalance that disturbs the normal functioning of the ovaries. It appears that the ovary becomes resistant to the follicle stimulating hormone (FSH) and so fails to produce eggs every month. Occasionally the pituitary gland sends out high levels of FSH and ovulation occurs. However, this change in the normal cycle eventually leads to less estrogen being secreted by the ovaries and there is an alteration in the normal menstrual pattern.

Sudden cessation of periods is rare. By far, the majority of women continue periods for a few months, then miss a few, on and off, then go longer and longer between periods until they eventually stop. A guideline is that if you are over 50 and your periods stop for 6-12 months,

There are a large number of symptoms associated with menopause and they may include any or all of the following. Non-physical symptoms often associated with menopause include:
▲ Depression
▲ Irritability
▲ Tearfulness and inability to cope
▲ Loss of libido
▲ Insomnia

Physical symptoms include:
▲ Hot flashes

▲ Night sweats

▲ Itchiness of the perineum - vaginitis
▲ Vaginal dryness
▲ Pain on intercourse

▲ Fatigue and lack of energy
▲ Aches and pains, as a result of the bones softening

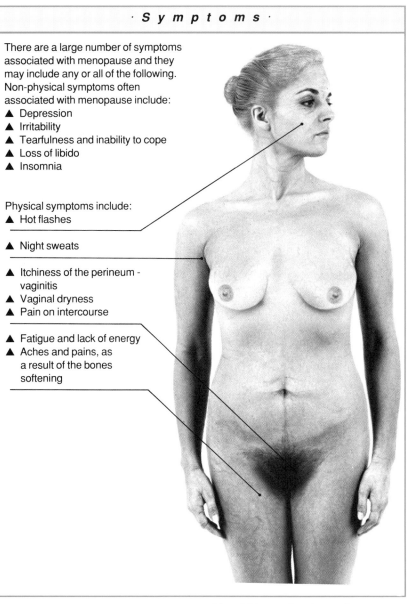

then it's likely they have stopped for good.

An artificial menopause with the accompanying symptoms will result after a total hysterectomy when the ovaries as well as the uterus is removed. Your physician should inform you of this, and prepare you for treatment to relieve symptoms.

Should I see the doctor?

By far the most common symptoms are night sweats and vaginal dryness. These can lead onto other symptoms such as insomnia and lack of desire. However, if any of the symptoms trouble you, or if you feel sad and depressed at the realization that you are no longer fertile, see your doctor right away.

It is never normal to have frequent heavy periods nor the passage of blood clots during menopause. Heavy bleeding or painful periods are not symptoms of menopause, so see your doctor if you experience these symptoms.

What will the doctor do?
By far the majority of women manage to cope with menopause. However, a doctor's unsympathetic attitude may make women view it as something to be suffered and beyond treatment. This is not so. Hormone therapy can replace the estrogen and progesterone so that the symptoms disappear. This treatment is almost 90% effective. If you feel your doctor isn't being very helpful or sympathetic, or won't let you try hormone therapy, go to another doctor.

Alternative methods of treating menopausal symptoms include dietary means. Calcium levels need to be kept up both before and after menopause because one of the after effects is a thinning and softening of the bones – osteoporosis. So plenty of calcium and Vitamin D is recommended.

You will need to watch your diet carefully. With the end of the protective effects of the female hormones, women are at equal risk with men from heart disease. Plenty of exercise and low-fat and low- sugar diets with healthy combinations of foods will keep this problem at bay.

Some emotional problems cannot be treated with hormone therapy and your doctor may prescribe tranquilizers and counseling to get you through the roughest patch.

What can I do?
Never view yourself as over the hill. Keep up your self respect and self assurance with your work, or retrain or get involved in volunteer activities. This is often the time in your life when your children leave home, adding extra stress when you may be least capable of coping with it.

On the other hand, many women experience a new lease of life once they are freed of reproductive responsibilities. We hear all the time about women who really come into their own in middle age. Women who have a positive view of menopause suffer fewer symptoms, less seriously. Remember that it marks the end of a phase of your life, and the beginning of another. It should not be a time for sadness and regret; it should be a time for looking forward to enjoying new interests.

MENORRHAGIA

This term describes menstruation when blood flow is unusually heavy. This may be a single bout of flooding, a period that goes on for a long time (say more than seven days) or very frequent periods so that the blood loss in any given month is excessive. On average only about 50ml (1.5–2 fl oz) of blood is lost at a single period; much of the vaginal secretion is mucus and the lining of the uterus.

What causes it?

This condition is common as women approach menopause when the lining of the womb (endometrial tissue) becomes extremely thick and there is consequently a heavier blood loss as the endometrial lining is shed. The recent fitting of an IUD can cause heavier periods for a few months afterwards. Fibroids may cause heavy bleeding because they increase the surface of the womb and its lining. A rare cause is an hormonal imbalance but this is most often characterized by irregular heavy flow.

If the rate of blood flow continues over several days for several periods, then anemia may develop, which if left untreated could become severe.

· S y m p t o m s ·

▲ Blood flow during menstruation so rapid and excessive that several sanitary pads must be worn at the same time

▲ Pallor, fatigue and breathlessness indicating anemia

Should I see the doctor?

If your periods change and become longer or much heavier than they were previously, see your doctor to check for the underlying cause.

What will the doctor do?

Your doctor will question you about your normal menstrual cycle and examine you for any abnormality of the uterus such as fibroids and for

signs of anemia. You may be given a blood test to determine if you are anemic and this will be treated with iron supplements to raise the iron content in your blood.

If you have an IUD fitted, your doctor may remove it or fit another device if it is not right for you.

The basis of treatment for menorrhagia where there is no disease of the uterus is hormone therapy aimed at preventing the build-up of endometrial tissue prior to menstruation. This is often the combined contraceptive pill unless you were already on the pill or it is unsuitable for you, in which case another drug will be prescribed. Danazol is a drug used to inhibit the over-production of the pituitary hormones. This can have unpleasant side-effects. If fibroids or some other cause is suspected, you will be given a D and C to scrape out the uterine lining. This is highly successful and used frequently as the first surgical remedy.

If the menorrhagia is grossly debilitating, there may be suggestion that the uterus is removed – an operation known as a hysterectomy. You should not agree to this operation without the fullest discussion with your gynecologist and your partner and only then after careful consideration. This surgical procedure is often performed and not always necessarily. You must consider a number of factors such as whether

you want to have children in the future.

What can I do?

If you have just one period with heavy bleeding, rest if you can and use absorbent sanitary pads with tampons to minimize embarrassment. Take a sensible precaution, particularly if you have had problems with anemia before, of increasing the iron content in your diet; liver, egg yolks and dark green leafy vegetables are rich in iron. To increase absorption of iron, take it with foods rich in Vitamin C. Cooking in iron pots also helps increase the iron content of food.

SEE ALSO

ANEMIA
BLEEDING
CERVIX PROBLEMS
CONTRACEPTION
DILATATION AND
   CURETTAGE
ENDOMETRIOSIS
FIBROIDS
HYSTERECTOMY
MENOPAUSAL PROBLEMS
PELVIC INFLAMMATORY
   DISEASE

METRORRHAGIA

This means bleeding between periods. It is sometimes called breakthrough bleeding. Except for the 10% of women who have a little spotting at the time of ovulation, metrorrhagia is always abnormal, particularly if it relates to intercourse. It may be a symptom of benign conditions such as cervical erosion or a cervical polyp. It may be because

an IUD has become dislodged or it may be the sign of a threatened miscarriage if you were pregnant. It is also a symptom of malignant conditions such as cancer of the cervix or uterus. If you ever have any spotting of red or brown blood between your periods, consult your doctor immediately.

MENSTRUAL PROBLEMS

Menstruation is a normal part of a woman's life. There aren't many things that can go wrong, and most of them are heralded by some change in your normal pattern so it is important to look at your personal cycle rather than be perturbed by facts and figures relating to the "average" woman.

The discharge we pass at menstruation is a mixture of mucus, blood and parts of the lining of the womb. It may seem like a lot but on average it is only about 50ml (1^1/$_2$-2 oz.). Disturbances of your normal cycle can be produced by various things, including stress, jet travel and the method of birth control you use. Menstruation can be controlled or completely suppressed with the contraceptive pill. There are many myths surrounding menstruation, both cultural and religious, such as not washing your hair or having sexual intercourse but there is no reason why you should not carry on during your period as you would at any time of the month. The changing levels of your hormones can induce difficult physical and emotional symptoms which are grouped under the umbrella heading of *premenstrual syndrome*.

However, there are disorders that you should be alerted to if you notice changes in your normal cycle. The most common disorder is painful periods when you have to rest or even go to bed every month, thus disrupting your normal life. This is *dysmenorrhea*. If your periods never start at all or stop suddenly, this is *amenorrhea*. The most common reason for amenorrhea when previously you had a normal cycle is, of course, *pregnancy*. This may also be the result of a change in your lifestyle. For example, extreme control of weight gain, *anorexia* or *bulimia*, may cause monthly periods to stop. Infrequent periods, fewer than 11 in a year, is known as *oligomenorrhea*.

If your periods are very heavy or very frequent, this is known as *menorrhagia*. Such loss of blood can result in anemia with symptoms of fatigue, listlessness and pallor.

MENSTRUAL PROBLEMS

Any change in the nature of your periods may indicate some problem in your womb or the surrounding area, such as *fibroids*, *endometriosis* or *pelvic inflammatory disease*.

Pregnancy brings about the most predictable changes in your cycle. There is a complete cessation of periods during pregnancy; this is one of the first symptoms. After the birth, your periods may take from 6 weeks to a year to return, especially if you breastfeed your baby.

The last period, *menopause*, usually occurs between 45 and 55 years of age and although this may be accompanied by distressing symptoms, it is no risk to your health.

There is a serious though extremely rare syndrome associated with menstruation that all women should be aware of. This is *toxic shock syndrome*. The major factor in avoiding this is to pay attention to hygiene during menstruation.

Bleeding from the vagina which occurs at times other than your period should be treated immediately.

MISCARRIAGE

Sometimes called spontaneous abortion, this refers to the loss of a fetus before 28 weeks of pregnancy. After this time, the death of the fetus is known as a stillbirth.

Spontaneous abortions are much more common than generally thought. Many occur that go undetected and many, if detected, go unreported. Up to a third of all first pregnancies miscarry but a second normal pregnancy usually follows. If you exclude early, unrecognized miscarriage, spontaneous abortion occurs in about 15 percent of all conceptions. Doctors feel that an abortion that occurs during the first trimester has done so for a very good reason, and it is usually as well that the pregnancy didn't continue.

What causes a miscarriage?
A spontaneous abortion can result because of parental, fetal or combined factors. These include:
- Defect in the egg or sperm resulting in an abnormal fetus
- Hormonal deficiency, particularly insufficient production of progesterone, the hormone that is basic to the maintenance of the pregnancy
- Abnormally shaped uterus which cannot carry a pregnancy because of some anatomical problem
- Uterine fibroids
- Incompetent cervix in which the cervix opens rather than remaining closed until labor begins; this is often the result of an unskilled induced abortion or a previous rapid labor
- Placental insufficiency; the placenta fails or does not develop properly and so cannot nourish the fetus
- Uncontrolled diabetes or severe high blood pressure
- Rhesus incompatibility
- Maternal infections – bacterial or viral such as syphilis or rubella

· S y m p t o m s ·
- ▲ Bleeding from the vagina
- ▲ Mucus in the vaginal blood
- ▲ Backache
- ▲ Abdominal cramps
- ▲ Fading of the physical symptoms of the pregnancy

Should I call the doctor?
If you know you are pregnant, or think you might be and experience any vaginal bleeding and/or cramping pain at any time, call your doctor immediately. While waiting for your doctor, go to bed and keep your feet raised. Wear a sanitary pad if necessary. Do not flush away any of the discharge as your doctor will want to examine it.

What will the doctor do?
With a threatened abortion, you will be advised to go to bed for 24 hours to wait and see. Bedrest increases the flow of blood to the uterus. Sometimes hormone treatment is given. The explanation for this may be vague and refer to a hormone imbalance. This means that hormones of pregnancy have failed to suppress the next menstrual period. Low hormonal levels usually lead to a miscarriage. In all cases, you will be advised to rest. An ultrasound scan will determine whether the fetus is still alive or whether there is any material left inside your uterus.

In some cases of miscarriage there may be a large loss of blood necessitating a blood transfusion.

If some products of conception remain after an incomplete abortion, you will need to be admitted to hospital for a D & C to remove it. If there is a missed abortion, the fetus will have to be removed surgically or by an induced labor.

If you habitually miscarry, you will have tests to find the specific cause. These include a hystero-salpingogram to check on the condition of your uterus and fallopian tubes. Your doctor will examine the aborted fetus and placenta as well in order to treat you accordingly. In some cases, you may be referred to an infertility expert.

If you have a septic abortion, you will be given antibiotics in large

TYPES OF MISCARRIAGE
Not all miscarriages are the same, and medical staff recognize the following:
- Threatened abortion is one that does not invariably lead to the loss of the fetus. There is spotting of blood but the cervix is closed.
- Inevitable abortion is where virtually nothing can prevent the expulsion of the fetus. It is accompanied by more severe vaginal bleeding and pain because your uterus is contracting.
- Complete abortion occurs when the fetus and placenta are expelled.
- Incomplete abortion happens when the fetus is expelled but some of the products of conception remain.
- Missed abortion occurs when the fetus dies in the uterus but remains there.
- Recurrent or habitual abortion is when three or more miscarriages have occurred at the same time and for the same reason in each pregnancy.
- Septic abortion happens if the abortion is followed by an infection. A high temperature and abdominal pain are the symptoms.
- Induced abortion is any termination of the pregnancy by medical means.

MISCARRIAGE

doses to combat infection which is the most frequent cause of maternal death following abortion. A D & C will be essential to remove the infected material. Infertility can result from such an infection.

What can I do to cope with the loss?

Whatever the reason for the miscarriage and whatever treatment your doctor decides to prescribe, the emotional effects of miscarriage can be devastating. As well as the natural feelings of grief, you will probably feel very angry that your body has let you down. The one emotion you must try to combat is guilt. It is not your fault and although you may feel like hiding yourself away, and perhaps punishing yourself, this is not the way to get back to normal. Try not to isolate yourself and try to be positive about what you can do in the future.

Anxiety is one of the emotional factors which can result in a failure to conceive. Your doctor should give you an honest answer as soon as possible about whether you can successfully carry a baby to full term without medical treatment. If so, keep trying, but also try not to get anxious about it. If you have some problem that can be treated, don't waste time being depressed but seek treatment.

You can usually resume sexual intercourse within three weeks, when the bleeding has stopped and the cervix has closed. You will probably be advised to wait for two menstrual periods before trying to conceive.

SEE ALSO:

ABORTION
CERVIX PROBLEMS
DIABETES MELLITUS
DILATATION AND
  CURETTAGE
HYSTEROSALPINGOGRAM
RHESUS INCOMPATIBILITY
RUBELLA
SYPHILIS
TERMINATION OF
  PREGNANCY

MOLES

Moles are pigmented birthmarks or nevi. Nearly every adult has one or two moles even if they are in their simplest form, the freckle. In some people with the tendency to develop moles, however, only a few are present at birth but new nevi appear during childhood. They can take various shapes and forms. Some moles have hairs growing out of them.

What are they caused by?
Moles are made up of dense collections of pigment cells or melanocytes. If these cells accumulate deep in the dermis rather than in the upper layers of skin or epidermis, they look blue. A common type of blue mole is called a mongolian spot and this type is most common among Mediterranean and black races.

The major problem with moles, aside from any concern about appearance, is that pigmented moles may become malignant and develop into a malignant melanoma, the most serious form of skin cancer.

Should I see the doctor?
Moles as a general rule should be left alone. If you already have moles, they may tend to become more deeply pigmented with time. However, if any of the following signs occur you should seek advice from your doctor as soon as possible:
- the mole enlarges
- the mole becomes darker in color
- the mole weeps, crusts or bleeds
- the outline of the mole becomes less distinct and irregular or it develops a black margin
- the mole becomes itchy
- a new mole appears
- in the elderly, large dark freckles appear.

If the mole is on the sole of your foot, or on your waistline, or where your bra strap might rub, you may want it removed. See your doctor.

What will the doctor do?
If your mole has changed character in even the smallest detail, your doctor will arrange for you to have a biopsy to find out if malignant change is present. The mole will be removed and examined for cancerous cells.

If there is some sign of cancer, the entire area will be excised and a skin graft may be used to cover the area. Radiation therapy might be necessary to prevent the spread of the disease.

If the mole is in an awkward place on your body, your doctor will arrange for its removal under general anesthesia.

What can I do?
If there are hairs growing from your mole, cut them back, pluck them or have them removed by electrolysis.

There are special ranges of cosmetics for camouflaging birthmarks. Visit your pharmacist to find the appropriate one for your skin type.

Moles can be excised for cosmetic reasons, but the scar may be about three times the diameter of the mole and you may not find this desirable.

SEE ALSO:

BIOPSY
BIRTHMARKS
COSMETIC SURGERY
RADIATION THERAPY
SKIN CANCER

MOOD CHANGES

Everyone experiences variations of mood. This is a normal, emotional response to life so we should expect them, learn to live with them, and deal with them. Mood changes show up differently in different people. Some will describe themselves as moody and confess to feeling fluctuations of temperament even throughout a single day. Others are quite untemperamental; they seem universally placid and little interferes with their steady good humor. At certain times of life, mood changes which are pronounced and out of character may be a symptom of some depressive illness or hormonal imbalance. During pregnancy, after childbirth, before menstruation and at the menopause many women complain of moodiness and depression.

Depending on the reason for your moodiness, you will probably be treated with either anti-depressives, hormone therapy or sleeping pills.

Whenever you are feeling positive emotions, try to preserve your feelings of happiness and contentment and concentrate on them. When you feel dragged down in mood, remember the good times. Prepare for changes in your life, such as menopause, by reading about the symptoms so you will be well prepared and not dismayed by any fluctuations of mood.

If you are unable to make a diagnosis from this chart consult your doctor.

NATURE OF THE PROBLEM	PROBABLE CAUSE
Your period is due	This could be part of the *premenstrual syndrome.*
You are over 45 and your periods are becoming irregular	This could be the onset of menopause (see *Menopausal problems*).
You have recently started a new brand of the contraceptive pill	Some brands can cause *depression*. Return to your clinic or doctor and suggest a change.
You have recently had a baby	This could be the "baby blues". If your baby was born more than a month ago, this could be *postpartum depression*. See your doctor immediately.
You have difficulty sleeping, are worried, and unhappy and your mood changes are cyclical, accompanied by other symptoms that interfere with your normal life	You could be suffering from *depression*. If your moods swing wildly from elation to misery, you could be suffering from manic depression. See your doctor right away.
You experience sudden changes of mood when you feel panic stricken	This could be a panic attack due to *anxiety*.

MORNING SICKNESS

Although this has passed into the language as "morning sickness", it may occur at any time of the day or night and throughout the day. It rarely causes actual vomiting and is often experienced as severe nausea with retching. It is most common during the first three months of pregnancy – the first trimester – and then it usually stops.

Some unlucky women suffer from these feelings of nausea and retching throughout pregnancy. However, there is no reason to suppose that having suffered from morning sickness during one pregnancy, you will suffer it in subsequent pregnancies.

· S y m p t o m s ·

- ▲ Feeling of nausea
- ▲ Retching
- ▲ Vomiting
- ▲ Intolerance of certain foods

What causes it?

It is not known precisely what causes nausea in pregnancy. It is most likely the effect of the increase in your circulating hormones. Added to this is the feeling of hunger. The sudden rush of hormones can have a direct effect on the lining of the stomach, producing a feeling of nausea. First thing in the morning, your blood sugar levels are low anyway and this is the major cause of true morning sickness. Sometimes, at other times of the day, the sensations may be triggered by the smell of tobacco smoke or frying food.

What is the treatment?

Because the first 12 weeks are a vital time in the growth and development of the fetus, you should not take any medication for morning sickness unless your doctor thinks it advisable. If your morning sickness is very serious, and you are vomiting several times a day and are unable to keep food down, you may suffer from dehydration and mineral imbalances.

NAUSEA REDUCING SNACKS

Here are some foods that you can have ready to damp down the feelings of nausea during the day. It is better to eat small snacks often rather than two or three main meals.

- ◆ Slices of toasted wholemeal bread or bread dried in the oven
- ◆ Hard cheese
- ◆ Nuts and raisins
- ◆ Dried apricots
- ◆ Green crisp apples
- ◆ Carbonated water with a slice of lemon or lime
- ◆ Fruit cake; wholemeal flour and wheatgerm give added nutrients
- ◆ Raw vegetables cut into lengths, for example, tomatoes, celery, carrots, young green beans, lettuce
- ◆ Natural yogurt, sweetened with honey, if necessary
- ◆ Fruit sorbet
- ◆ Fresh juice made into frozen ice cubes to suck
- ◆ Water crackers
- ◆ Sesame thin biscuits
- ◆ Commercial muesli bars

Your doctor may then help you by prescribing anti-nausea drugs which are known to be safe if used in the early weeks of pregnancy. You may feel you would rather persevere and try the self-help measures (below) rather than take medicines at this time.

What can I do?

There is no doubt that food provides relief from these irritating symptoms. Ironically at this time of feeling nauseous, you need to think about food a lot. You must keep yourself well nourished for your own and the baby's sake and you need to plan and prepare your snacks so the symptoms are kept at bay.

The following tips should help in combating nausea and obviate the need for medications.

- ◆ Keep a glass of milk by your bed and take it with a cookie or dry toast as soon as you wake in the morning. This will raise your blood sugar level.
- ◆ Avoid the triggers such as fried foods or smoke-filled rooms.
- ◆ Nutritious forms of carbohydrate are good to combat the nausea. Try slices of wholemeal bread, rice, potatoes and raw vegetables (see above).
- ◆ Rest so that tiredness doesn't exacerbate your nausea.

- ◆ Talk to other women who have suffered from morning sickness. Once you hear how others have experienced the same and it passed, you may come to terms with it, because it will go away.

> **SEE ALSO:**
>
> NAUSEA AND VOMITING
> PREGNANCY PROBLEMS

MOUTH PROBLEMS

The mouth is inhabited by many species of bacteria, but they are held in a delicate balance and should rarely present a problem unless you interfere with that balance. For example, sucking too many cough lozenges can lead to an overgrowth of the yeast that causes oral thrush (See *Yeast Infection*).

Smoking upsets this delicate balance too; it stains your teeth, and causes unpleasant bad breath (see *Body odors*). If you smoke a lot, the lining of your mouth and tongue can thicken as a reaction. This is known as leukoplakia or smoker's keratosis. It will disappear once you stop smoking. Another cause of bad breath is pyorrhea, a chronic infection of the gums (see *Gum Disease*). In fact, the most significant cause of tooth loss is not through tooth decay, but through diseases of the gums.

Cold sores generally appear on the lips and are unsightly and painful. They are caused by a virus similar to that which causes *genital herpes* and therefore it is inadvisable to have any oral/genital contact if you have either herpes infection.

Aphthous ulcers
These may reach such a large size that to the untrained eye they look malignant. They are extremely painful and last 10–14 days no matter what treatment is applied. However, steroids in a special base which clings to the gums and cheeks despite saliva may be effective. They are usually caused by some snag on the lining of the mouth, from a pitted tooth or a fingernail.

Oral lichen planus
This most commonly affects middle aged and elderly women and may also be present in the skin. It shows itself as a change in the lining of the mouth and the sides of the tongue; this change could be an outbreak of white pimples or shiny red patches. The cause is usually poor oral hygiene and a steroid drug will be prescribed. Although the tongue is subject to many different changes in texture, if any condition fails to improve in three weeks, see your doctor. Quite often this could be a symptom of another condition, such as *anemia*, when the tongue can become dark red and smooth.

MULTIPLE PREGNANCY

Bearing more than one child at a time tends to run in families. While the most common multiple pregnancy involves two babies, a multiple pregnancy can be triplets, quadruplets or quintuplets, particularly with the advent of fertility drugs used for infertile or sub-fertile couples. These are used to stimulate the ovary, but careful monitoring should prevent unnecessarily large numbers of babies, although the incidence of twins is increased with fertility drugs. In vitro fertilization techniques involve the transfer of more than one embryo to give a better chance of success. However, no more then three or four embryos would be transferred at a time.

Twins are born once in every 80 pregnancies, and it is this kind of pregnancy that I will be discussing here. Twins are either identical, formed from one fertilized egg splitting in two so that their genetic makeups are identical and they share the same amniotic sac and placenta, or fraternal, formed from two separate eggs each fertilized by a different sperm. These twins are no more alike than other brothers and sisters. They usually have their own placentas.

When should I suspect twins?

If you have a family history of twins (usually twins skip a generation) or if you are bigger than your dates suggest, or if an alpha fetaprotein blood test reveals raised levels at around 18 weeks when levels should be lower, a multiple pregnancy will be suspected.

What will the doctor do?

Even if there is no reason to suspect twins, with modern prenatal screening they will usually be detected by half way through your pregnancy. They can be spotted on ultrasound scan by eight weeks and the doctor should pick up two heart beats, particularly when using an electronic fetal stethoscope.

With advancing pregnancy, two or more heads can be felt as well as multiple arms and legs.

Once a multiple pregnancy is confirmed, you will have special care, with an emphasis on avoiding anemia. You are more susceptible to the anemia caused by insufficient folic acid. Your blood, therefore, will be checked regularly as well as your blood pressure. Your blood pressure must remain low so that your uterus doesn't go into labor prematurely – as is often the case with multiple pregnancy.

What will the birth be like?

Your labor may be somewhat longer than normal, though not necessarily more painful. Because the babies will need to be born in the hospital, you may be admitted before your due date. The danger is to the second baby who must be born quickly after the first.

You are likely to lose blood during the birth and require a transfusion. If one of the babies is in the breech position, your doctor may decide to deliver the twins by Caesarean section. This should be discussed beforehand so you can prepare yourself.

What can I do?

You should eat little and often to feel comfortable and keep your weight down. Eat salads and light snacks because you must avoid excess weight gain. Eat foods rich in iron such as egg yolk, liver and green leafy vegetables. You should

TYPES OF TWINS

There are two kinds – binovular or uniovular. Binovular twins are fraternal, and can be of different sexes; uniovular twins are identical and are always of the same sex.

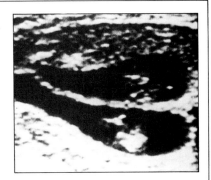

Twins
Ultrasound has proved an invaluable tool in establishing the presence of twins at an early stage of pregnancy.

Identical twins develop from one egg that splits into two. They share the same placenta but have their own cords and sacs. Fraternal twins each have their own placenta and are only as genetically similar as any two siblings of the same parents.

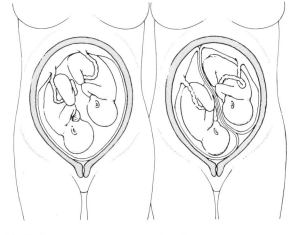

Identical   Fraternal

not neglect taking the supplements of folic acid prescribed by your doctor.

The main problem for you will be the size of your uterus which will crowd out your other organs causing such nuisances as heartburn, breathlessness, hemorrhoids, varicose veins, frequent urination and abdominal discomfort. If you notice any of these symptoms or swelling of your hands, ankles or face, alert your doctor immediately.

Rest as much as you can to keep your blood pressure down and prevent yourself becoming overtired. The heavy uterus puts more strain on your body than a single pregnancy. Don't stand up when you can sit down, and don't sit if you can lie down especially on your side.

Don't lift heavy loads; this increases the pressure inside your abdomen and strains muscles and joints. Always pay particular attention to posture. You can avoid backache this way.

You can take out insurance against having twins; this must be done before the eighth week of your pregnancy. However, insurance is not usually granted if you have taken a fertility drug, or if you have a history of twins in your family.

SEE ALSO:

ANEMIA
BREECH BIRTH
CAESAREAN SECTION
PREGNANCY PROBLEMS
PRENATAL CARE
ULTRASOUND
VARICOSE VEINS

NAIL PROBLEMS

The eyes may be the mirror of the soul but doctors feel that the nails are the mirror of the body. It takes nine months for a nail to grow from under the cuticle at the root to the fingertip and any health problems are indicated in the nails with pits, ridges and marks. If you're someone who constantly picks at the cuticles or presses them back, your nails will grow with minute ridges formed every time you press the cuticle far enough back to interfere with the nail root. Certain diseases show up in the nails as minute pits, for example, liver disease and psoriasis. Others show up as white marks, like cirrhosis of the liver (see *Alcoholism*).

When the body is traumatized, whether it's physical or emotional, there will be some sign of upset in the nails. With a profound infection or a surgical operation, nail growth may be disturbed and a broad ridge will appear in the nail coincidental with that event. Worry, anxiety, over-work or a protracted period of *insomnia* can also show up in the nails as lines and ridges. Quite often if you suffer *hair loss*, the nails may be affected as well, producing lines of weakness and pitting.

The greatest worries for women are thinning, weakness, cracking and splitting. All kinds of lotions and potions are applied to nails to strengthen them but usually the cause is not within your control, not even improving your diet or eating iron or calcium-rich foods will help. The health and strength of your nails depends on two main factors – a healthy blood supply and the use of detergents. The bed of the nail is rich in capillaries, but if these are shut down to conserve heat, then nail growth is impeded and distorted. For example, the nails are nearly always weakest in winter because the finger ends are often cold as there is insufficient circulation to the fingertips, and this naturally affects nail growth.

Strong biological detergents are de-fatting and as they are used almost universally by women several times a day, they soften and weaken the nail, encouraging cracking and splitting. The simple expedient of wearing rubber gloves for all household tasks will do more than any lotions to keep them strong.

NAIL PROBLEMS

Infections with fungi such as those that cause athlete's foot, cause thickening and painful lifting from the nail bed. As the fungus lies in the growing nail itself, it takes nine months to grow out. Anti-fungal medication will therefore need to be taken for nine months in severe cases. Monilia, which also causes thrush, commonly affects the nail folds down the side of the nails. This nearly always occurs in skin that is wet and sodden. Once the monilia is flourishing in the nail folds, painful abscesses can form. The only treatment is with an anti-fungal ointment.

If you pick at your nails or allow them to become wet and soft, you may develop a whitlow, an infection with staphylococcus aureus which forms painful collections of pus around the edge of the nail. Your doctor will have to lance it for you.

Psoriasis, with its peeling skin, *arthritis* and thickening and pitting of the nails, is an upsetting condition. Nails become a problem because they catch on everything, reducing manual dexterity. This condition of the nails is very difficult to treat; often the best you can do is keep them trimmed.

A blood blister usually results under the nail if you bang your finger or catch it in a door. This is painful because the collection of blood cannot expand under the rigid nail plate. An emergency self-help treatment is to release the blister with a sterile needle.

Clubbed fingers are a symptom of chronic lung disease. The fingernails curve round the ends of the fingers and the cuticles disappear. The reason why this should show up in lung disease is not known but it may appear early on in the illness.

NAUSEA AND VOMITING

Vomiting most commonly occurs when your stomach is irritated enough to contract and throw up the contents. There may be abdominal cramps depending on the cause of the vomiting. If so, don't take aspirin for the pain as this only irritates the stomach more.

Nausea is the sensation of impending vomiting and you should follow the same treatment of small sips of plain water only. Occasionally vomiting can be a symptom of some malfunction in the nerve signals from the brain, or in the inner ear.

If you are unable to make a diagnosis from this information, consult your doctor.

NATURE OF THE PROBLEM	PROBABLE CAUSE
You have missed a period and feel ill all day or just in the morning	This may be *morning sickness*, one of the first symptoms of your pregnancy.
You also have severe abdominal pain on the lower right side	This could be appendicitis. Call your doctor right away.
Nausea is accompanied by flashing lights, tingling down one side of your face and a blinding headache	This could be migraine. Lie down in a darkened room and take painkillers. See your doctor for a diagnosis.
You experience these symptoms when traveling	You probably suffer from travel sickness. Take anti-sickness pills before traveling.
You have recently received a blow to your head	You could have a brain injury. Get help immediately.
You have *diabetes mellitus*	You may be hypoglycemic. Drink milk or juice to raise your blood sugar level.
The vomiting follows suddenly and you have eaten within 2-4 hours	The food may have been spoiled and you could have food poisoning, or you may be allergic to some new food or have taken in chemicals. If you also have *diarrhea* and/or a *fever*, you could have dysentery or gastroenteritis. See your doctor if the vomiting continues for more than 48 hours.
You have drunk a lot of alcohol or eaten too much rich food	You probably have gastritis, inflammation of the stomach lining. Sleep it off and drink lots of water. (see *Alcoholism*).
Your skin and the whites of your eyes are yellowish	You could have jaundice as the result of a disorder of the liver or *gallbladder disease*.
You felt dizzy before you vomited	This could be a disorder of the inner ear (see *Fainting*). Consult your doctor for a diagnosis.
You are taking drugs or some form of medication	This may be a side effect. Discuss this with your doctor, and remember that alcohol taken with certain drugs can cause nausea and vomiting. If you take a contraceptive pill, and you suffer an attack of vomiting, your protection may be affected. Use another form of birth control until you start a new packet.

NIPPLE PROBLEMS

Nipples come in all shapes and sizes and rarely cause serious problems to health. The nipple is surrounded by an area of pink or brown skin known as the areola. Each nipple has about 15-20 ducts from which the milk emerges during lactation. Self-examination of your breasts is a simple check on your health which you should carry out at least once a month for life. In addition to the problems treated here, there are some that may develop during breastfeeding.

INVERTED NIPPLES

Because it contains muscle, the nipple becomes erect when you are cold, sexually excited or breastfeeding. Some women's, however, do not protrude so they do not have these abilities. Inverted nipples are not unhealthy, except if they were previously normal (see below), and are usually a minor abnormality of development. However, if you are planning to breastfeed, an inverted nipple must be corrected during pregnancy because the baby will not be able to get purchase on the nipple and feed successfully.

Any inversion of a nipple where previously there was not a problem may be a symptom of breast cancer, so contact your doctor immediately.

What is the treatment?

You can usually correct an inverted nipple by the simple technique described below, which can be done even if you are not pregnant.

If you are pregnant, your breasts will be examined and any inversion of the nipples noted during your first thorough physical examination at the prenatal clinic. If the condition needs treatment, you will be advised to wear breast shields under your bra from about week 15 of your pregnancy. You will need to build up the number of hours you wear them each day – a few hours at first increasing to several hours during

the last trimester. The round glass or plastic shields are not uncomfortable to wear, and your nipple will be gently drawn through the hole in the shield by suction. If you wear the shields during your pregnancy and then put your baby to the breast as soon as possible after the birth, you should have no problems with breastfeeding.

If your nipples are flat and you want to ensure that breastfeeding goes successfully, you can try an exercise known as the Hoffmann technique. Place a finger either side of your areola and stretch the nipple; repeat this with your fingers above and below the nipple. Do this exercise a couple of times each day during your pregnancy.

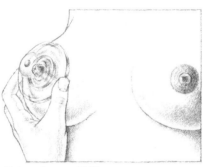

Using a breast shield
You can improve flat inverted nipples by wearing breast shields under your bra. Made of rubber or plastic they have a hole through which the nipple is gently pulled by suction.

DISCHARGE FROM THE NIPPLE

If you are not pregnant and not lactating, you should consult your doctor immediately if you notice a discharge, crusting or bleeding from the nipple. Seek immediate medical advice if you notice any scaling of the skin around the nipple, changes in the nipple texture – other than the enlargement of the Montgomery's tubercles on the areola, one of the first signs of pregnancy when the

pigmentation changes to a darker skin color.

Discharge of milk or a whitish substance from a non-lactating woman is known as galactorrhea. However, if the discharge is any other color it may be a symptom of a growth and should be investigated.

What will the doctor do?

Because any abnormal discharge from the nipple is usually a symptom of an underlying condition, your doctor will examine your breasts and try to take a sample of the discharge.

Investigations will reveal whether you have a small benign tumor in the nipple duct or whether the discharge is a symptom of a malignant tumor.

CRACKED NIPPLES

Cracked nipples are in rare cases a symptom of a growth but in general this problem only relates to breastfeeding. However, persistent eczema of the nipple, particularly if you are over 50, may be a sign of Paget's Disease of the nipple. This is a feature of breast cancer in which the tumor starts in the milk ducts of the nipple, causing itching and burning.

What should I do?

You should consult your doctor immediately if any eczema persists for three to four weeks and ask for a biopsy to be performed. If a cancer is confirmed, it will have to be surgically removed.

SEE ALSO:

BENIGN BREAST DISEASE
BREASTFEEDING PROBLEMS
BREAST CANCER
BREAST OPERATIONS
BREAST SELF-EXAMINATION
BREASTS AND BREASTFEEDING
GALACTORRHEA

NUMBNESS AND TINGLING

Numbness and tingling are common if you get up from an awkward position because pressure on a nerve means the blood supply is temporarily cut off. If it occurs for no apparent reason, this could indicate a more serious problem.

In the condition known as hypothyroidism, the accumulation of mucus-like substance makes your skin swollen and puffy. If this occurs in the wrists, for example, the pressure on the nerves that run through your wrists can cause numbness and tingling in the fingers. This also arises when there is fluid retention because of hormonal changes, such as during pregnancy and at menopause.

If you are unable to make a diagnosis from this information, consult your doctor.

SITE AND NATURE OF PROBLEM	PROBABLE CAUSE
You feel numb when you wake from sleeping or getting up from a chair.	If you sit in one position for a long time, pressure on a nerve can cause numbness, sometimes so severe that it results in temporary paralysis. Your sensations should return to normal in a couple of minutes as your circulation gets going again.
The tingling occurs when you are nervous or anxious	You may be unconsciously over-breathing. Concentrate on your breathing and take deep rather than shallow breaths.
The numbness occurs in your hands but your neck is stiff, and you are over 50	This could be cervical spondylosis. This form of *arthritis* affects the bones and joints of the neck which put pressure on nerves and blood vessels.
The numbness is only in your hands and is worse at night and/or pain shoots up your hand from the wrist	This could be *carpal tunnel syndrome*.
You have other symptoms such as weight gain with a loss of appetite, you feel cold all the time and your skin is dry and puffy	Your thyroid gland could be under-active, producing swollen tissues in your wrists (see *Hyperthyroidism*).
Tingling and pain only affects one arm, and this is the arm you play racket games with	This could be a *sports injury* caused by the way you hold your racket.
Numbness only affects one side of your body and you experience blurred vision, loss of movement in a limb, confusion and difficulty speaking	There may be a temporary interruption of blood flow to your brain. Call your doctor immediately.
The numbness comes and goes regularly, and you have a blind patch in your vision	This could be multiple sclerosis. See your doctor right away.
Your fingers or toes go white, then blue, then red when cold	You may have a hypersensitivity to cold. This could be *Raynaud's phenomenon* and it is most common in those with poor circulation, or if you are taking beta blocker drugs for your blood pressure (see *Hypertension*), or if you use pneumatic drills all the time.
It only affects one foot and you have pain down the back of your leg	This could be sciatica caused by a slipped disc. Consult your doctor.

OBESITY

Obesity is caused by eating too much. If you weigh more than 20% over the average for your height and frame, you are termed obese. As women start off with more body fat than men, they are at a certain disadvantage, and in our society more women than men are obese.

What causes it?
Hardly anyone is obese because of a glandular abnormality. Some obese people have a slow metabolism which means they need to eat very little to settle the equation of energy taken in (food eaten) minus energy used (calories expended) equals fat deposited (weight gain). Research has shown that some obese people conveniently forget a lot of the food they have eaten, others eat food absentmindedly, as though just to keep their jaws moving, and others engage in compulsive eating patterns.

Obesity as a result of compulsive eating need not be seen as an example of a weak character and lack of self control; it may be a woman's way of coming to terms with her life, how she views herself and how others view her.

Undoubtedly obese people eat too much and just as importantly, the wrong foods. Some foods are richer in calories than others and they add very little to the nutritional value of your diet. The foods containing the most calories are fats, notably animal fats; they are also not good for health.

What happens to your body?
When you're fat, you put a strain on your heart, lungs and joints. Obesity can lead to heart disease, worsening varicose veins, high blood pressure, gallbladder disease, diabetes and hernias. By losing weight, you immediately put yourself in a lower risk category.

· S y m p t o m s ·
▲ More than 20% over the average weight for your height and frame

Should I see the doctor?
If you are overweight and uncomfortable, and this is making you unhappy, talk to your family doctor.

What might the doctor do?
You will probably be examined and if your health is at risk, your doctor will advise you how to lose weight. There are surgical procedures to help the grossly overweight but they are quite drastic. The best approach with the highest success rate is with self-help groups, like Weight Watchers.

What can I do?
If you don't want to lose weight, don't complain and stay fat. If you are unhappy, and compulsive eating is one of the ways you cheer yourself up, and you want to lose weight, start today. You can either join an established group such as Weight Watchers or join a women's group where other women who have the same experience can help you to work through your fears and feelings in group sessions or individual counseling. In this way you can come to terms with your size and shape.

In tandem with the group sessions, you will need to take in less food and take more exercise. You will need to overcome your indolence and lack of willpower in

WEIGHT GUIDE

Use this chart to check your actual weight against the healthy weight for your height. Rule a line across from your height (on the left) and a line up from your weight (on the bottom). If the point where the lines meet is in the central colored band, your weight is healthy for someone of your height.

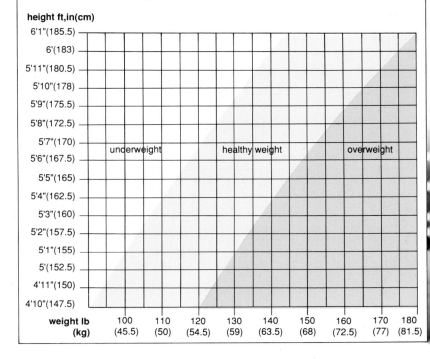

height ft,in(cm)

6'1"(185.5)
6'(183)
5'11"(180.5)
5'10"(178)
5'9"(175.5)
5'8"(172.5)
5'7"(170)
5'6"(167.5)
5'5"(165)
5'4"(162.5)
5'3"(160)
5'2"(157.5)
5'1"(155)
5'(152.5)
4'11"(150)
4'10"(147.5)

underweight   healthy weight   overweight

weight lb 100   110   120   130   140   150   160   170   180
(kg)   (45.5) (50) (54.5) (59) (63.5) (68) (72.5) (77) (81.5)

order to use up the calories. If you exercise for half an hour every day, you can use up 500–1000 calories. As 500g in weight equals about 3500 calories, you can lose 450g (1 lb) per week by exercising every day. Exercise can be addictive if you try hard enough. You may find you enjoy the feeling of achievement after swimming or a brisk walk. Exercise can make you feel confident; you will find your body feels better and you hold yourself better. If willpower is a problem, try a group activity such as gym classes or dancing.

Develop a more sensible diet; eat high-fiber, low-fat foods and avoid cakes and sweets as much as you can. They contain only empty calories. Don't allow yourself to run short of essential minerals and vitamins. Rather than embarking on a "diet," create new eating habits for life – cut out certain foods and cut down on others.

If you have a sweet tooth, try to deny it. If you can't do without sweetness in food, use artificial sweeteners. Learn to cook with natural forms of sugar, such as dried fruits and fruit juices. Gradually you might be able to change the sensitivity of your palate.

Substitute different foods for favorite treats: use low-fat yogurt instead of cream; substitute polyunsaturated fats in cooking for

FAT IN PREGNANCY

Fat is laid down on the upper arms and upper thighs during pregnancy as fat stores to provide the energy to make milk when you're breast-feeding. This fat gradually reduces during the first 4–6 months of breastfeeding – breastfeeding uses up about 600–800 calories per day. The important considerations after your baby is born are to keep eating a healthy diet to provide the nutrients for you and your baby and to exercise to strengthen your internal organs. Exercise in the first few weeks should be specially planned to firm up your pelvic floor muscles and your abdominal muscles. After that, a normal active life and breastfeeding should bring your figure back to normal.

butter or saturated fats; cook with unrefined products such as whole-wheat flour – this way you'll feel fuller and not want more to eat again inside an hour.

Weigh yourself regularly and if your weight increases by say 5lbs, cut back immediately on food and increase your exercise and watch your weight go down again.

Some women regulate their weight without constant weighing. Put on your tightest skirt or jeans every week to check that they're comfortable. This may be difficult premenstrually, for example, but as a quick barometer of your weight, it's less obsessive than constant weighing.

Unfortunately there is no known way of spot reduction, so if you're worried about your thighs or upper arms for example, you'll have to take off weight generally to reduce the size of the larger parts of your body.

DIETS AND DIETING

Dieting isn't really about food; it is more a matter of eating. On the whole, diets aren't a lasting solution. The way to lose weight is to change your eating habits for the rest of your life. Going on a diet does nothing to solve this. The failure rate of diets is extremely high, hence the plethora of them. And many of them are dangerous. In any case the success of a diet depends on cutting down the number of calories you eat. Most active women can lose weight eating less than 1500 calories a day. Those who have a sedentary lifestyle need to eat less than 1000 calories per day, and those who have a slow metabolism may need to eat less than 800, and even then the weight loss will be slow so you'll need to keep to this regime for several months.

SEE ALSO:

ANOREXIA NERVOSA
BULIMIA
DIABETES MELLITUS
EATING PROBLEMS
GALLBLADDER DISEASE
HEART DISEASE
HYPERTENSION
NUTRITION AND DIET
VARICOSE VEINS

OSTEOARTHRITIS

Osteoarthritis is quite different from rheumatoid arthritis and usually begins in late middle age. It is said to be the natural aging process of joints, which in some people occurs earlier in life than it should. Predisposing factors are past injuries, such as fractures and sprains, and too great a strain on the weightbearing joints due to overweight. In contrast to rheumatoid arthritis, osteoarthritis affects the large central weight-bearing joints of the body such as the hips and the knees.

Other joints, which take a great deal of strain during life, such as the spine, are also affected. Both the neck (cervical) and lower back (lumbar) regions can be involved. Osteoarthritis may cause pressure on the nerves in the back giving rise to pain down the arms and numbness and tingling in the fingers. In the lumbar region, pressure on the nerves can lead to sciatic pain spreading down through the buttocks and the back of the leg to the feet.

Heberden's arthritis mainly affects women but has a genetic component. This degenerative disease of the last joints of the fingers is characterized by bony nodular enlargements that are often painful.

The pain in ostoeoarthritis is less after resting and gets worse as the day progresses. The stiffness is caused because the joints are simply wearing out and because new bone may have formed along the edges of the joint preventing smooth, frictionless movement. In osteoarthritic joints there is no true inflammation as there is in rheumatoid arthritis, and swelling of the joint is caused by new bone laid down in an effort to stabilize and strengthen a joint which is becoming worn out. Osteoarthritic joints are therefore "cold"; there is no destructive inflammatory process inside them and they are not as rapidly destroyed.

Should I see a doctor?
Because osteoarthritis is a natural part of aging, you are bound to have

---

· Symptoms ·

Usually only occurring in one or two joints:
▲ Recurring pain
▲ Stiffness
▲ Swelling
▲ Joints are knobbly
▲ Inability to move a joint

---

it in some of your joints though you may not notice it. You should seek a diagnosis in the first instance, in case you have some other form of arthritic disease. Try the self-help measures unless the swelling and pain makes life difficult, when you should see your doctor for relief.

What will the doctor do?
Your doctor may arrange for you to have X-rays and blood tests to diagnose the disease. The aim of treatment in osteoarthritis is to relieve pain and strain on the joints. Pain relief is accomplished by the use of myriad painkilling drugs. Some of them have unpleasant side effects and you should report this to your doctor right away. The most common side effect with anti-inflammatory drugs is stomach irritation. Reduced strain on the joint can mainly be achieved by weight loss.

If the pain is severe, your doctor may inject a steroid directly into the joint.

It must be said that osteoarthritis is in no way as serious or as debilitating a disease as rheumatoid arthritis and very often doctors are prepared to let the condition progress, particularly if it involves the knees or hips, without radical intervention. In the latter, hip replacement is the best option, easy to perform and giving excellent results. Hip replacement is constantly being improved and, in many cases, changes the life of the sufferer. The joints are made of metal or a combination of metal and plastic. Knee replacement is more difficult and more complicated. It is much less commonly performed than hip

---

replacement but techniques are improving all the time.

What can I do?
◆ Keep your weight at a sensible level.
◆ If you are overweight, you should try to lose some to take the pressure off your weightbearing joints.
◆ For immediate relief try a hot water bottle wrapped in a towel, placed on the affected joint. Heat is soothing and will help you keep the joint moving.
◆ A cold compress might also work. A plastic bag filled with ice cubes is one homemade method.

The exercise you need to take will depend on the joint affected by the arthritis. You do need to exercise the joint or the muscles will become weak because you're not using them. Move your joints slowly through their normal full movement without putting stress on them.

Try not to do exercises that cause you to twist or turn or jolt your limbs such as jogging. The best exercise is swimming in warm water.

Maintain the exercise program even when the symptoms fade. This could prevent an early return of the condition.

There are no dietary means to combat this natural process; a good diet that keeps your weight down is the best diet.

For pain, take acetaminophen or aspirin. Don't take any of the wonder drugs advertised to kill arthritis pain; some of them have had devastating effects. If there is an apparent cure, this is more likely a period of remission. The swelling will usually return again.

If you take the prescribed doses of aspirin with food, the possible effects of stomach irritation will be lessened.

PAIN RELIEF

The mainstay of analgesic therapy for osteoarthritis is a group of drugs known as the non-steroidal anti-

FIBROSITIS

Also called fibromyalgia, this is sometimes mistaken for a form of arthritis, but it is the muscles and tendons, not the joints, that are stiff and painful.

Fibromyalagia doesn't present a serious threat to health; but it can be debilitating for two to three days. It's a common cause of chronic aches and pains in women in middle age, who may be encouraged to believe that the non-specific pain is in their imagination.

Treatment includes the avoidance of stress if the pain is the result of an emotional problem that is causing tension in the muscles; improvement in general physical fitness; local anesthetic sprays for instant relief, heat treatment, massage and painkillers such as acetaminophen.

inflammatory drugs (NSAIDs). There are many potent painkillers in this group – several of them under different brand names.

Osteoarthritis, despite its name, does not involve inflammation of the joint. Nonetheless, the NSAIDs are used for the treatment of pain relief because they are effective and have lower incidences of side effects than other drugs such as aspirin.

Despite the fact that aspirin can cause serious side effects in 30–40% of patients taking it, it is still used as a first-line therapy for pain relief in both osteoarthritis and rheumatoid arthritis. For the large number of patients who cannot tolerate aspirin , the NSAIDs are a good and effective alternative. None of them can halt the progress of the disease; all of them are symptomatic remedies. They do not get to the root of the problem which for osteoarthritis is virtually impossible.

The newest of the NSAIDs, however, have a very low ulcerogenic potential and cause gastrointestinal side effects in very few patients. The NSAIDs are not in the main dangerous and can be taken for long periods of time. There are many brands of these drugs on the market, each vying with the other in making extravagant claims. None of them provides a cure, let alone a miracle cure and you should ask your doctor to explain what the possible side effects are before you start taking a course of these drugs.

SEE ALSO:

ARTHRITIS
AUTOIMMUNE DISEASE
HIP REPLACEMENT
MENOPAUSAL PROBLEMS
OSTEOPOROSIS
RHEUMATOID ARTHRITIS

OSTEOPOROSIS

Osteoporosis is a wasting of bone. The interior of the bones is gradually reabsorbed by the body and is not replaced at the usual rate so that although the bones remain the same size, they contain less calcium and their structures are weakened.

Osteoporosis is found more often and earlier in women than in men. It is predominantly due to aging – not a process of normal aging, but an age-associated disorder – and occurs more frequently as women get older. One out of five post-menopausal women experiences this gradual softening. If the bones of the back become affected, this leads to back-ache and thinning and flattening of the spine and vertebral discs.

As osteoporosis leads to weakening of the bones, there is a tendency for post-menopausal women to sustain more fractures as they get older. The most common are the wrist and hip.

What causes it?
All bones are subjected to osteoporosis with time. However, in women estrogen is an important contributor to the healthy calcium balance and sturdy protein architecture of the bones. When estrogen supplies fall calcium may not be properly incorporated into bone tissue.

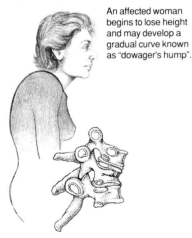

An affected woman begins to lose height and may develop a gradual curve known as "dowager's hump".

Estrogen levels fall in the menopause so that bones thin, become weak and are more likely to fracture.

This also gives rise to aches and pains in the bones and joints. Poor calcium absorption or an inadequate amount of calcium and protein in your diet will lead to osteoporosis. Calcium and phosphorus harden and maintain healthy bones, and Vitamin D is essential for efficient absorption of these minerals.

Should I see the doctor?
If you are post-menopausal and you feel low back pain or spasms in your back, consult your doctor.

What will the doctor do?
Your doctor will send you for an X-ray analysis to see if there is any thinning of the bones. Although you can't reverse the process of osteoporosis, these bone changes can be arrested.

Hormone replacement therapy (HRT) with estrogen and progesterone combined can stop the weakening of your skeleton. To abolish bone loss completely, HRT must be continued for a year or more. If HRT is stopped within six months, the bones will be exactly the same as if you'd never taken these protective hormones.

In tandem with this hormone therapy, it will be necessary to include more calcium in your diet. Your doctor will prescribe calcium tablets and advise you to increase your protein intake as well as getting plenty of exercise.

Estrogen therapy cannot repair weakened bones but it does prevent the condition from getting any worse. HRT should always be accompanied by calcium and Vitamin D supplements. HRT or calcium on their own are not effective. After age 65, however, hormones become less important and calcium and Vitamin D alone are probably sufficient.

What can I do?
If, as you approach menopause, you have symptoms such as hot flashes, night sweats, vaginal dryness, loss of libido, sleeplessness and irritability, go and see your doctor and discuss the possibility of receiving HRT, particularly if you are having aches and pains in muscles, bones and joints.

FRACTURED WRISTS AND HIPS

A Colles fracture is one at the lower end of the forearm, just above the wrist, which involves both bones of the forearm, the radius and the ulna. This fracture is usually sustained when a woman trips and falls, using her outstretched hands to break the fall. The jolt as her lower arm takes her weight is often sufficient to fracture the radius and ulna. The fracture is extremely simple to treat; the bones are first aligned and then immobilized with a Plaster of Paris cast that extends from just below the elbow to the root of the fingers. After about three weeks the bones will have knitted and the plaster can be removed. It is essential to keep the fingers moving during the healing period.

A fractured neck of femur is usually sustained when a woman slips and falls and sits down with her legs underneath her. If the neck of femur is subject to osteoporosis, it doesn't take much force to snap it. Healing will not occur without a two- or three-week hospital stay, and in very old women, immobilization in hospital can sometimes lead to pneumonia with its complications. For this reason, fractured neck of femur can be a fatal condition.

BONE LOSS AND FRACTURES

All bones deteriorate with age. The graph below left shows the % decrease in bone materials and minerals between men and women, and on the right the % increase in fractures over a similar period.

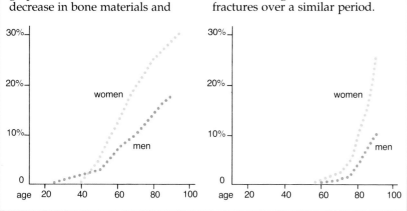

A special X-ray examination (bone-density) can be performed on certain bones of the body, particularly those of the fingers, hands and wrists, and compared to standard X-rays to show whether or not the bones are losing calcium and protein, becoming thin and soft. Against a standard scale, therefore, bone density of each individual person can be measured and read off a pre-determined scale. Treatment is started and bone density investigations can be repeated as treatment progresses. Return to normal bone density can then be plotted. This technique is used to ensure the effectiveness of various treatments for osteoporosis and also to chart recovery. This particular kind of investigation was pioneered by Professor Nordin of Leeds University in Great Britain.

What can I do to prevent osteoporosis?

It's been found that osteoporosis can be prevented if women take regular exercise from the age of 35 onwards. It is important that this exercise is weight-bearing and therefore must be done in the upright position. So walking, jogging, cycling, playing tennis and squash are all useful. Eating a balanced diet with plenty of calcium and Vitamin D is essential. Sources include cheese and milk, sesame seeds, legumes, almonds and seaweed. As Vitamin D promotes the absorption of calcium from the intestine and increases its efficiency to strengthen bones, get plenty of sunshine and eat oily fish, eggs and fortified foods such as margarine.

Falls can be minimized if you pay attention to safety features in your home such as good light in dark passages, non-slip surfaces, no loose linoleum or carpet and grit on outside pathways if it is icy.

SEE ALSO:

HIP REPLACEMENT
HORMONE REPLACEMENT
   THERAPY
MENOPAUSAL PROBLEMS

OTOPLASTY

This means any operation to change the shape of the external ear or to reconstruct an ear absent or severely defective from birth, or damaged by disease or injury. The operation may be very simple as in the procedure, commonly done in children, to pin back ears which protrude unduly from the head, or it may be very difficult when much of the tissue is absent or destroyed and both cartilage and skin must be taken from another part of the body.

Why is it done?
Most otoplasty operations are minor and are done to correct protruding ears. Most ears stand out from the head because the concha or bowl is large or because the fold in the upper part of the ear is not properly formed.

Ears that appear unduly large or prominent in infants and children may become less so with time and growth of the head, but adults who continue to be bothered by their appearance often have it done if they cannot minimize any embarrassment by simply growing their hair long. In some cases, ears can stand out at right angles to the head.

How is it done?
When ears stand out prominently at right angles to the head, this is usually due to an actual malformation in the cartilage skeleton of the ear rather than to simple malplacement. Because of this, an attempt to pull back the ear simply by removing an ellipse of skin from the back of the ear and then stitching up the opening, will fail, for the elasticity of the cartilage will soon stretch the skin. Permanent correction will be achieved only by a properly planned procedure in which an elliptical skin incision is made on the back of the ear and a crescent of cartilage removed in such a way as to allow the main cartilage to fold back into a normal position. This operation calls for experience and judgment, but the results are usually excellent.

CORRECTING PROTRUDING EARS

Real embarrassment and severe distress can be the result of greatly protruding ears. However, not until the age of five, when the ears are fully developed, should they be pinned back.

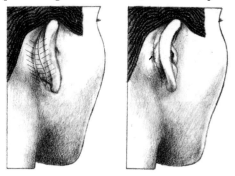

The ears can be pulled flat against the head by removing a strip of skin from behind the ear and sewing together the two raw edges.

Alternatively, skin can be removed from the back of the ear and from the adjacent area of the scalp, and the two raw surfaces brought into contact so that they fuse permanently together. Some doctors perform this operation on an out-patient basis, under a local anesthetic. A dressing holds the ears flat against the head and the stitches are removed after five days or so. This operation, too, can give good results. There is bound to be discomfort for the first two weeks, and it is important to maintain firm pressure for several days by padding and the wearing of a firm turban bandage, to avoid bruise formation. This can lead to pain, infection, destruction of cartilage and distortion of the ear. Fortunately, this complication is rare and the bruising from minor bleeding under the skin soon absorbs. The discomfort settles quickly. After healing, incision lines are invisible or inconspicuous.

The less common condition of "lop ear," in which the upper border of the pinna is folded down, is also caused by a defect in the cartilage skeleton and requires internal reconstruction.

Otoplasty may be necessary for loss of tissue from disease, such as cancer, or burning or mechanical injury. In these cases, plastic construction, using tissue flaps or free grafts, is necessary and it is very difficult to achieve cosmetically good results. Some surgeons use a shaped silicon rubber skeleton as a basis on which to fashion skin flaps.

SEE ALSO:

COSMETIC OPERATIONS
COSMETIC SURGERY

OVARIAN CYSTS

The majority of cystic growths in the ovary are benign. Sometimes a few cysts can be considered normal when the ovary is described as a cystic ovary. This common condition is known as polycystic ovarian syndrome and is due to an hormonal imbalance. If the ovaries are enlarged because of many small cysts, this can be a reason for failure to ovulate resulting in infertility. While overall nearly 75% to 85% of cysts discovered are benign, more often than not, the medical usage of the word "ovarian cyst" indicates a malignant growth.

What causes it?
In women of childbearing age, a cyst may result when, instead of bursting and releasing an egg, a follicle continues to grow, accumulating fluid and producing the hormone estrogen. As the cyst expands, the ovarian tissue stretches out and may eventually become a thin layer which completely surrounds the cyst. Some cysts grow larger than 8cm (3in) in diameter and are filled with thick jelly-like material which hardly ever escapes into the pelvic cavity.

The cells making up a cyst are extremely primitive. They are the cells from which a baby grows and

therefore have the potential to grow into any tissue of the body. It is not uncommon for ovarian cysts to contain teeth, hair, bone and cartilage. If teeth are present, they can often be seen on X-ray. Because the cells are primitive, they also possess the potential to develop into cancerous cells.

Quite often a large ovarian cyst can be felt by external examination of your abdomen. However, it is impossible to tell if it is malignant or not without further investigation. The likelihood of the cyst becoming malignant increases as you get older.

· S y m p t o m s ·

- ▲ Abdominal swelling leading you to believe you are putting on weight
- ▲ Change in your normal menstrual cycle
- ▲ Breathlessness
- ▲ Frequency of urination
- ▲ Pressure on the veins of the lower legs causing varicose veins and swollen ankles
- ▲ Infertility
- ▲ Amenorrhea

Should I see the doctor?
While ovarian cysts are small they have few symptoms; many disap-

pear by themselves and you may never know you had them, but as they get larger you may notice the swelling and think you are putting on weight or be disturbed by a change in your normal menstrual cycle. If you don't see your doctor for a diagnosis, pressure symptoms may arise as the cyst presses against your lungs, bladder and major blood vessels.

An ovarian cyst rarely causes vaginal bleeding unless it is producing a lot of estrogen. Very rarely the stalk of the cyst may become twisted or rupture, causing symptoms of severe abdominal pain. This requires an emergency operation.

What will the doctor do?
Your doctor will examine you externally and if a swelling is felt, a diagnosis can only be confirmed by ultrasound scan, X-ray or surgery. This involves an internal examination by laparoscopy using a fiberoptoscope. This method is not suitable for taking a specimen to check for malignancy because of the risk of seeding the peritoneal cavity with suspected malignant cells.

If a cyst is diagnosed, it will probably be surgically removed, whether it is malignant or not.

If your condition is diagnosed as polycystic ovaries, your doctor will treat the symptoms or refer you for infertility treatment if you wish to conceive.

What happens during surgical treatment?
During the operation, a small piece of the cyst is taken out, freeze dried and rushed to the pathology laboratory to be examined. The surgeon can then proceed with removal of the cyst, fully aware of the seriousness of the situation should the cells prove to be cancerous.

If the cyst is benign, it will be removed and the ovary left in place. The surgeon will always look at the other ovary because cysts some-

---

A FUNCTIONAL OR "NORMAL" CYST

Quite often, part of the ovary, the corpus luteum, contains abnormal amounts of fluid. When this

produces severe pain, the fluid must be removed by an incision and the cyst area stitched over.

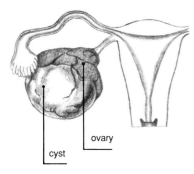

cyst

ovary

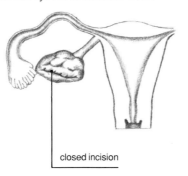

closed incision

OVARIAN CYSTS

times occur in both.

If a diagnosis of malignancy is made, the cyst, ovary and fallopian tube will be removed. The second ovary will also need to be inspected. If the ovary appears clear, microscopic examination of the tumor will determine if it is slow-growing or not. If it is, the surgeon may decide to leave the second ovary in place; if not, the second ovary and fallopian tube will also be removed.

What can I do?

Discuss all the possibilities before you have the operation. Ask whether it is necessary to have both ovaries removed if the tumor turns out to be malignant. Ask about hormone therapy, and how long you will need to take it. Also find out about what happens with premature menopause. Never allow yourself to be in the position of going into the operating room without being satisfied in your mind that you can cope with any surgical eventuality. The surgeon's advice may depend on whether you are still of childbearing years or if you have finished your family.

What is the outlook?

If the cyst and one ovary was removed, everything will be as normal, with secretion of female hormones, menstruation, ovulation and a normal menopause.

If both your ovaries are removed, it will be necessary for you to undergo hormone replacement therapy if you don't wish to go through premature menopause. You can continue with the hormone therapy until the approximate time when your menopause would have occurred naturally.

SEE ALSO:

AMENORRHEA
HORMONE REPLACEMENT
  THERAPY
INFERTILITY
LAPAROSCOPY
MENOPAUSAL PROBLEMS
OVARIAN PROBLEMS·
ULTRASOUND

OVARIAN PROBLEMS

The ovaries are the female gonads, glands that produce the female hormones as well as storing a life's supply of ova. Because the ovaries are deep within the pelvic cavity, any growths are quite difficult to notice. Ovarian tumors are slow-growing and usually don't produce symptoms until they are quite large. Though *ovarian cysts* are relatively common, less than 5% become cancerous. The usual symptoms include changes in the menstrual cycle (most often lengthened but occasionally shortened), *menorrhagia*, abdominal lumps or pressure and *infertility*.

Inflammation of the ovaries, such as with a *sexually transmitted disease* like *gonorrhea* and, very rarely, as a result of the mumps virus, will be felt as local pain.

If your periods become scanty and less regular, physical examination or *laparoscopy* may reveal enlarged ovaries with many cysts. This condition is known as polycystic ovary syndrome or Stein-Leventhal syndrome. These cysts are a result of hormonal imbalance and are characterized by a difference in the production of your female sex hormones. One early symptom may be *amenorrhea*. With some disorders of the ovaries, certain hormonal changes cause identifiable symptoms such as increased body hair, obesity and deepening of your voice. This is because testosterone has risen in your blood. Polycystic ovaries are a common cause of infertility.

Any malignancy in the ovary itself is rare – about 6% of tumors are cancerous. Few women under the age of 40 have cancer of the ovaries, nor do those with children. However, any abnormality in post-menopausal women is a cause for concern and should be investigated immediately. Laparoscopy will diagnose the affected ovary and an operation will be carried out to remove it and often the uterus, if affected. This operation is a *hysterectomy*. In some cases, the other ovary may be affected.

Radiation therapy treatment and anti-cancer drugs will follow the operation to prevent the disease recurring or to slow down its spread. Any fluid that develops on the tumor will be drawn off from time to time. This is known as paracentesis.

PAINFUL INTERCOURSE

Any pain or discomfort with sexual intercourse, whether because of a local genital problem or pain deep in the pelvis, can be described as dyspareunia. It can vary from mild discomfort or tightness to exquisite pain which prevents intercourse altogether. Psychological factors are by far the commonest cause of dyspareunia. Inhibitions about the sexual act, resentment, anger, fear or shame and anticipating that sex will be unsuccessful are all causes of disturbed psychological attitudes affecting sex.

Are there physical reasons?
There are several medical conditions that must be eliminated first, however. These include vaginal infections, pelvic inflammatory disease, endometriosis, prolapsed uterus, urinary tract infection, irritation of the vulva (pruritis vulvae), hemorrhoids, hormonal deficiency at the menopause or after childbirth causing dryness in the vagina, and painful perineal scars after an episiotomy.

· S y m p t o m s ·

▲ Pain during intercourse; either externally or deep in the pelvis during thrusts of penetration
▲ Lack of desire or inclination for sex
▲ Involuntary closing of the legs and vagina to prevent penetration (vaginismus)
▲ Dryness in the vagina

Should I see the doctor?
If you experience physical pain during intercourse or for some reason you are loath to permit your partner to penetrate your vagina, see your doctor.

What will the doctor do?
Your doctor will examine you to check for any underlying disorder. If you have an infection, antibiotics should clear it up. If the discomfort is the result of poor stitching after childbirth, your doctor may advise you to wait another couple of weeks, or to have the area restitched. This depends on how recently you have given birth.

If your problem is not a physical one, your doctor will refer you to a trained sex therapist who will try to uncover the reasons for your fear of sexual intercourse. However, if your relationship is no longer a loving one, sex counseling will not help. You cannot heal a broken relationship with sex and you should admit this from the outset.

What can I do?
Don't keep quiet about your expectations and preferences. You have to take responsibility for your own pleasure. Try to discuss this with your partner and try not to feel guilty about ordinary sexual practices. The only prerequisite for good sex is loving your partner, and if you do, all your sexual problems should be resolved. If your problem has a physical cause, find other ways of showing affection.

Forget labels. No woman is frigid. If you label yourself or are labeled frigid, you may become anxious and lose hope.

Remember also that even if you are aroused by your partner, unless you have sufficient clitoral stimulation and your vagina lubricates sufficiently to make penetration easy and comfortable, you won't experience good sex. You may find you need to use a lubricating jelly.

SEE ALSO:

CYSTITIS
ENDOMETRIOSIS
EPISIOTOMY
HEMORRHOIDS
MENOPAUSAL PROBLEMS
PELVIC INFLAMMATORY
  DISEASE
PERINEAL TEAR
PROLAPSE
PRURITIS VULVAE
SEXUAL PROBLEMS
VAGINISMUS
VAGINITIS

PAINFUL URINATION

If you feel pain or a burning sensation when you urinate, this is either a urinary tract infection or an irritation of the skin of the vulva.

The female urethra is short, about 4cm (1¹/₂in) in length and is susceptible to infection because of its proximity to the vaginal opening. Any bacteria can therefore penetrate and cause infection. *E coli* is one such bacterium which causes the painful and recurring urinary tract infection, cystitis. The urethra itself is a muscular tube with a complex lining and if infection lodges here, the inflammation makes the passage of urine painful and sometimes bloody.

Though the bacteria normally live in the intestines and around the anus, this should cause no problems unless through reasons of poor hygiene, or bruising, or other infection, they ascend the urethra.

During pregnancy, the problem is with frequent urination – micturition. The weight of the enlarged uterus causes pressure to build up when only a little urine is in the bladder. The hormonal changes cause a general relaxation of muscle which may mean that some urine is retained in the bladder and urethra. This can also lead to infection, but regular prenatal checks on urine will catch any symptomless infection.

If you are unable to make a diagnosis from this information, consult your doctor.

NATURE OF PAIN	PROBABLE CAUSE
You are suffering from low abdominal pain, frequency of urination and your urine is cloudy	This could be an infection in your bladder such as *cystitis*.
You are thirsty all the time and losing weight	You may have developed *diabetes mellitus*.
You have pain in the small of your back and/or a fever	This could be a kidney infection. Consult your doctor right away.
You have recently had sexual intercourse very regularly	You may have bruised your urethra. Consult your doctor for a diagnosis.
Your vulva is itchy and there is a vaginal discharge	This could be a *yeast infection*. If the discharge is green and smelly, this could be *trichomoniasis*, a sexually transmitted infection.
Your vulva is itchy	This could be *pruritis vulvae*. In younger women this is usually an allergic reaction to soap powders or manmade fibers. In older women this may be a symptom of menopause, when hormone levels cause the vagina to become dry. By scratching the vulva, the perineal skin becomes irritated further and burns on urination.
You have fairly constant pain and symptoms of a urethral infection	You may have a *prolapse* where a bulge in the front wall of the vagina irritates the urethral lining.
There is pain on urination and perhaps a discharge	You may have contracted a *sexually transmitted disease* such as *gonorrhea* when either the vagina or the urethra is infected, usually within a week of intercourse. This disease can be symptomless in women and may go unnoticed.
You seem to have constantly recurring bladder infections	This is more common after menopause. See your doctor for a different antibiotic if the treatment is not working.

PALPITATIONS

Palpitations are the sensations you experience when your heart beats strongly or irregularly or more rapidly than usual. This is a normal aftermath of strenuous exercise or when you are nervous or afraid. However, if they occur when you haven't been exercising, they may be a symptom of a disorder.

In some cases, anxiety about heart disease may actually cause the palpitations to be more noticeable.

Atrial fibrillation is when the muscular contractions of the two atria are disordered and they beat much too fast – 400 pulsations per minute. As the ventricles can only beat at about 140 per minute, this lack of co-ordination obviously reduces the amount of blood pumped out by the heart. There is a less severe condition, known as atrial flutter, when the muscle fibers contract at about 300 pulsations a minute. Often these two conditions, which are fairly common, cause no problem and no symptoms. If they do, there may be palpitations and dizziness. The conditions are usually the result of coronary artery disease, rheumatic fever or in the event of a high fever. They cause problems if the ventricles fail to cope. As they often can, the palpitations will only be noticed some of the time. Your doctor will probably refer you for an electrocardiogram to diagnose the condition.

If you are unable to make a diagnosis from this information, consult your doctor.

NATURE OF THE PROBLEM	PROBABLE CAUSE
You are anxious, and this is a common condition with you	If you have an intense awareness of your heart beating, this is probably *anxiety*.
You are losing weight and you feel the heat more than before and your palms are sweaty	This could be an overactive thyroid gland (see *Hyperthyroidism*).
The palpitations occur on exertion but are accompanied by pain in your chest	This could be a sign of *heart disease*.
You smoke heavily	This could be a reaction to nicotine which speeds up the heart rate.
You also feel tired, short of breath and weak	You could be suffering from *anemia*.
You feel that your heart has "missed a beat"	This may indicate some disorder of your heart rate. See your doctor as soon as possible.
The palpitations are accompanied by dizziness and perhaps *fainting*	This could be atrial fibrillation or flutter and you will need to have treatment to correct the underlying condition that causes this disorder. See your doctor immediately.
You are suffering from *heart disease*	This could be a reaction to the drugs that you have been prescribed for your condition. See your doctor to decide whether it is necessary for you to change your medication.

PAP SMEAR

The Pap smear, named after the doctor who originated it, is a procedure that takes place during a pelvic examination and is used primarily to detect cancerous and pre-cancerous cells on the cervix.

Why is it done?
This is a routine screening procedure which should be performed on all sexually active woman when they begin having intercourse. For the average women, a Pap smear every two to three years is recommended, but it is important to check with your gynecologist about how often you should have a smear. Women who are from low socio-economic populations, who have frequent and multiple sex partners, or have family histories of uterine, cervical or vaginal cancer, are high-risk and should be tested at least annually. Women who were exposed to DES in utero should have a Pap smear every six months. The test is also vital for those who have had a genital herpes infection as this carries a higher risk of cancer. It is also used to diagnose urogenital viral infections and sexually transmitted diseases.

How is it done?
The smear should be part of a pelvic examination. A warmed speculum is passed into the vagina to separate the walls so the doctor can see the condition of your cervix. A wooden spatula or cotton swab is wiped across the cervix and the smear is transferred to a glass slide before being fixed and sent to a laboratory for analysis. Sometimes more than one smear is taken from different parts of the vagina as well as the cervix. The results should be available within six weeks.

You should not be menstruating or have had sexual intercourse 24 hours before your test. Blood and semen make the results unreliable.

What happens next?
The results of a smear test are classified into four or five categories. Negative gives you the all-clear, some mild dysplasia means you may have some infection and should be screened more regularly, and a positive smear test, though not always indicating cancer, means there is a detectable change in the cells necessitating further investigation.

With mild dysplasia you will probably be required to have a regular smear every few months.

If your test is positive you may be referred for colposcopy. This gives a clear magnified view of the suspect area, and enables cells to be removed for more tests.

The next step is a biopsy. A simple biopsy allows for a further small number of cells to be examined. A cone biopsy can offer treatment as well. The entire layer of suspect cells is removed under general anesthetic and examined. This may be done with a scalpel or a laser beam. If cancerous cells are discovered, treatment will be given for cervical cancer.

The major debate at present is how often women should be screened for cervical cancer and how quickly the results should be received. The test is simple and quick. However, the system is only as good as the procedures notifying women of their results or reminding them that their next smear is due.

PERFORMING A SMEAR TEST
Normally carried out as part of an internal examination, it should be done annually over age 40.

spatula
speculum
cervix

A speculum is inserted into the vagina and then opened to provide a clear view of the cervix. Using a spatula, the doctor or nurse will remove some tissue from your cervix and smear this onto a glass slide. The fixed and stained cells will be sent to and examined in a specialist laboratory.

SEE ALSO:

CERVICAL CANCER
COLPOSCOPY
CONE BIOPSY
DES
GENITAL HERPES
PELVIC EXAMINATION

PELVIC EXAMINATION

Internal and external investigations make up a pelvic examination which is a routine diagnostic check on the health of your pelvic organs. All women have them, and they should be done regularly after the age of 18 (or at the onset of sexual activity) when such diseases as cervical cancer and the presence of growths can be detected with this form of screening.

Women tend to have mixed feelings about pelvic examinations, especially with male gynecologists. Although they are uncomfortable, particularly if you have had no children, they are not painful. As women become more interested in the health of their bodies, some have established self-examination groups to keep a check on their own internal organs. With a speculum, flashlight and mirror some idea of what is normal for your vagina and cervix can be gained, particularly if you look at someone else. This is important in knowing your body and to break down taboos, though a diagnostic judgment would be very difficult with the untrained eye.

Try to schedule any pelvic examinations between periods, unless of course the examination is to try to sort out any bleeding problems.

Why is it done?
Pelvic examinations are done as a matter of routine in women's health clinics and as a diagnostic check on symptoms such as irregular bleeding, pelvic pain and bladder problems. The most common reason for a pelvic examination is as a means of determining if you are pregnant or not. Other reasons include:

◆ As a general check before you are prescribed any form of contraception: the contraceptive pill, fitting of an IUD, diaphragm or cervical cap.
◆ If a Pap smear is being done.
◆ If you have had any bleeding after intercourse.

◆ To check on any unusual or smelly vaginal discharge so that a sample can be taken for laboratory investigation.
◆ Irregular or unusually heavy menstrual bleeding or bleeding between periods.
◆ If you have any pain during intercourse (dyspareunia).
◆ If you suspect that you might have contracted a venereal disease with any symptoms of pain when passing urine or sores on the genital area.
◆ If your mother took the drug DES while she was pregnant with you.

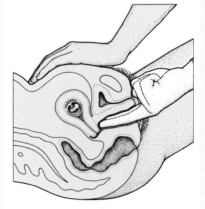

Bi-manual examination
The size, shape, position and tenderness of the uterus, ovaries and fallopian tubes can be felt by placing the first and middle fingers inside the vagina and pressing down on the abdomen.

How is it done?
You will need to remove your lower garments and lie on your back with your knees bent and legs apart. Some doctors put your legs in stirrups or have you lying on your side with the upper knee bent up.

An internal examination is usually made up of two parts. Your doctor will do a preliminary manual examination by placing one or two fingers inside the vagina and the other hand on top of the abdomen. In this way, the doctor can roll a

cyst, for example, between two hands and get some idea of size, shape and texture. There should also be a visual check on your vulva to spot any abrasions or lumps.

The speculum examination is an integral part of an internal pelvic examination. The speculum is a plastic or metal instrument shaped rather like a duck's bill, which is inserted into the vagina to separate the walls of the vagina so the cervix can be examined. Before use it should be lubricated and warmed. If it feels icy cold you are more likely to tense your muscles.

The speculum is inserted with the blades closed. Once inside your vagina, the blades are gently opened so that a visual check can be made, with the aid of a flashlight, of the cervix and the walls of the vagina.

While the examination is being done, you should relax as much as possible. Open your pelvic floor muscles and relax your jaw, neck and hands.

In some cases, it may be necessary to examine your rectum too. The doctor will insert a finger in your vagina and one into your rectum. You may feel as though your bowels are going to move. They won't.

PELVIC INFLAMMATORY DISEASE

This is a general term used to describe the chronic inflammation of any of the pelvic organs – the uterus, fallopian tubes or ovaries. Irrevocable scarring of the fallopian tubes and ovaries is the most serious complication that can arise because it quite often causes sterility. Other complications of pelvic inflammatory disease, or PID, include scarring and continuous pain during intercourse making it impossible (dyspareunia).

At one time, the commonest cause of this disease was tuberculosis. Now it is gonorrhea.

Some infections are complicated by the use of intra uterine contraceptive devices which may also be contributing factors.

Should I see the doctor?

PID must be treated early to prevent long-term problems. The symptoms of an acute infection are close to those of other pelvic disorders such as an ectopic pregnancy and the discomfort and pain should alert you to the fact that there is something wrong. A chronic infection may only cause recurrent mild pain and sometimes backache. But both forms must be investigated. Don't wait for it to go away, see your doctor as soon as possible. If you have an IUD, go to your clinic immediately.

What will the doctor do?

You will be examined and given a Pap smear to identify the organism causing the infection. Your doctor will probably prescribe antibiotics and complete bed rest. Eat well and don't have sexual intercourse during the course of treatment.

If antibiotics are not suitable for you, you may have to have more treatment. If PID develops into a chronic infection, it can be difficult to eradicate. You may need investigative laparoscopy to confirm the diagnosis. In severe cases, for a long-term infection, hysterectomy can be the only course of action, though you should go through any alternatives fully before agreeing to this operation.

What can I do?

Don't let any vaginal discharge continue for any length of time without full investigation and treatment. Because PID can recur, have a full check-up to confirm that your infection has been completely eradicated.

If you suspect that you might have a venereal disease, or your partner may do, go to a sexually transmitted diseases clinic right away.

· Symptoms ·

▲ Abdominal pain
▲ Back pain
▲ Persistent menstrual-like cramps
▲ Vaginal spotting of blood
▲ Tiredness
▲ Pain during and after intercourse

▲ Foul-smelling vaginal discharge
▲ Flu type symptoms of fever and chills
▲ Sub fertility or infertility

area of pain

SEE ALSO:

CONTRACEPTION
ECTOPIC PREGNANCY
GONORRHEA
HYSTERECTOMY
INFERTILITY
LAPAROSCOPY
PAINFUL INTERCOURSE
PAP SMEAR
SEXUALLY TRANSMITTED
  DISEASES

PELVIC PROBLEMS

For the purposes of this entry, pelvic problems relates to the pelvic genital organs, not the pelvic intestinal organs. In the female, the pelvis can be thought of as a funnel, the sides of the funnel being formed from the pelvic floor muscles, with an opening at the lower end through which the vagina, the rectum, and the urethra pass. You can see that if the pelvic floor muscles stretch, slacken or sag, any or all of the pelvic contents will drop and press onto the pelvic bones; some, if the muscle weakness is great, even prolapsing into the genital area itself. If the muscles primarily supporting the rectum weaken, the rectum may turn inside out and drop down making bowel movements difficult and painful. The same may happen with the walls of the vagina, and even the cervix, which may be so prolapsed that it appears at the vaginal opening. A kinking in the urethra would cause *urinary problems*, and if the bladder wall is prolapsed there will be *incontinence*. An added danger with a *prolapse* of the urethra or the bladder is the possibility of an infection from the vulval area, ascending first into the bladder causing *cystitis* and thence upwards to the kidney.

For the sake of the health of the pelvic organs it is essential to treat all *sexually transmitted diseases* promptly. Certain STDs can ascend from the vagina to the cervix and even to the pelvic cavity causing *pelvic inflammatory disease* and *infertility*. Any problem that causes scarring can lead to other disorders such as ectopic pregnancy.

An *ovarian cyst* may be symptomless until it is quite large. *Endometriosis* is a cause of painful periods and can be quite difficult to treat, though modern hormone remedies can be of some benefit to everyone. *Fibroids* are benign tumors of the muscular wall of the uterus. They can be as small as a pea or as large as your fist and can vary from one to 50. Quite often they are symptomless; sometimes if they protrude into the uterine cavity they can result in a *miscarriage*. If they are very numerous and causing *menorrhagia*, it may be necessary as a very last resort to consider a *hysterectomy*. A manual *pelvic examination* can often pinpoint the area of concern so that further tests can be taken.

PERINEAL TEAR

The perineum is the triangular area of skin, muscle and membrane situated between the vaginal opening and the rectum. During childbirth, the tissue stretches to allow the baby's head to pass through the vagina. If the labor is too rapid and the tissues have not stretched naturally and slowly, the tissue may tear as the head crowns.

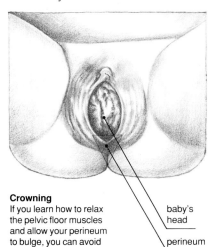

Crowning
If you learn how to relax the pelvic floor muscles and allow your perineum to bulge, you can avoid a tear.

baby's head

perineum

If the doctor thinks the perineum will not stretch sufficiently to let the baby's head through without tearing, an episiotomy may be performed under a local anesthetic.

Until recently, an episiotomy was standard practice and was performed at most first births. It was felt that a tear involving the perineum and underlying muscle healed badly and left weaknesses, possibly creating a tendency to prolapse. Recent research, however, has shown that stitched tears heal more quickly and less painfully than cuts and that episiotomy involves a higher risk of infection and does not prevent prolapse.

What will the doctor do?
Perineal tears are graded according to their depth and severity as first, second or third degree and they will always be stitched as they tend to heal slowly and awkwardly, often

leaving flaps of skin. The stitching is done under a local anesthetic and takes some time, as it is done in layers – the deeper muscles are stitched first and the superficial muscles separately from the skin and other tissue. The stitches dissolve in 5–6 days.

How can I avoid a tear?
Doctors and midwives use their judgments about whether to perform an episiotomy or to let the perineum take the strain. If the doctor talks you through the labor and particularly the transition period when the urge to push is often too great to resist, the tissues should thin out slowly and gradually.

Conducting labor in a more upright position also reduces the likelihood of a perineal tear because the pushing is not uphill. Tears are far less common among women in cultures where labor and childbirth are in an upright position. There are useful exercises known as Kegel exercises (see index) which you can do during

your pregnancy to learn to stretch the perineal tissues and help the vaginal area to bulge out easily without straining and pushing. Keeping up the pelvic floor exercises also helps.

Stitches always cause some discomfort so be prepared for pain when sitting down, passing urine or moving your bowels. Sit on a rubber ring and have plenty of warm salt baths to prevent infection and soothe the area. Dry your perineum with a hair dryer and change your sanitary pads frequently so the area doesn't become soggy and damp. If you feel sore and swollen, an ice bag or a sanitary pad soaked in witch hazel may give relief. The discomfort may remain for weeks and prevent intercourse.

SEE ALSO:

EPISIOTOMY
LABOR

UPRIGHT LABOR POSITIONS
Squatting makes your pelvic joints more flexible; relieves back pain and strengthens the thigh and back muscles.

Half squat
Holding something secure, lower yourself so weight is on one leg at a time.

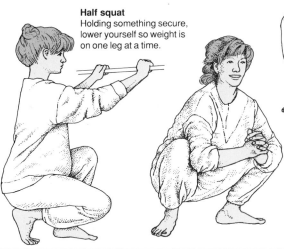

Practicing squats
Stand with your back against the wall and slide down onto a pillow.

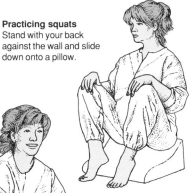

Full squat
Keep your back long and straight and get down as low as you can. Try to get your heels on the ground. Pressing your elbows against your thighs increases the stretch.

PHLEBITIS

Literally this word means inflammation of a vein. To the medical profession, phlebitis means inflammation of a superficial vein, that is one lying near the surface of the skin. It does not apply to a deep-vein thrombosis when the inflammation is in the larger, deeper veins. Phlebitis is therefore more accurately called superficial thrombophlebitis (thrombus meaning blood clot).

Thrombophlebitis is slightly more common in women because of its association with childbirth, the contraceptive pill and varicose veins. It nearly always occurs because of a local infection, such as a boil or an abcess, or because of injury. It appears like a tender, firm, red streak in the skin. This is because the blood clot has strongly adhered to the wall of the vein. There is therefore no danger of part of the blood clot breaking away and forming an embolus and causing thrombosis elsewhere. This happens with deep-vein thrombosis when the risk of pulmonary embolism is always present. Superficial thrombophlebitis is therefore uncomfortable but not dangerous.

· S y m p t o m s ·
▲ Tender, red, firm streak under the skin
▲ Itchiness over the hard swelling
▲ If there is infection, you may have a temperature

Should I see the doctor?
If you have a boil or any other skin disorder, and the area becomes painful and hard and swollen, see your doctor. This may also be the case if you have recently had any intravenous treatment. If the site becomes sore and red, see your doctor in case of infection. Varicose veins are sometimes the site for this disorder.

What will the doctor do?
If there is infection, your doctor will first treat this with antibiotics, local antiseptic and antibiotic creams. As the infection is brought under control, the blood clot will dissolve, shrink and eventually disappear without trace.

If the blood clot is large, it may leave a small scar which can be felt as a lump. However, even if the clot was large enough to block the vein completely, no harm is done. The network of veins in the upper layers of the skin is so vast that new channels open up to do the job of the obstructed vein.

What can I do?
It may be more comfortable to compress the affected area with an elasticated bandage. This causes blood to flow more quickly, thus preventing more clots from forming. The medical treatment should affect a cure within two weeks.

If the area is itchy, use a zinc and castor oil cream to relieve the irritation.

SEE ALSO:

CONTRACEPTION
DEEP-VEIN THROMBOSIS
VARICOSE VEINS

PHOBIA

This is a paralyzing, irrational fear of a situation, an object, animal, person or element. The onset of the phobia may be unexpected although it is usually associated with a depression or intense anxiety. However, there are certain times of life when phobias may appear as part of normal development. In the very young for example, sudden loud noises cause extreme fear. As children grow older, it's accepted that they will be fearful of any object, such as a snake, which moves towards them rapidly with a jerking or swerving movement. Fear of animals or the dark is common in pre-school children. In old age, we begin to have phobias about cancer, heart disease and death. There are other fears that are often the butt of jokes such as fear of thunder and lightning or sharks.

Why do they arise?
Research has shown that people who suffer phobias may be different from people who don't – the so-called phobic personality. The natural feelings of anxiety appear to have a greater physical effect on phobics than on other people. Even mild anxiety, which we all experience say when boarding an aircraft, may bring an increased heart rate, palpitations, shaking and sweating in a phobic. These are termed panic attacks. Nearly all phobics are aware that they are behaving unreasonably but are unable to control their fear.

What types of phobias are there?
In addition to agoraphobia (see box), the following have been recognized: acrophobia, fear of heights; ailurophobia, fear of cats; arachnophobia, fear of spiders; aquaphobia, fear of water; brontophobia, fear of thunder; claustrophobia, fear of enclosure; cynophobia, fear of dogs; equinophobia, fear of horses;

microphobia, fear of germs; murophobia, fear of mice; mysophobia, fear of dirt; ophidiophobia, fear of snakes; pyrophobia, fear of fire; thanatophobia, fear of death; xenophobia, fear of strangers; zoophobia, fear of animals.

Should I see the doctor?
Many people suffer from phobias that they can easily avoid, such as sharks and horses for example. However, if the symptoms arise and cause panic attacks, and you feel they are irrational or physically difficult to come to terms with, making normal life impossible, talk to your doctor.

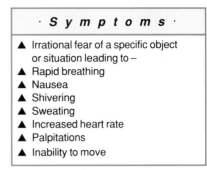

· S y m p t o m s ·

- ▲ Irrational fear of a specific object or situation leading to –
- ▲ Rapid breathing
- ▲ Nausea
- ▲ Shivering
- ▲ Sweating
- ▲ Increased heart rate
- ▲ Palpitations
- ▲ Inability to move

In the case of others, it is important to distinguish between behavior which is phobic, and behavior which is only eccentric. A woman who refuses to go outside is not necessarily ill. If she is a housewife, she may decide

PSYCHOLOGICAL TREATMENTS FOR PHOBIAS

In addition to the various behavioral therapies described below, other methods for treating phobias include hypnosis, meditation and psychoanalysis.

Desensitization is an attempt to combine the phobic situation with a pleasurable experience. For example, if you are afraid of cats, start by looking at pictures and then slowly build up to being able to stay in a room alone with a cat and stroking it and then allowing it to sit on your lap.

Modeling is a technique in which the phobic is exposed to the phobia with people who are entirely fearless. With repeated instances of exposure, the phobic learns to imitate the behavior of others until she behaves herself in the observed normal, natural way.

Flooding must be orchestrated by a professional. It involves exposure to the phobia, frequently for long periods until the phobic becomes so accustomed to the experience

that it causes no fear and you find that there is no cause for fear.

Logotherapy works on the basis that instead of trying to control your fears, you exaggerate them and make them as bad as you can. Having faced your worst fears, you may gradually cease to be haunted by them and be able to take a less fearful view of the everyday world.

Cognitive manipulation involves talking to yourself and telling yourself repeatedly that you are not afraid. This type of therapy requires technical support sometimes in the form of a monitor that allows you to hear your own heart rate. You can hear your heart rate speed up as you approach the phobic situation. The therapy involves repeating this experience but replacing your heart rate with a recording of a normal heart rate and trying to match this. Eventually you may be able to control your body so that your heart rate is lowered and the fear of the situation should subside.

that this role devalues her and so is attempting to draw attention to it by withdrawing her labor.

What will the doctor do?

Your doctor may prescribe anti-depressants or treat you for anxiety by suggesting relaxation exercises or, in some cases, tranquilizing drugs. If the panic attacks are severe, you may be referred to a psychotherapist either on an out-patient basis or in hospital. The most successful techniques to get rid of phobias, including the treatment of agoraphobia, are those which involve behavioral therapy.

What can I do?

The obvious way to treat a phobia is to avoid the situation. If this is unsatisfactory from your point of view because it involves great restriction on your life, try desensitization which is the only behavioral therapy you should attempt on your own. In any event you would be wise to talk to a professional before you try to cure yourself in this way.

Don't think of yourself as being different, inadequate or inferior. Talk about the phobia openly if you can so your friends and family understand and you won't find yourself in the position of having to react first and explain your behavior later.

Ask your medical advisors to put you in touch with a self-help group; such groups work well and will help you to realize that you are not unusual; they have a high success rate.

AGORAPHOBIA

Agoraphobia is a fear of open spaces and quite commonly this fear is great enough to keep a woman prisoner in her home, a place which provides a barrier against the outside world. More than 90% of agoraphobics are women, and, although the exact cause of this and other phobias is not known, psychologists have put forward reasons such as self-defense, for example.

Agoraphobia is common after a marriage, and may be seen as some sort of proof of dependence on the man and the home.

Treatment involves using the desensitization method of therapy; the agoraphobic is coaxed out with a friend on a public outing that gives her pleasure, such as shopping, a theater trip or a walk in a garden or park. This form of treatment is usually accompanied by exercises and relaxation. In time, the expeditions can be undertaken alone, perhaps with a walkie-talkie system so that someone can give guidance and encouragement at all times.

SEE ALSO:
ANXIETY
DEPRESSION

PLACENTA PREVIA

This is a rare but serious complication of pregnancy of unknown cause. In a normal pregnancy, the placenta is attached to the upper segment of the uterine wall but if it attaches itself anywhere on the lower segment, it prevents this part of the uterus expanding during the birth and sometimes blocks the cervix. In addition, the placenta will peel off in labor, causing serious bleeding in the mother and reducing the blood supply and therefore oxygen to the baby. If the placenta peels off before labor, this is known as placenta abruptio.

Placenta previa occurs in about one in every 100 pregnancies. However, because of improved prenatal screening of pregnant women, this condition rarely goes undetected.

· S y m p t o m s ·

▲ Bright red blood from the vagina with no pain.

Should I see the doctor?

If at any time during a pregnancy, or even a suspected one, you experience any bleeding, consult your doctor at once.

What will the doctor do?

The doctor will normally perform an ultrasound scan in the case of bleeding, but if bleeding hasn't occurred and a routine ultrasound scan has confirmed placenta previa (after 28 weeks it can be seen clearly), you will receive meticulous medical attention. From the 32nd week, you will probably have to remain in hospital until your delivery.

In most cases, your doctor may decide to deliver your baby by Caesarean section. Otherwise you will go into labor as usual although there will be a lot of bleeding before the onset of labor and more when labor starts. You may need a blood transfusion depending on how much blood you lose during delivery.

What are the risks?

You are more likely to have a premature labor with this condition with inherent risks to the baby. However, you will be monitored more frequently because you will be in hospital, and any fetal distress will be picked up as soon as possible.

There is no reason to suppose that you will have this condition again with subsequent pregnancies. However, your medical history will alert your medical advisers and you will be closely monitored.

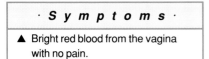

Position of the placenta
In a normal pregnancy, the placenta is positioned high up in the uterus. But in placenta previa, it develops near, or sometimes over the cervix.

Normal placenta   **Placenta previa**

SEE ALSO:

BLEEDING
CAESAREAN SECTION
LABOR
PREGNANCY PROBLEMS
ULTRASOUND

POSTNATAL CARE

During the first days and weeks following the birth of your baby, you will experience still more changes in your body and mental state. Much of what follows pregnancy and birth inevitably seems like an anti-climax. You need to be prepared for this and learn about what is going to happen to you. Don't set your standards too high; you'll be surrounded by family and friends with lots of advice – be easy on yourself and progress at your own pace.

BREASTFEEDING

In the first few days after your baby is born, your breasts are going to take something of a battering, so it's worth looking after them as breastfeeding gets going. The nipples are delicate and they need time to toughen up; you'd be wise to increase the length of time on each breast gradually. At first, two minutes on each breast will give your baby sufficient colostrum.

Eighty per cent of the food is taken during the first five minutes and this is when most babies suck strongly. Armed with this knowledge, you need not be afraid of keeping feeding times on the short side to prevent your breasts becoming sore.

Soreness can develop quickly if the breast is pulled from your baby's mouth rather than released. The way to do this is to insert your finger into the corner of your baby's mouth and gently ease her off the breast; gently pressing down her chin will do the same thing.

SIX WEEK POSTNATAL CHECK

All mothers are seen six weeks after delivery for an examination to see if the breasts are healthy and the genital organs are returning to normal. The following checks are made:
- a full examination of the breasts and nipples
- examination of a urine specimen
- weight check

- check on blood pressure
- examination of lochia (vaginal discharge from the shrinking and healing uterus), if still present
- pelvic examination to feel the size and consistency of the uterus and make sure that it is shrinking satisfactorily and to visualize the cervix, assess its progress back to normal amd make sure that there are no tears
- inspection of an episiotomy wound to make sure that healing is satisfactory

The postnatal check is also a time when you can voice any of your worries to your doctor. If there are questions about yourself or the baby you wish to ask, make a list of them before you go along to the clinic, and make sure that you get satisfactory answers. If you have experienced a mild depression since the birth of your baby and it is not getting better, or it is getting worse, make sure that you mention this matter to your doctor. Postpartum depression treated quickly has a very good chance of disappearing in a short time. The longer you leave postpartum depression untreated, the longer it may last.

GETTING BACK TO NORMAL

For the three to six weeks following delivery there will be a discharge from your vagina, even if you had a Caesarean section. This is the vagina draining itself and is called lochia. It starts off red, then brown to white and back to normal vaginal discharge. You will need to wear sanitary pads or towels (not tampons) and change them frequently.

You should try to urinate as soon as possible after delivery. Pour warm water over yourself if the urine stings because of any stitches. You may need to urinate frequently in the first few days; this is the way your body eliminates any excess fluid.

Don't worry about your first bowel motion. This doesn't normally occur

for about two days after delivery. Eat high-fiber foods (lots of fruit) and drink plenty of water. Moving around also helps to get your bowels going. If you had stitches for any reason, bathe frequently and sit on a rubber ring to relieve pressure.

You may experience afterpains for the first few days. This is the uterus contracting back to its pre-pregnant size. The faster and harder it contracts down, the less likelihood there is of postpartum hemorrhage and an excellent sign that you are getting back to normal. These pains are normally experienced most strongly when you are breastfeeding. Both the contracting down and the cessation of lochia occur more rapidly if you breastfeed.

POSTNATAL EXERCISES

As soon as possible after delivery try your pelvic floor exercises (see below). Having learned them during pregnancy, you should be prepared to continue exercising every time you pass urine by arresting the flow. This way you will strengthen the pelvic

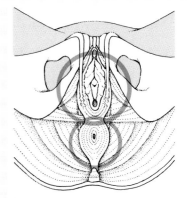

The pelvic floor muscles
These lie in two main groups forming a figure of eight.

floor, firm up the vagina and prevent a prolapse.

Within a few days of delivery, there will be many physical and emotional changes. Your uterus will shrink back to its pre-pregnant state, your breasts will fill with milk and any stitches will heal. You can help yourself by starting postnatal exercises right away. Your abdominal muscles won't contract back immediately and they will appear to sag. This is normal but that doesn't mean you won't want to correct the condition as quickly as possible. Most women take at least three months to return to their previous shape, so don't panic either, just work on your figure as much as you can.

You can start to exercise before you even get out of bed. The two main areas to concentrate on are your pelvic floor and your abdominal muscles. When you're resting, lie on your stomach with pillows under your hips. This encourages your pelvic organs to return to their normal positions. This will probably be uncomfortable when your milk comes in and your breasts engorge.

To strengthen your abdominals, lie on the bed, with your knees bent and your hands flat on your stomach. Squeeze your buttocks together and press your back into the bed. Combine this exercise with the Kegel exercises.

While still in bed you can circle your feet to encourage circulation in your ankles and feet and reduce swelling. You can start gentle curl up exercises on the bed, building up to sit ups by the second week.

Kegel exercises

The pelvic floor muscles are special muscles in a woman. They support the organs in the pelvis – the uterus, bowel and bladder. Making these muscles strong and keeping them that way, is essential for long-term enjoyment of sexual intercourse, avoidance of a prolapsed uterus or stress incontinence.

One of the ways to practice pelvic floor exercises, known as Kegel exercises, is to halt the flow of urine several times when emptying your bladder.

◆ Lie down on your back, legs bent and apart.

POSTNATAL EXERCISES

Your postnatal exercise routine should start within days of delivery and you should exercise for about five minutes several times a day for

at least three months. Your hospital physical therapist will set out a basic routine for you.

With your hands on your stomach muscles to feel them tighten, raise your pelvis at the same time as you draw up your pelvic floor muscles.

Start with gentle curl ups by running your hands up your thighs to reach your knees. Curl down slowly with your arms crossed in front of you and feel your abdominal muscles tighten.

◆ Draw up the pelvic floor muscles, concentrating on the vaginal sphincter.
◆ Hold and relax.
◆ Make sure you're not just tightening your buttocks.
◆ Think of the pelvic floor as a lift and draw it up slowly little by little.
◆ Release in the same smooth way.
Once you get the knack, you can do it while sitting down or standing wherever you are.

During sexual intercourse, grip your partner's penis with your vagina, hold and then relax. Your partner will be able to tell when you are squeezing; if he can't, practice some more.

REST

The most important consideration is to get enough rest. Never ignore signs of tiredness; you will need all your strength when you get back into

your normal routine. Tiredness will be almost inevitable and you may lose your confidence and not enjoy the early weeks if you don't get enough rest. One reason you will feel fatigued is that the volume of blood drops by about 30% at delivery and your muscles are relatively deprived of oxygen as a result, making you feel weak.

SEE ALSO:

BREASTFEEDING PROBLEMS
CAESAREAN SECTION
EPISIOTOMY
INCONTINENCE
NIPPLE PROBLEMS
PERINEAL TEAR
POSTPARTUM DEPRESSION
PROLAPSE

POSTPARTUM DEPRESSION

This is a term used to cover anything from the feeling of weepiness around the third or fourth day after childbirth – the baby blues – to a psychotic condition with delusions and hallucinations. As there has been so little research into this form of depression, the exact cause is not entirely clear and certainly not straightforward. The baby blues are common but the true postpartum depression is extremely rare. The problem at both levels seems to arise for both emotional and physical reasons.

What causes it?

There is no question that postpartum depression is partly caused by the wide disparity most women experience between their expectations of life after the birth of their babies, and the reality of having to cope with helpless, demanding infants.

Physically there are the changes too in the level of circulating hormones which descend into a trough after the high levels of pregnancy, and then increase with the arrival of another set of hormones which initiates the milk flow. Added to this is the sort of birth you had and how it compared to what you were expecting and the treatment you received in the hospital.

If your family are supportive and uncritical, you will probably be happier and be able to learn to look after your baby without the anxiety caused by being critically observed. Women who live far from their families, or without a supportive partner, or who have experienced a bereavement during their pregnancies are more likely to suffer this depression postnatally.

Is it serious?

The enormous swing in hormonal levels which occurs before menstruation and during pregnancy makes most women tearful, irritable, indecisive and anxious. After childbirth, these feelings usually subside as the domestic routines become more organized and you learn to cope with the stresses of parenthood and the night feeds. If the depression deepens and continues, it does not represent the normal depressive illness which may be the aftermath of pregnancy. Instead, it may herald a severe psychological disturbance that could continue for some time. The need to identify this early is essential, or you may suffer a huge shock because the happy event you and your partner were anticipating turns sour.

· S y m p t o m s ·

- ▲ Tearfulness
- ▲ Irritability
- ▲ Extreme tiredness and fatigue
- ▲ Insomnia
- ▲ Lack of interest or inability to look after yourself and the baby
- ▲ Feeling of inferiority and inadequacy
- ▲ Marked changes of mood from deepest depression to elation
- ▲ Feeling of terror
- ▲ Contemplation of suicide or harm to the baby

Should I see the doctor?

If you suffer any depression, no matter how minor, seek help, whether from your doctor or community organization.

What will the doctor do?

Your doctor will initiate the counseling and support from professionals as well as family and friends which will help in the organization of a routine to relieve the real and imagined pressures.

If the depression continues, your doctor may decide to prescribe a course of anti-depressive drugs to help you get back to normal quickly.

If you are one of the small number of women whose depression stretches into months, there are usually two outcomes. Most commonly the depression does not warrant hospital admission; it can be treated by your family doctor or by a psychiatrist with anti-depressants and counseling. For severe postpartum psychosis, you will be hospitalized, preferably in a mother and baby unit. The mainstay of treatment is anti-depressants but electroconvulsive therapy (ECT) is also used today with a high success rate. Support for the family as a whole is essential. This depression is hard on you but your partner may develop psychological difficulties too and you will both need to be reintroduced to family life after your treatment is over.

What can I do?

Read up as much as you can about postpartum depression before you give birth so you can recognize any symptoms. Once you are at home alone with the baby, the interrupted nights and demands of an unpredictable human being can dominate your time so you must plan to avoid any build up of stress and tiredness. You can prevent things from getting on top of you by being very clear about priorities.

Forget about minor concerns like the housework, cooking or ironing. Allocate chores to your partner, family and friends. Whenever anyone asks if they can do anything, point them towards the washing or ironing, or hand them the shopping list. Don't plan to sell your house and move just after the baby arrives. Put aside all grand schemes until you're more used to each other.

Don't be ashamed of feeling low when you thought you'd be thrilled. If you feel negative about the baby, talk to someone about it. Don't bottle these emotions up. Time on your own is an absolute necessity. Try to put away some time each week in which you can feel independent with a life of your own. Enjoy yourself when you are away from the house. Give yourself a treat: a new hair-do, have lunch out with a friend, go to a movie. Don't make motherhood the only reason for your existence.

Give your partner time alone with the baby so he can be involved, too.

BABY BLUES

Most women experience some feeling of depression and weepiness around the third or fourth day after delivery. These baby blues classically start with the first flow of milk. The baby blues can spoil your enjoyment of your baby if you don't recognize that this is a normal reaction and that things will get better. Usually no medical attention with drugs is necessary, although after consideration your doctor may prescribe a short course of sleeping pills if you are not getting enough rest. You'd be right to expect the baby blues as almost every woman has some reaction after the birth.

Make certain to ask your doctor to explain any aspects of baby care that you don't understand.

Don't fall into the trap of thinking you will get better soon if your depression stretches on over weeks. Talk to someone quickly about your fears and go to your doctor. The longer you are untreated, the longer it will take for you to get better. Postpartum psychosis can recur so prepare yourself during your next pregnancy and make sure your doctor and support services know about your past medical history. An optimistic attitude and good preparation will reduce the chances of a recurrence.

If you are in hospital, do try to have the baby with you. Even though you may feel he or she is responsible for your condition, any separation will be damaging in the long term.

Through mothers' groups organized by hospitals or community groups such as the La Leche League, new parents can meet together. This is often a good place to air your concerns about your reaction to parenthood. The social pressures to be the smiling perfect mother are never the reality so be true to yourself and don't try to live up to other people's views of what you are or should be.

SEE ALSO:

ANXIETY
DEPRESSION
INSOMNIA
MOOD CHANGES

PREGNANCY PROBLEMS

PROBLEMS	SYMPTOMS	SELF-HELP TREATMENT
Abdominal pain	Cramp-like or dragging pains on one side only can occur when you're sitting or lying down. This is round ligament pain caused when the ligaments that support the uterus stretch.	A hot water bottle or heating pads will relax muscles. You shouldn't take any painkillers as the pain is likely to be sporadic anyway.
Backache	Ligaments become more flexible in preparation for labor and the increased weight combined with bad posture leads to low back pain. If your baby is in the posterior position with its head pressed against your sacrum, you may have a backache labor (see Backache).	Action depends on the cause. Try to concentrate on good posture, and watch your footwear. High heels are foolish. Check your mattress and exercise to strengthen your spine. If the baby is in the occipito posterior position, get down on all fours to take the pressure off your back.
Bleeding gums	If your gums bleed after brushing or eating hard foods, this could be gingivitis. Your gums are thicker in pregnancy because of the hormones and the softer margins allow food to collect at the base of the teeth. If bacteria grows and multiplies this can lead to tooth decay and gum disease.	Brush your teeth regularly and use dental floss to keep your gums healthy. Visit your dentist every six months.
Constipation	Relaxation of the muscles of the intestine can lead to sluggish bowel movements and feces dry out making your stools hard and painful to pass.	Take plenty of dietary fiber and lots of fluids. Regular exercise helps prevent constipation too. Always open your bowels when you feel the need to. Don't take laxatives (unless prescribed by your doctor); use natural laxatives like dried fruit and bran.
Cramp	Pains in the calf, thigh or foot, which are usually felt at night. Why cramps should be more common in pregnancy is not known but it could be either low calcium levels or not enough salt in the diet.	Massage the affected part firmly; if the cramps are in the leg, flex your foot hard, pushing your heel away from you. See your doctor if the cramps persist.
Cravings	Desire for certain foods, often quite irrational, is thought to be something to do with progesterone levels. Often tastes change too. Some flavors, formerly enjoyed, may be quite unacceptable. Sugary and sweet foods often become favorites.	Eat whatever you feel like, but make sure the foods aren't low in nutrients or fattening.
Fainting	Dizzy, spinning sensation as the demands of the uterus for increased blood supply temporarily deprive your brain of blood.	If you feel faint, lie down with your feet slightly elevated and your head flat. Avoid standing for long periods and don't rush around.
Flatulence	A sluggish intestine allows a build up of wind that you may have more difficulty expelling.	Avoid problem foods such as fried foods. Peppermint and a soothing hot milk drink might help. Try not to gulp air; gum chewing causes you to take in air, for example.
Fluid retention	Swelling in the hands, feet and face because your body retains fluid in pregnancy. The fluid stagnates in the lower parts of your body.	Rest with your legs up and avoid standing so fluid doesn't pool in your legs and hands. Take it easy in hot weather. Avoid very salty foods; salt causes fluid retention. Mention noticeable edema at your prenatal clinic.

PROBLEMS	SYMPTOMS	SELF-HELP TREATMENT
Frequency of urination	Urgent need to empty your bladder, even small amounts, throughout the day and night, is caused by pressure of the uterus on the neighboring bladder. Increased blood supply to the pelvis causes the bladder to become irritable and empty itself more frequently.	Don't drink too much just before going to sleep; avoid coffee, which is a diuretic, last thing at night. Rock backwards and forwards when you're passing urine to empty your bladder thoroughly.
Heartburn	Burning sensation behind your breastbone, sometimes accompanied by a sour taste in your mouth because the valve at the entrance to your stomach relaxes and allows acid to reflux into the esophagus (see Digestive problems).	Avoid troublesome foods such as acidic fruits and fatty foods. Have a hot milk drink before going to bed. Raise the foot or head of the bed to prevent reflux. Lose weight; obesity and overeating can also result in heartburn. Try not to take antacids; speak to your doctor before taking any medication.
Hemorrhoids	These may be felt as an itchiness and pain around the anus, and they may prolapse after delivery. The pressure of the baby's head in late pregnancy obstructs major blood vessels, impairing the return of blood from the pelvic organs and causing ballooning, rather like varicose veins in the lower legs. Constipation, which increases pressure, makes them worse.	Eat a high-fiber diet to keep your stools soft and easy to pass. If the hemorrhoids itch, apply soothing cream or ice packs. Don't have hot baths, this increases the blood flow and makes them more itchy. After delivery, if they prolapse, they can be manually pushed back. They will soon disappear.
Incontinence	Urine leaks when you laugh, cough or jump about because your bladder capacity is reduced and the pelvic floor muscles can't stop urine leaking through.	Empty your bladder often, and avoid constipation and anything that increases internal pressure, such as lifting. Do your pelvic floor exercises assiduously (see Postnatal care).
Insomnia	The baby's metabolism knows no day or night and the kicking may disturb you, preventing sleep. The baby is more alert if your blood sugar levels are high. The need to empty your bladder often and night sweats can also keep you awake.	Wear natural fibers in bed to avoid overheating at night. Have a good book, a soothing night drink or a television in the room to relax you so you don't fret about the lack of sleep. Doctors rarely prescribe sedatives unless your sleeplessness is leading to exhaustion.
Morning sickness	This can occur throughout pregnancy and not just in the morning. The feeling of nausea is usually made worse by the smell of food or other things such as tobacco smoke.	Eat little and often. Try nutritious snacks (see Morning sickness) to combat the rising nausea. Don't get overtired.
Nasal discomfort	Your nose may feel congested or stuffy, and you may have nose bleeds. The mucous membrane in the nose softens and thickens under the influence of the pregnancy hormones.	Don't use a nasal spray and treat your nose gently. Avoid dry, dusty environments.
Pelvic pain	Pain in the groin and on the inside of your thighs can be felt when you're walking. This is because the baby's head is pressing on the nerves, particularly towards the end of pregnancy.	Rest with your body supported on pillows. Don't take painkillers as the pain is usually sporadic. Try gently rocking to ease the discomfort.

PREGNANCY PROBLEMS

PROBLEMS	SYMPTOMS	SELF-HELP TREATMENT
Pigmentation changes	During pregnancy your body makes more of the melanocyte-stimulating hormone. Pigmented areas are made worse when exposed to strong sunlight. The skin around the nipple darkens, you may notice a line down your abdomen (linea nigra) and a mask-like darkening of the skin (see Rashes).	Use a sun block in strong sunshine. Don't bleach your skin; the pigmentation marks will fade after delivery.
Rashes	If you are too heavy, the folds of your skin could become hot and sweaty and develop rashes if you don't keep yourself clean and dry. This is most common under the breasts and in the groin.	Keep yourself clean and well dried. Apply talcum powder to folds of skin and don't allow yourself to get overweight.
Rib pain	Exquisite pain and soreness under the breast, usually on the right side. This is known as costal margin pain and occurs towards the end of pregnancy as the uterus rises.	Prop yourself up so the ribs aren't compressed. The pain will disappear at about week 36 when the baby drops into the pelvic cavity.
Stretchmarks	Silvery marks on the abdomen, thighs and breasts are caused by excess weight and your skin type and elasticity.	No cosmetic lotion will have any effect. The marks are unavoidable. They will fade and become smaller after delivery. Avoid sudden excess weight gain.
Sweating	Night sweats and general feeling of warmth – your own central heating system – are a result of the increased blood supply that causes the blood vessels beneath the skin to dilate.	Wear light natural fibers and don't exert yourself too much.
Tiredness	Fatigue, unrelated to the amount of sleep you are getting, is common in pregnancy. It can also result from carrying excess weight, lack of fitness and exercise, insomnia, or poor nutrition because of nausea.	Sleep or rest whenever you can. Eat small meals often to keep up your energy levels. Get other people to do the work and be sensible about your workload at home and at work.
Vaginal discharge	Increase over the normal white discharge results from a thickening and softening of mucous membranes throughout the body, including the vagina and cervix. Any brown bloody discharge could be cervical erosion.	If the discharge is very heavy, wear a panty liner for comfort. Don't do anything else. See your doctor if you notice any brown discharge (see Cervix problems).
Varicose veins	Dark purplish veins, usually in the lower leg, which may be itchy. Tendency to varicosity runs in families, but if you are overweight or the baby's head presses on major blood vessels and causes blood to pool in the legs or vulva, these veins will balloon and itch.	Put support hose on before getting out of bed. Elevate the foot of your bed slightly. Do exercises to improve the circulation in your feet and legs and don't stand around too long allowing the blood to stagnate in your legs. For varicose veins on the vulva, sleep with your bottom on a pillow or wear a sanitary pad.
Visual disturbances	Contact lenses may be uncomfortable because of retention of fluid causing the eyeball to change shape slightly.	Consult your optician, you may have to stop wearing contact lenses during pregnancy.

PREGNANCY TESTING

Most women know they are pregnant before the clinical test confirms their suspicion. The simplest positive pregnancy test is a missed period. Shortly after this, you may notice that your breasts are tender and larger, you need to urinate more frequently and you may feel nauseous.

On your first visit to your family doctor, you will have an internal pelvic examination. If your uterus is enlarged, and there is a softening of your genital organs, and with a speculum examination the cervix takes on a characterisic purplish velvety look, you are pregnant.

How do tests work?

Detecting the presence of the pregnancy hormone human chorionic gonadatrophin (HCG) is the most common test. The developing placenta begins to produce this hormone to prevent menstruation and protect the pregnancy. For the test to be reliable, urine needs to be tested for HCG two weeks after the missed period; that is approximately six weeks after the first day of the last period. For an earlier result, HCG can be detected in a blood sample, although this is more expensive.

Some of the older pregnancy tests involved the use of high-dose hormone tablets which were really a way of making the uterus bleed (a withdrawal bleed) if a fetus was not present. If a fetus was present, and it was female, there was the possibility that the hormones could produce masculinization. Because of this danger, hormone pregnancy tests have largely been superseded.

HOME KITS

There are several home kits that you can use to confirm a pregnancy before you visit the doctor. They also rely on the detection of HCG in your urine. The advantage of a home kit is that you know right away whether you are pregnant or not, and if you are, you can immediately start to look after your unborn baby by eating well and avoiding all drugs and chemicals. This is a dangerous time when toxins can cross the placenta, pass into the fetal circulation and damage the developing embryo.

For best results, take a sample of your first urine of the day. This contains the highest amount of HCG. The tests work by either dipping an indicator stick into the urine and checking the color, or adding a chemical to the urine and waiting for a change. Read the manufacturer's instructions carefully.

Some of these home kits are expensive but if the test is done two weeks after the missed period, it will be about 95% accurate. There is always the possibility that a pregnancy test will give you a false negative but such is the accuracy of these latest high technology pregnancy tests that this is a very rare occurrence. If your pregnancy test comes up negative and you really believe that you are pregnant, simply do a repeat test yourself, making sure you use a concentrated urine sample taken first thing in the morning, or get a second one done at a laboratory. False positives are extremely rare although they will follow up to a week after an abortion.

SEE ALSO:

PELVIC EXAMINATION
PREGNANCY PROBLEMS

PREMENSTRUAL SYNDROME

More widely known as PMS, this disorder is characterized by a group of symptoms – emotional, mental and physical which affect about 75% of all women in the days just prior to or early in menstruation.

What causes it?
PMS usually has three major components: depression, aches and pains and changes in mood. The exact cause is still not known but it seems that the symptoms are in some way linked with the production of the female hormones estrogen and progesterone which both start to fall off at different rates in the days prior to menstruation. As both these hormones are crucial to our metabolism, mood and level of activity, it is not surprising that an imbalance could give rise to the array of symptoms repeatedly reported by women premenstrually, and now regarded seriously by the medical profession.

What are the characteristics of the syndrome?
Any number of the symptoms form part of the syndrome and in most cases all can be remedied, often by the same treatment.

In severe cases, PMS has been quoted as causing serious personality changes, even giving rise to criminal tendencies. Such crimes as shoplifting are 30 times more common among women premenstrually than at other times.

Dr Katharina Dalton in her book *The Menstrual Cycle* advocates that progesterone deficiency is a common cause of PMS. Her studies showed that the PMS symptoms were only present when progesterone should be in the bloodstream and temperature charts confirmed that PMS sufferers did not have raised temperatures, which is a sign of lack of progesterone. Also, these symptoms manifest themselves at times when hormonal balance is

disturbed, such as after pregnancy, after taking the contraceptive pill and at puberty.

> ## · S y m p t o m s ·
>
> ▲ Fluid retention – feeling of being bloated, heavy breasts, thickened waistline, puffy face, hands and feet, causing headaches and pain especially in the breasts and abdomen
> ▲ Changes in mood – irritability, loss of temper, tearfulness
> ▲ Depression often leading to suicidal feelings and violence towards oneself

Should I see the doctor?
If your symptoms are severe enough to disturb your normal life every month and the self-help measures don't alleviate them, go to your doctor to get medical treatment.

What will the doctor do?
Your doctor will question you about the symptoms and possibly ask you to record your symptoms over a period of one month. It is difficult to find out if you are one of the women who suffers from the progesterone deficit, so your doctor may decide to try progesterone on a trial basis and look for improvement. Progesterone is only soluble by mouth in an artificial form so you will probably be offered suppositories. You will probably be recommended to take up to four 400mg doses per day but as the individual needs of patients differ, the treatment will be tailored to your specific needs wherever possible. To help with this, note down on your menstrual chart how much progesterone you need each day to affect your symptoms.

The treatment should be started four days before you expect the

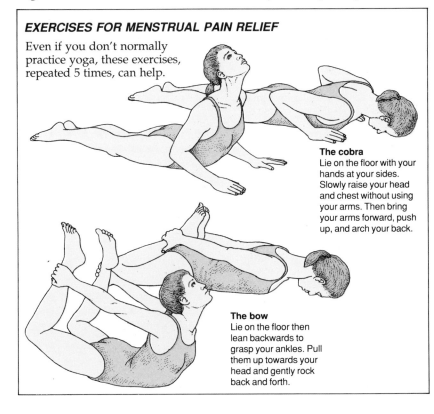

EXERCISES FOR MENSTRUAL PAIN RELIEF
Even if you don't normally practice yoga, these exercises, repeated 5 times, can help.

The cobra
Lie on the floor with your hands at your sides. Slowly raise your head and chest without using your arms. Then bring your arms forward, push up, and arch your back.

The bow
Lie on the floor then lean backwards to grasp your ankles. Pull them up towards your head and gently rock back and forth.

symptoms. Suppositories will absorb the drug into your system in 20 minutes; the level will drop within a few hours and be back to normal in 24 – so spreading, say, four throughout a 24-hour day is an ideal regime.

The risks from progesterone therapy are virtually nil. The only contraindication to its use would be pregnancy or suspected pregnancy. Injections of progesterone are also available but this may not be as convenient as they may need to be administered daily. For cases where symptoms are severe and progesterone deficiency is diagnosed, a progesterone implant which lasts up to 6-18 months is a convenient form of medication.

If fluid retention is the basis of your problem, diuretic drugs may be offered. These drugs are taken for about 10 days before a period.

Hormone therapy in the form of a drug called aldactone is sometimes prescribed. This affects the water balance, thus relieving symptoms relating to fluid retention. Another hormone treatment is the contraceptive pill but as this is made from artificial progesterone, the therapy may not work and may even make the symptoms worse or spread them less severely throughout the month.

What can I do?

PMS is a recurring syndrome tied to your menstrual cycle so there's not a lot you can do to reduce its frequency. You can be prepared for it, however, and keep a diary or chart so that you can start the treatment that works for you before the symptoms occur. In that way you won't be taken by surprise and you'll have a record for your doctor to monitor the therapy. Eat little and often to keep your strength up and if there is any problem with constipation, keep plenty of high-fiber foods in your diet. Try to get plenty of rest to prevent the tiredness becoming more real and if at all

possible limit stressful situations. Talk about your feelings to anyone who will listen, and make sure your family knows to what extent you are affected.

About a third of women who suffer from PMS benefit from dietary measures during the premenstrual period. Some of these measures are controversial. For example, Vitamin B6 (pyrodoxine) has helped some women to reduce the tension and fluid retention. I am not in favor of self medication so always check with your doctor on the level of B6 that is safe. Not all women respond to B6 and so you must consult your doctor. If you overdose yourself there could be unpleasant side effects such as numbness in your fingers. Tablets of 50mg taken twice daily three days before the symptoms is the recommended dose.

If you are given a diuretic drug, you will urinate much more often. These drugs can flush important minerals out of the system so you should watch your diet at this time. Water-soluble vitamins should be supplemented – Vitamins C and B – and increase your intake of foods rich in minerals such as potassium (fruit, seafood, nuts and beans).

To help prevent fluid retention, cut salt out of your diet as far as you can. Salt absorbs water and so increases the possibility of retention. Reduce your fluid intake if possible from about 10 days before your period, though strong black coffee is a diuretic so that can be drunk regularly.

For pain such as that associated with dysmenorrhea, try aspirin which is a drug that inhibits prostaglandin production. Excessive prostaglandin is believed to be the cause of the contraction-like pains experienced during menstruation. If severe pain is the only symptom, ask your doctor to prescribe a course of anti-prostaglandin therapy to see if this works for you.

Exercises can be helpful; deep breathing and relaxation techniques bring relief of tension and improve insomnia. Swimming will often do the same.

SEE ALSO
DEPRESSION
DYSMENORRHEA
MOOD CHANGES

PRENATAL CARE

Proper monitoring and advice before a baby is born can ensure a healthy baby and the best delivery possible. From the time you find out you are pregnant until you go into labor and give birth you should be well looked after by your own doctor or at a prenatal clinic. Prenatal care, on a regular and frequent timetable set out at the beginning of your pregnancy, ensures that every possible complication is discovered and treated or avoided. This information is gained by a careful record of your personal and family medical history and regular checks on you and the growth of your baby. This care should begin as soon as you suspect or know that you are pregnant, certainly within the first twelve weeks of pregnancy.

What happens during checks?

Whether you attend your doctor's office, your local health clinic or the hospital clinic, the care will be essentially the same. You will have tests regularly or at specified times during your pregnancy (see opposite) to keep a constant check on your health and that of your baby. Other tests which will be carried out only if indicated will be amniocentesis, alpha fetoprotein (AFP) screening and fetoscopy.

How is the information recorded?

Everything will be recorded on a prenatal file which will become bulkier and bulkier as your pregnancy advances. It carries information about you and your partner's past medical history and any family medical history which needs to be taken into account, such as the incidence of twins. To determine the estimated date of delivery (EDD), you'll be asked about your last menstrual period and the nature of your periods, and whether you were using any means of contraception. The history of past births is noted. Doctors can also gain valuable information about possible problems if you tell them about such factors as your

WHAT DOES PRENATAL CARE PROVIDE?

Good prenatal care is a form of preventive medicine. Its acceptance by parents has led to a significant fall in maternal and perinatal mortality. There are many elements to good prenatal care –
1. To keep a check on the mental and physical health of the mother.
2. To check that the baby is developing normally in the womb.
3. To detect problems that may affect the baby's growth and development after birth.
4. To prepare the mother for feeding her baby.
5. To educate the mother and father about pregnancy and labor so they can make choices about it and enjoy the experience.
6. To advise on nutrition and exercise programs to help with the birth and regain health and fitness afterwards.

working conditions, whether your job is sedentary and when you intend to give up work before the baby is born. If your medical advisers talk to you in words you don't understand, ask them to explain. Don't allow yourself to remain in ignorance. If certain subjects aren't covered, bring them up.

PRENATAL VISITS AND CLASSES

Whenever you attend the clinic, you should take a list of questions and problems so you don't forget to ask.

You should also discuss with the medical staff the sort of labor and birth you want. For example, if you want to try to give birth without painkilling drugs, ask the nurse to put this in your notes. Mention if you feel strongly about such matters as having a routine episiotomy, fetal monitoring and artificial rupture of your membranes.

This is the time to ask the staff about the hospital policy regarding natural versus medically assisted childbirth. A guided tour of the delivery and birthing rooms in the hospital will help you to see if the baby will be rooming in with you, whether the hospital has a birthing stool, for example, or a delivery suite with music, cushions and a cosy atmosphere for labor.

Enroll in prenatal classes either at the hospital or through a local

support group. These classes combine health education and an exercise regime to help you prepare for the birth and regain your shape afterwards. You will be taken through the relaxation and breathing techniques for natural childbirth. Your partner should be welcome too and he can help you practice these methods in preparation for labor.

SEE ALSO:

AMNIOCENTESIS
EPISIOTOMY
FETOSCOPY
GENETIC COUNSELING
INDUCTION
LABOR
PELVIC EXAMINATION
PREGNANCY PROBLEMS
PREGNANCY TESTING
TOXEMIA OF PREGNANCY
ULTRASOUND

PRENATAL TEST	PURPOSE	SIGNIFICANCE
Height and shoe size	To assess the size of your pelvis and pelvic outlet.	Very small feet or height can suggest a small pelvic outlet and consequently perhaps a more difficult delivery. Your doctors will be alerted to the possibility of a *Caesarean section*.
Weight	To follow the growth of the fetus.	A loss of weight will be investigated although it can be normal during the first trimester if you suffer from *nausea* and *morning sickness*. Sudden weight gain may suggest pre-eclampsia.
Breasts	To check for lumps and the condition of your nipples.	If your nipples are retracted and you wish to breastfeed, you will be advised to wear a breast shield and perhaps do exercises or just wait and see. The nipples may correct themselves during your pregnancy (see *Nipple problems*).
Heart, lungs, hair, eyes, teeth, nails	To check on your general physical health.	You may need advice on diet and special dietary supplements. Dental visits will be encouraged.
Legs and hands	To look for varicose veins and any edema in your ankles, hands and fingers.	Cases of extreme puffiness can be a sign of pre-eclampsia. Advice on how to alleviate *varicose veins* will be given.
Urine (MSU)	To test for possible urinary infection or kidney infection. After cleaning your vulva with a sterile pad you pass a sample of urine into a sterile container. Catch only the mid-stream urine (MSU), not the first drops.	An existing kidney infection will be treated with antibiotics.
Urine	1. To test for protein in case your kidneys aren't coping. 2. To test for the presence of sugar (glucose); if found repeatedly you may have diabetes. 3. To test for ketones; this may be a sign of diabetes.	1. Protein in the urine late in pregnancy is a sign of pre-eclampsia (see *Toxemia of pregnancy*). Bed rest will be prescribed. 2. Pregnancy can unmask *diabetes* which must be treated and stabilized. It may go away after delivery only to return in later pregnancies. 3. Presence of ketones indicates that the body is short of sugar. You may be treated for diabetes.
Internal examination	To confirm the pregnancy and check that the uterus is the size it should be according to your dates. To take a Pap smear to exclude any disease of the cervix. To check for pelvic abnormalities. To check that the cervix is tightly closed.	Pelvic abnormalities may require elective *Caesarean section*. If you have ever had an active infection of *genital herpes*, let your doctor know. This can cause serious problems for the baby if delivered vaginally. The cervix may be incompetent and may require a suture to allow the pregnancy to proceed to term (see *Cervix problems*).
Fetal heart beat	To confirm that the fetus is alive and that the heart and heart rate are normal.	Check on the health of the fetus and listen for more heart beats in case of a multiple pregnancy.

PRENATAL CARE

Abdominal palpation	To assess the height of the fundus (the top of the uterus) and the size and position of the baby.	Gives a guide to the length of the pregnancy and the way the fetus is lying in the womb. This is significant after the 32nd week. For example, if the fetus is still in the breech position, the doctor may try external version or prepare you for a *breech birth*.
Blood pressure	This is a measurement of the pressure at which the heart is pumping blood through the body. The test is done to assess if it is normal or not. The reading is made up of two numbers: the top one is the systolic pressure when the heart contracts, pushes out blood and beats. This can be heard when the arm band is tightened. The bottom number is the diastolic pressure, the resting pressure when the heart rests between beats.	*Hypertension* (high blood pressure) can indicate a number of problems. including pre-eclampsia. Bed rest and perhaps hospitalization will be prescribed if it rises.
Blood tests	1. To find your ABO grouping. 2. To find your Rhesus blood group. 3. To check your hemoglobin level. This is a measure of the oxygen carrying substances in your red blood cells. Normal levels measured in gm are between 12 and 14gm. 4. To find the alpha fetoprotein level – a special test at 16 weeks. 5. To detect the presence of German measles antibodies and the AIDS virus. 6. VDRL, Kahn and Wasserman tests for the presence of *syphilis*. 7. To detect sickle cell disease and thalassemia, both forms of anemia found in dark skinned people and inhabitants of the Mediterranean countries.	1. Blood group needed in case of a transfusion. 2. Prepare for the possibility of *Rhesus incompatibility*. 3. Pregnant women have more circulating blood but if your Hb level drops below 10gm, you are suffering from *anemia*. You will be encouraged to eat more iron-rich foods and given supplements of iron and folic acid. Raising Hb levels means that more oxygen is carried to the baby. 4. AFP is a substance found in the blood of a pregnant woman. The levels vary during pregnancy, but are low between 16 and 18 weeks. Raised levels at this time may indicate a neural tube defect or other brain abnormalities. Also shows if you are carrying more than one baby. However, the test must be repeated and backed up in case your dates are wrong as AFP levels rise as pregnancy progresses. 5. If you have no immunity to *rubella*, you will be warned not to come into contact with a case of German measles. You may be given a gamma globulin injection to protect you. The *AIDS* virus can severely affect the baby. 6. A STD must be treated before 20 weeks. After this time it can be transmitted to the baby. 7. This can affect the baby and your pregnancy. Extra folic acid will be prescribed and, depending on your condition, a blood transfusion may be necessary for you during the birth.
Ultrasound	Useful for determining fetal age, position and expected date of delivery.	Performed as a matter of routine now in pregnancy and appears to be safe for mother and baby.
Amniocentesis	To take a sample of the amniotic fluid to check for any problems, usually done at 18 weeks.	This is not a routine test and is only performed if indicated.
Fetoscopy	To check for brain disorders and abnormalities such as cleft palate. The fiber optic is passed into the amniotic sac to view the fetus directly.	This is a major intervention and is only performed if absolutely necessary.

PROLAPSE

Another name for prolapse is "pelvic relaxation" and it occurs when the pelvic muscles become weakened and allow one or several pelvic organs to protrude and drop out of position. This becomes noticeable when pressure inside the abdomen is increased, such as when straining to open your bowels, coughing, or lifting heavy weights. The most commonly affected organ is the uterus. But the bladder, rectum, urethra and vagina may also prolapse. If one or more organs drop, the vaginal wall may be pushed as far as the opening. If the uterus prolapses, the cervix may protrude.

Are there different types?
If the rectum bulges into the vaginal wall it is called a rectocele; if it is the urethra, this is called a urethrocele; and if the bladder drops into the front vaginal wall, it is called a cystocele.

Why does it happen?
Prolapse is nearly always caused by earlier injury to the pelvic floor muscles, cervix or supporting tissue of the uterus during labor, especially if you had a rapid delivery or were allowed to go on too long in labor (this is less common today), or if your babies were large.

Should I see the doctor?
If you have severe backache or pelvic discomfort, or if you are having difficulty voiding or trouble with bowel movements, consult your doctor as soon as possible.

· S y m p t o m s ·

- ▲ Backache
- ▲ Dragging down feeling in the pelvis
- ▲ Pain on intercourse or inability to achieve orgasm if the vagina is slack
- ▲ Stress incontinence
- ▲ Frequency of urination (urethrocele)
- ▲ Discomfort on moving the bowels, difficulty in defecating (rectocele)
- ▲ Frequency of urination and cystitis-type symptoms of pain and burning when passing urine (cystocele)

What will the doctor do?
Your doctor will give you an internal pelvic examination and ask you about your deliveries, for example if your babies were larger than normal, or if the second stage of labor was allowed to go on too long, or if the cervix was allowed to tear.

If you are in middle age, the tissues lose their strength after the menopause and the damage that occurred years before in childbirth can still result in a prolapse.

What is the treatment?
If the prolapse is mild, your doctor will recommend that you keep up a daily routine of Kegel exercises (see index) to strengthen your pelvic floor muscles.

If infirmity makes surgery impossible, or in less severe cases, you may be fitted with a ring pessary which is placed high in the vagina. This should not be worn for long

periods, however, because it can erode the thin tissue simply by friction.

Correcting a severe prolapse is usually done by hysterectomy. The uterus and the torn stretched muscle, including the cervix, can be removed. In some cases, surgical repair may be possible via the vagina.

If you are overweight, this can cause the prolapse to be more troublesome, so your doctor will advise you to lose weight.

What can I do?
If you suffer from backache, avoid standing for long periods and maintain good posture. Wear a tight girdle to counteract the dragging feeling in your pelvis.

If you have difficulty with sexual intercourse, you and your partner may need to explore other ways of achieving sexual pleasure.

Wear light sanitary panty liners if you are troubled by leakage of urine when you play sports or run, or when abdominal pressure is increased. If the stress incontinence becomes more severe and a source of embarrassment, see your doctor for treatment.

The most important preventive treatment is being conscientious about pelvic floor exercises during pregnancy. Re-starting them immediately after the birth of your baby, whether you have stitches or not, can pre-empt the development of a prolapse.

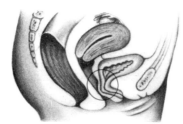

Urethrocele
This is a bulge of the lower front wall of the vagina which contains the urethra. If it irritates the urethral lining, it leads to a frequency of urination

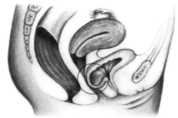

Cystocele
This occurs when the bladder bulges into the upper front wall of the vagina

---

SEE ALSO:

CYSTITIS
HYSTERECTOMY
INCONTINENCE
LABOR
OBESITY
PAINFUL INTERCOURSE

PRURITIS VULVAE

This describes an itching feeling of the skin anywhere around the genital organs and the rectum. Once scratching starts, it is difficult to stop so the itch may recur during the day. If you continue to scratch for several days, the condition may become chronic and the scratching cause thickening of the vulval skin. The cycle of itching, scratching and itching becomes difficult to break. It often occurs in girls before they begin to menstruate and in older women after menopause. There are no dangers directly associated with the condition but if white patches of abnormal skin, known as leuko-plakia, form in the irritated area, there is a slightly increased risk of developing cancer of the vulva.

What causes it?
Pruritis vulvae is the name given to this itchiness of the vulva when no other obvious cause can be found. For example, if the itching is accompanied by a thick discharge, you could have a vaginal infection such as yeast infection.

If, as menopause approaches, or when an artificial menopause has been induced by surgical removal of the ovaries, the levels of hormones – particularly estrogen – diminish, this can lead to dryness and scaling of the linings and the skin of the genitalia. A consequence of this is tingling, itching and scratching. The condition is sometimes referred to as vaginitis. The lubrication of the vagina and the health of the skin around the vaginal opening, the labia and the genitalia is closely bound up with the healthy secretion of female hormones.

Other reasons for itchiness of the vulva are diabetes and an allergy to talcum powder, vaginal deodorants, nylon tights or synthetic panty hose. However, if none of these factors apply, the reason for the itching is usually emotional. Anxiety about a sexual involvement or lack of confidence in relationships could be the cause.

> ### · S y m p t o m s ·
>
> ▲ Intense itchiness of the vulva
> ▲ Urgent need to scratch
> ▲ Sensitive skin in the vulval area
> ▲ Dryness and scaling
> ▲ Scalding and burning when passing urine – scratching causes minute tears and urine irritates these abrasions

Should I see the doctor?
If the itching persists and you are unable to resist scratching, see your doctor right away. If you decide to try the self-help measures below first and there is no improvement in a week or so, see your doctor.

What will the doctor do?
Your doctor will examine you to exclude obvious reasons for the irritation. If you are over 45, this condition is quite common and your doctor may suggest that you have some form of hormone therapy such as estrogen suppositories or hormonal creams to apply to the area.

For the symptoms on the skin, your doctor may suggest antihista-mine pills to reduce the itching sensation and a mild sleeping pill if the itchiness is severe. Itchiness is quite often worse at night when you are warm and the skin heats up. Your doctor might recommend a steroid or hormone cream to apply to the affected area to relieve irritation.

What can I do?
If the area is dry, use an emollient cream regularly to keep the skin well lubricated. Cut down on soap when washing the area and avoid hot baths; this warms the skin and sets up the itchiness. Shower instead. Avoid scented soaps, douches, talcum powder, vaginal deodorants, bath oils and wear only cotton or natural fibers against your vulva. Wash with warm water after passing urine.

Use a lubricant such as a water soluble jelly during intercourse.

If all medical causes of the itching are excluded, you will need to be honest with yourself. If pruritis vulvae is an expression of your sexuality, then you must treat it by sexual means. Face up to the facts about your sexuality. You may be denying your need for a sexual relationship and affection or you may be afraid of such an involvement. Try to be more sociable and outgoing and bolster your confidence by making more friends and avoiding isolation. Ask your doctor to put you in touch with a self-help group or a therapist who specializes in sexual problems.

> **SEE ALSO:**
>
> DIABETES MELLITUS
> HORMONE REPLACEMENT
>   THERAPY
> ITCHING
> MENOPAUSAL PROBLEMS
> PAINFUL INTERCOURSE
> SKIN PROBLEMS
> VAGINAL PROBLEMS
> VAGINITIS
> YEAST INFECTION

RADIATION THERAPY

Radiation therapy is treatment with either X-rays or radioactive materials. Its commonest application is in the treatment of malignant disease. Radiation therapy is lethal to cells that are rapidly dividing. Cancer cells are growing at a much faster rate than normal body tissues and are therefore more sensitive. The aim of radiation therapy is to destroy cancer cells while leaving normal cells intact and with modern techniques this can be achieved.

Gamma radiation interferes with the most basic physiological processes going on within cells and is at its most powerful when the chromosomes divide to produce new cells. Therefore with radiation treatment, cell division is prevented and the tissue cannot heal itself, repair itself or replace worn-out cells so that it eventually dies.

Why is it done?
Radiation therapy is usually chosen as treatment for squamous cancer of the skin, tumors of the upper air passages, mouth, tongue and lip. Tumors vary in their degree of radiosensitivity and those of the skin are extremely sensitive to X-rays so it is often the treatment of choice. Other tumors are less so when surgery and chemotherapy (see overleaf) are the mainstays.

In stage one cervical cancer, radiation therapy is as effective as surgery. Even in the later stages of cervical cancer it is usually the preferred treatment.

It is very often used as a supplement to surgical treatment and here it is particularly effective for cancer of the breast, tumors of the ovary and thyroid.

How is it done?
From research and experience, radiation therapists are aware of the various kinds of tumors that are sensitive to X-ray therapy and how radio-sensitive each tumor type is. On the basis of a league table of radio-sensitivity, the dose of

radiation therapy which will destroy the tumor and prevent spread can be established.

For each tumor, therefore, a total dose of radiation therapy can be calculated. This is nearly always split up into several doses, often separated by a week or more between sessions. The number of sessions is dependent upon the size of the dose and the size of the tumor. Treatment programs are usually spread over three or six weeks. Treatment can be on its own or after surgery to remove the tumor.

What is the procedure?
Radiation therapy administers gamma radiation and this radiation can be given in different ways.

◆ In a narrow X-ray beam from an X-ray transmitter – if the beam is very narrow it can be centered on a particular organ or tumor, for instance, a small breast cancer or an ovarian tumor. It can be given in a wider beam to cover a larger area into which a cancer may have spread.

◆ As a radioactive implant – this is inserted inside the organ and as it "decays" it gives off gamma radiation slowly and steadily thereby killing off the tumor. This is a form of radiation therapy which is quite often used in advanced breast cancer.

◆ As several radioactive needles – these can be inserted in larger, more diffuse tumors. The radioactive material is contained in small needle-shaped parcels or in wires, and radioactivity is given off over a carefully measured period of time in a sufficiently high dose to eradicate the tumor.

◆ As radioactive isotopes – given in liquid form by injection for certain kinds of tumors. This is particularly useful in thyroid tumors where radioactive iodine 131 is given by injection into the blood and is taken up by the thyroid gland. Once the radioactive iodine has been incorporated into the gland as it manufac-

tures thyroxine, the radioactivity inside the gland will kill off the tumor.

What are the side effects?
All forms of radiation therapy work by giving off gamma radiation. If uncontrolled, this form of radiation is harmful and dangerous. It is the type of radiation that causes various types of serious illness and death after an atomic or hydrogen bomb is exploded.

The area of skin immediately over the tumor may become burned by the X-rays; the symptoms and treatment are exactly the same as for sunburn. X-rays also affect the whole body, even though they are given to one particular site, and so it's common to feel nauseated, even sick for 24 – 36 hours after a treatment with X-ray therapy. Appetite is also depressed, though eating should return to normal within two to three days.

There are certain tissues in the body which turn over more rapidly than others. These include the bone marrow which produces blood, hence one of the first effects of excessive radiation is suppression of the bone marrow, leading to anemia. A second tissue is the lining of the mouth, the gullet, stomach and intestines and this accounts for bleeding gums, vomiting and diarrhea which is seen with a heavy dose of gamma radiation.

Ulceration of the mouth and throat about seven to ten days after starting treatment may occur if the face, throat or mouth is being treated. Regular mouthwashes and gargles are therefore essential during treatment to minimize pain on eating, speaking and swallowing. The cells in the hair follicles are also rapidly dividing and a large dose of gamma radiation makes hair fall out.

DEEP X-RAY THERAPY

The term deep X-ray therapy is used to describe rays of a special type which carry gamma radiation

RADIATION THERAPY

through the body wall and deep into internal organs. Not all X-rays are powerful enough to penetrate the body to this extent. Indeed there are some very "soft" X-rays called Grenz rays which only penetrate the top few millimeters of the skin and are used for treating certain skin cancers.

One form of radiation therapy is DXT or deep X-ray therapy. DXT is nearly always given in the form of a narrow beam that is centered on a tumor. Special precautions are taken to make sure that there is a minimum scatter of X-rays.

CHEMOTHERAPY

Chemotherapy is the term used for treatment of cancer with anti-cancer drugs or cytotoxic agents. The words chemotherapy, anti-cancer drugs and cytotoxic drugs are synonymous. All cytotoxic agents are poisonous to cells and eventually kill them. They work by interfering with basic chemical processes going on in the cells, and prevent them from metabolizing – using oxygen and producing energy. When cells can do none of these things, they die. Cytotoxic anti-cancer drugs don't all work by attacking the same chemical processes; they may attack a chemical chain-reaction at any link in the chain, but they all have the same overall effect.

When is it used?

Except in leukemias and certain lymphomas, chemotherapy is rarely used as the first line of treatment. It is nearly always used as back-up to surgery or radiotherapy.

Doctors know from experience that certain chemotherapeutic agents are particularly effective with certain tumor types. For instance, malignant melanoma quite often responds to cyclophosphamide and so this drug would be used early in treatment.

Chemotherapeutic agents are often used as a cocktail, one, two or even more being used together in an attempt to damp down cancer cell growth. Nearly all the agents are cytotoxic and interfere with cell growth. They do this by antagonizing crucial growth factors such as enzymes and vitamins. One whole class of anti-cancer agents is folic acid antagonists which prevent cells from using folic acid in their vital metabolic processes, thereby starving them to death.

Certain cancers are treated with surgery and/or radiation therapy or chemotherapy alone but often both agents are used to produce a more powerful anti-cancer treatment and also to have a two-pronged effect on the major aspects of a cell's health, metabolism and repair. A commonly used technique is a course of radiation therapy, followed by a short recovery period, then a course of chemotherapy.

SEE ALSO:

BREAST CANCER
CANCER
CERVICAL CANCER
HYPERTHYROIDISM
LUNG CANCER
MASTECTOMY
OVARIAN PROBLEMS
SKIN CANCER
UTERINE CANCER

RAPE

Rape is defined as forcible sexual intercourse with an unwilling partner. The term "statutory rape" is applied to sexual intercourse where the victim is under the legal age of consent or is not capable of giving consent due to mental incompetency. Currently, twenty-three states in the U.S. recognize marital rape but in the majority of states, a husband cannot be prosecuted for raping his wife.

In recent years, there has been a considerable increase in reported rape cases. It is difficult to know whether this reflects a genuine increase in incidence or a greater willingness on the part of victims to report the crime. Nevertheless, rape is still one of the least reported of all crimes; it is estimated that 70% of rapes go unreported. Studies have clarified the nature of the crime revealing that, contrary to popular belief, rape most often occurs between people who already know each other, and is not always accompanied by physical violence.

The present rape laws and the judicial system are still biased towards men making many women feel that they cannot take on the burden of reporting their rapes to a police system not always sympathetic to victims, and following up a rape charge to a court case.

Some studies suggest that rape is often primarily an aggressive rather than a purely sexual act. The rapist may include forcible sex as just one among various other forms of aggressive behavior or he may be motivated by a profound hostility toward women, using rape to hurt, humiliate, or terrify. In other instances, rape is sexually motivated, but the rapist needs to use force to achieve sexual satisfaction. Other motives include the need to feel powerful or to prove masculinity. There is also evidence of a significant link between alcohol abuse and rape. Very few rapists have a true psychiatric illness.

What can happen?

If you are attacked, it may be a natu-

ACTION CHECKLIST

- Report the crime to the police. If you feel that you cannot do this tell your friend to do so on your behalf and then help you to report the incident together.
- Contact your doctor and ask to see him or her as soon as possible.
- If your doctor is not immediately available go to the nearest emergency room.
- Do not take a shower or bath.
- Take off the clothing that you were wearing but don't wash it. Put it in a bag and keep it for the doctors and police to examine.
- Try to remember details about the man who assaulted you.
- Keep a note-pad by you and

write down everything that you can think of. The police will be interested in more than physical features such as an accent, a tone of voice, certain words that were used, smells etc.
- Don't stay at home alone, particularly after you've just made your report to the police. Take your friend with you.
- Immediately after the rape don't stay at home by yourself. Always try to have a friend with you or if you can't, go and stay with friends or relatives.
- Contact the nearest rape crisis center or Women's Center for support and counseling.

ral instinct to defend yourself and attack the rapist. If the rapist is armed, it is never safe to to this so when in doubt, don't be violent, try to stay calm. Talk quietly and carefully to your attacker and remind him that you are a human being.

Avoid exciting him further by answering leading questions about your feelings. If he demands an answer, make it factual like "my arm is crushed". Try to concentrate on his features, looks, clothing, his voice, accent, particular words that he uses. If possible, switch your mind to something else and think of your plan of action after the rape. Start listing the things that you are going to do. A show of violence or paradoxically pain and weakness may make the rapist more violent, so try to control your feelings and emotions.

What are the physical effects?

You may sustain a variety of injuries, most commonly as a result of a beating or choking. Severe injury to the genitals is rare, but there may be swelling of the labia, bruising of the vaginal walls or cervix, and occasionally tearing of the perineum. You may suffer tearing and bruising of

the rectum so that there is bleeding.

What should I do?

Many women respond to rape with the desire simply to go home, have a bath, not talk to anyone and pretend it didn't happen. This is wrong on several counts. By law a rapist should be convicted and punished and you will be protecting other women by reporting your rape. Secondly, it will make it difficult to come to terms with the incident if you do not face up to it honestly. By far the best action is to contact someone who lives fairly close to you so that they can get to you quickly and ask them if they can stay with you for several days if possible. Warn them that you may not want them to leave you at all, even when you sleep.

What will the police/doctor do?

The doctor will make a general examination of your whole body to examine bruises, redness, cuts, and find areas that are painful and tender.

An internal pelvic examination is mandatory, partly to take samples of vaginal secretions to see if there are any sperm present or a chemical called acid phosphatase which is present in seminal fluid, and to note evidence of injury. Ask that you have tests done for sexually transmitted diseases including gonorrhea, genital herpes and AIDS.

Your mouth and anus will also be examined for injury.

Ask for a pregnancy test at the earliest convenient time. In the advent of pregnancy discuss with the doctor there and then the use of the morning-after pill or the possibility of an abortion.

Do your utmost to have a friend or relative with you when you are with the authorities, not just to act as a witness but to give you moral support.

Note down the names, addresses and telephone numbers and the jobs of the people who speak to you.

COPING WITH RAPE

For nearly all women the horror of rape and sexual assault does not end when the attacker leaves. You may have to cope with physical effects such as a vaginal discharge, itching and soreness of the perineum, yeast or trichomoniasis infection, bruises, swelling and tenderness of the genital areas and other parts of your body injured during the rape, cuts and lacerations that require daily dressing from a doctor or nurse.

Women differ in their emotional response to being raped but all are severely traumatized. All rape victims suffer psychological after-effects and most take a long time to feel anything like normal again, some never do and say that they are a completely changed person whom they have to get to know, and learn to live with all over again.

After such an experience a new identity has to be forged – that of being a rape victim. It's difficult to pin down what is different about a woman after rape. It's not just that her behavior is circumscribed and that she no longer walks home alone in the dark, or sleeps by herself in the house. Somehow she has become a different person with a different

awareness of things. She may feel that a new role has been added to her life and how does she cope with this new persona.

What is the therapy?
What many rape victims have to come to terms with is that they have been fundamentally changed by their experience and feel isolated and alone in a new identity.

In an attempt to find the best way to help rape victims, new research has shown that rape victims who try to relive their experience, to face up to the fear and terror caused during the rape, are better able to rehabilitate themselves back into a normal life than those who try to put the matter out of their minds. No person can go through this harrowing relearning without help and support from others which is usually a small, supportive family kind of group, nurtured by counselors and psychologists.

Most rape victims admit that it is easy to wallow in self-pity and the comfort of being a victim. What they have to do is to reconstruct their lives and take the initiative and responsibility for doing this.

No-one can do this alone but you

could help yourself through women's groups and through rape crisis centers. They are experienced in dealing with all the various reactions that you can feel after being raped; not only will they give you emotional comfort and support but they will not be soft on you. They will encourage you back into a normal existence.

PREVENTING RAPE

It has been strongly argued that the incidence of rape reflects a male-dominated society's attitudes toward women generally. The best long-term approach to the problem therefore lies through education and an adjustment of the emphasis on male sexual virility. There seems to be strong evidence that television, films, and pornography do promote violent sexual behavior and, in future, their subject matter may become subject to more restrictive legislation.

On a more practical note, research has shown that some women are more likely to be victims than others. Follow the advice set out below if you are in doubt about the type of behavior to exhibit.

AVOIDING RAPE
By your behavior you may put off a rapist or even avoid him altogether.

On the streets
◆ Don't venture out alone in areas where there is poor street lighting, where you know there is trouble or where youths hang out in gangs.
◆ Whenever you walk in the street, keep towards the edge of the curb where you are clearly visible and the street is better lit.
◆ If you suspect that someone is following you, leave the curb and walk into the middle of the street where there are cars, then run.

◆ If you are being followed and you think that a man may attack you, run into the middle of the road and scream.

By your car
◆ Always park by a street lamp.
◆ Never leave your car unlocked.
◆ Before you get into your parked car look into the back seat.

At home
◆ Make sure there are strong locks on doors and windows.
◆ Have a peep-hole in all of the outside doors.
◆ Before opening your door to a stranger, ask for identification.

RASHES AND SKIN CHANGES

Any discoloration or recognizable change to your skin may be the result of contact with an irritant or because of some internal disease. If you have a fever with the rash, this could be a childhood infectious disease – a more likely diagnosis if you have young children.

Skin rashes themselves are hardly ever serious but some can be symptoms of an underlying illness. Purpuric rashes are in the skin rather than on the skin because they show a disorder in the blood. You can detect a purpuric rash by pressing against the skin; it will remain visible.

Spots or skin problems can also result from hormonal changes.

Chloasma

This is a skin condition that looks rather like giant freckles. It usually covers the face and neck and appears in pregnancy and in women who take the combined pill. It is thought to be a reaction to the sex hormones estrogen and progesterone. The condition cannot be prevented because the tendency to develop chloasma is inherited. Women with dark skin may notice the opposite effect. They can develop white patches which also disappear soon after delivery of their babies.

There is another form of patchy skin pigmentation which may occur down the side of the face and neck. This is usually a response to the aromatic oils in certain kinds of perfume.

Chloasma nearly always goes away of its own accord when the high levels of circulating hormones in the body return to normal. Because of this there is really no need to seek medical advice. Doctors are understandably circumspect about any form of radical interference. However, if the reason for your chloasma is your contraceptive pill, you may decide to change it to a lower dosage to see if this makes any difference.

Chloasma can be made worse by sunlight so avoid direct sunlight during a pregnancy. Wear a sunblock

NATURE AND SITE OF RASH	PROBABLE CAUSE
It is a fine red/purple rash which remains when you apply pressure	This could be a purpuric rash. This is caused by a blood disorder and is not a problem on the skin. Consult your doctor.
You have a fever, dry cough, sore eyes and runny nose	This could be the measles. Check with your doctor.
You have recently started a course of medicine	This could be a drug reaction. Consult your doctor about whether this is a side effect of the particular drug.
You have swollen glands at the back of your neck	This could be German measles. Keep away from pregnant women as this is highly dangerous to an unborn child. If you are pregnant, contact your doctor immediately (see *Rubella*).
The rash is very itchy with blisters that scab over	This could be chickenpox. Apply calamine lotion, or have tepid baths with bicarbonate of soda in them if the itchiness is severe. Consult your doctor.
You have been out in the sun a lot and the rash is all over	This is probably a heat rash. However, if there are large weals, you could be allergic to certain ultraviolet rays. Consult your doctor.
You are pregnant, and the rash appears mainly on your face, rather like a dirty mark or a large freckle	This could be chloasma, which is a change in skin pigmentation as a result of the hormonal changes of your pregnancy.
You are pregnant, and you develop *acne*	Any eruptions of pimples or spots during pregnancy is the result of hormonal changes and is normal.
The sores are near to your mouth or on your lips and they tingle and sting	This is probably a *cold sore*.
You notice a new *mole* or any change in an existing mole	You should seek medical advice immediately. This could indicate a serious skin disorder (see *Skin Cancer*).
You detect warts around your genitals or anus	These are genital warts, a *sexually transmitted disease*, and should not be treated at home. See your doctor as the skin is too sensitive to be treated like warts elsewhere on your body.

RASHES AND SKIN CHANGES

NATURE AND SITE OF RASH	PROBABLE CAUSE
You have itchy, scaly skin, particularly on your hands	This may be the result of an allergic reaction to your brand of household detergent or cleaner. Apply moisturizing lotion, change your brand and wear rubber gloves and see if the skin heals. Often this form of eczema becomes worse with stress. Consult your doctor (see *Skin problems*).
The rash appears on your trunk where you experience a searing, burning pain	This could be shingles, a viral infection like chickenpox. Consult your doctor.
The rash is itchy and merges into the surrounding skin, particularly occurring in the skin folds	This could be a fungal infection. It is most likely athlete's foot if it occurs between the toes, or ringworm on the scalp or in the armpit.
The rash is raised red on a white base, and it is itchy	This is urticaria or hives, and is a symptom of an allergic reaction, usually to food. If you can pinpoint a new food, avoid it for a while. If the weals reappear, consult your doctor. If this reaction occurs on the face or mouth, this can be dangerous and affect your breathing. Consult your doctor immediately (see *Skin problems*).
Your hands are itchy and you can make out tiny grey lines and red spots	This could be a parasitic infection, scabies. This is highly contagious and the rest of your family can easily get it. Consult your pharmacist or doctor for the correct medication and apply the treatment immediately. You'll need to launder your bedding and clothes too.
There is puckering of the skin on your breast or any change in the areola	You should seek medical advice immediately. This could be a symptom of *breast cancer*.

and a hat to cover your face and neck. Use a makeup that contains a sunscreen. If you insist on sunbathing, you should wear a camouflage base to blend the patches in with the rest of your skin.

If you think you have a reaction to certain perfumes, don't dab on concentrated perfume with your fingertips. Use a spray eau de cologne instead.

If you are unable to make a diagnosis from this information, consult your doctor.

RAYNAUD'S PHENOMENON

Raynaud's phenomenon is a circulatory disorder when there is a hypersensitivity of the blood vessels in the hands and fingers to cold. When the hands are exposed to cold the skin goes through color changes. At first it is white, then blue and then red. When the fingers are white and blue, the skin is numb, but with the return of circulation, pain can be quite severe. When this numbness is not associated with any underlying condition, it is known as Raynaud's disease.

What causes it?

Normally when you are cold, your arteries contract to reduce the amount of blood reaching your skin and cooling you down too much. With Raynaud's phenomenon, the arteries which supply blood to your fingers go into vigorous spasm when you experience a drop in temperature. Blood no longer passes along the arteries, your skin turns white and you lose the sensation of touch. If the blood supply is so poor that oxygen is used up, the blood turns purplish blue and so does your skin tone. This is known as cyanosis.

Raynaud's phenomenon is most commonly seen in young adult women. It can be a symptom of a number of disorders. These include scleroderma, a rare autoimmune condition where antibodies attack many systems in the body.

Occasionally people who suffer from cervical spondylosis where there is pressure on the sympathetic nerves which supply the arm and its blood vessels exhibit this symptom. If you are taking beta-blocker drugs, this may be a side effect.

Very occasionally people who are sensitive to cold develop antibodies which make the blood clot when temperatures are very low.

Should I see the doctor?

If you notice any of the above, see your doctor for a diagnosis. You may be suffering from some other disorder for which this is a symptom.

· Symptoms ·

▲ Characteristic white, blue, red color change in the fingers – occasionally in the toes
▲ Pins and needles
▲ Ulceration as a result of the reduced blood supply
▲ Diminution in the sense of touch

What will the doctor do?

Vasodilator drugs, which cause the blood vessels to widen, may be prescribed though their success is not guaranteed. These drugs have the side effect of lowering the blood pressure, so their use has to be carefully judged, particularly in older people.

Surgery to sever certain nerves will produce an improvement until the nerves grow back again.

What can I do?

As treatment depends on the underlying cause, this may be a symptom you have to learn to live with. There are ways you can ease the numbness.

◆ Always protect your hands and fingers against exposure to cold with warm, loose-fitting gloves.
◆ Stay inside in very cold weather.
◆ Stop smoking as this will damage your circulation further.
◆ Alcohol is a vasodilator; have a little each day and see if this helps.

SEE ALSO:

AUTOIMMUNE DISEASE
ARTHRITIS
HEART DISEASE
NUMBNESS AND TINGLING
OSTEOARTHRITIS

RHESUS INCOMPATIBILITY

This is something we either have in our blood or we don't. We are all either rhesus positive or rhesus negative besides being in the standard ABO blood grouping. Special attention is always given to rhesus negative women during pregnancy because their blood might be incompatible with the blood of their rhesus positive babies.

What causes the problem?
When a rhesus negative woman becomes pregnant, the odds are the father of her child will be rhesus positive – 85% of the population are. The baby will therefore either be rhesus positive or negative. If the baby is rhesus negative, like herself, there is no problem. If, however, the baby is rhesus positive, antibodies in the mother's blood will regard the baby's blood as foreign, and will react.

With the first child there is rarely a problem as the maternal and fetal bloodstreams do not mix very much. (However, if the mother previously was transfused with rhesus positive blood before she became pregnant, there may already be rhesus positive antibodies in her blood.) But some blood from the baby can mix with the mother's blood, usually at birth when the placenta separates from the uterus. This sensitizes the mother to produce antibodies which remain in her blood and can cross the placenta to her next baby's body and start to destroy its blood, if it is rhesus positive.

Despite this chain of events, danger during subsequent pregnancies still may not be significant because antibodies haven't formed in large enough numbers. However, during prenatal checkups, rhesus negative mothers will have their blood tested constantly for antibodies and a check kept on whether they rise or not.

It is known that a certain level of circulating antibodies in the blood can damage the developing baby, but this is reached in less than 10% of cases. Finding out that you are

---

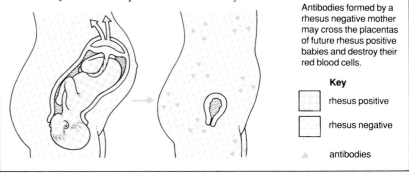
---

rhesus negative is therefore no reason for despondency because no harm will come to your baby – though you will receive extra care.

What will the doctor do?
If you have had a baby before, you will have been given an injection of anti-rhesus globulin protein which will destroy any of the baby's cells remaining in your blood, so that no more antibodies are produced. This should be done after every delivery and abortion and every invasive procedure during pregnancy (e.g. amniocentesis) where there is possible leakage of the baby's blood into your own. This ensures future babies are safe from rhesus incompatibility.

If you haven't had this treatment, you will be tested early in your pregnancy to see if you have the antibodies in your blood. Then you will have an amniocentesis to check for high levels of bilirubin in the amniotic fluid. If the levels are high, your baby may be given an intrauterine transfusion of rhesus negative blood. This is done using fetoscopy or ultrasound.

The baby at risk may be delivered early by Caesarean section and given a blood transfusion immediately after birth, particularly if jaundice is

advanced. This is done gradually with 9g ($^1/_3$ oz) of blood being withdrawn at a time with the same amount of fresh blood replacing it so that in 72 hours the antibodies and the bilirubin will have been washed out of the baby's system and the baby will no longer be in any danger. During transfusion, some of the pigments of damaged blood, which make your baby's skin appear a yellow color, will also be washed out and your baby will become a normal healthy color.

What can I do?
Make sure you always tell your doctor that you are rhesus negative whenever you have a blood transfusion, miscarriage or abortion.

SEE ALSO:

AMNIOCENTESIS
CAESAREAN SECTION
FETOSCOPY
PREGNANCY PROBLEMS
PRENATAL CARE
ULTRASOUND

RHEUMATOID ARTHRITIS

Rheumatoid arthritis is an auto-immune disease in which the body becomes allergic to the lining of the joints – the synovial membrane – and it produces antibodies to the synovium. These antibodies attack the synovial membrane which becomes inflamed and scarred and is finally destroyed, the joint along with it. The disease is most common between the ages of 45 and 60 and tends to run in families.

At the start of an autoimmune disease, the collagen throughout the body is affected. But depending on the nature of the specific disease contracted, the site of the collagen affected and its resulting symptoms will differ, and so produce symptoms indicative of the particular disease. In rheumatoid arthritis it is the collagen in the joints which is most acutely inflamed – the pain, stiffness, immobility and destruction of joints being the most obvious sign. There are nearly always some microscopic changes in other organs such as the lungs, arteries or kidneys.

· **S y m p t o m s** ·

▲ Inflammation of joints, most commonly in the hands, feet and ankles; the middle joint of the fingers is often spindle-shaped
▲ Muscular aches and pains
▲ Headaches
▲ Wasting of the muscles

What causes it?
All autoimmune diseases are caused by the same underlying disease process. Because of the allergic reaction in the collagen, chemical substances are released which cause inflammation and destruction; the collagen swells and disintegrates. Blockages of arteries, ulceration of the skin, a lot of fluid in a joint, weakening of muscles, damage to kidneys and collapse of a lung – all or any of these may occur in any of the collagen diseases. So, if you take a biopsy of an artery in rheumatoid

arthritis you will nearly always see damage to collagen in the wall of the artery, even though there are no symptoms referrable to this.

While this process is going on the joints are extremely painful, very swollen and stiff. If the disease is not treated promptly and radically, destruction of the joints can advance so that they become fixed and immobile.

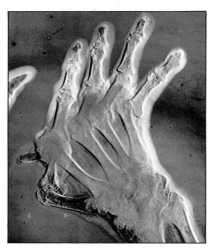

The woman is suffering from extreme rheumatoid arthritis in the joints of her fingers. This is referred to as polyarthritis when it affects more than one joint.

The natural history of rheumatoid arthritis is that it goes through periods of activity and inactivity. With each attack, however, the destruction of the joint can be worse. Eventually, in late middle age, most cases "burn out," leaving a patient severely disabled, even crippled, if attacks have not been treated properly.

Stiffness in rheumatoid arthritis is related to the acute inflammation inside the joint and swelling due to fluid inside the joint which in itself prevents movement. This stiffness is worse early on in the day and the severity of "morning stiffness" is used as an index of how severe the disease is. The longer morning stiffness takes to wear off, the more serious the stage of the disease.

Should I see the doctor?
If you notice this morning stiffness or you have vague muscular aches and pains, see your doctor, particularly if there are cases of rheumatoid arthritis in your family.

What will the doctor do?
Before a firm diagnosis can be made, your doctor may have to observe your progress over a couple of months. You will be sent for blood tests and X-rays to attempt to identify the form of arthritis you are suffering from.

There is no cure for rheumatoid arthritis but there is a great array of drugs which doctors use, both to damp down the inflammation in the joints and to bring relief of pain. One of the most potent is aspirin, with its anti-inflammatory properties, given in very high dosage. There are large numbers of aspirin-like drugs which have the same beneficial effects but fewer side effects. In the late 1940s and early 50s, steroids were thought to be the miracle cure for rheuma-toid arthritis but use of these drugs is limited to short courses because long-term use has many unwanted side effects.

Substances such as gold and quinine derivatives are also used to help to arrest the disease. In very severe cases, anti-cancer drugs may be prescribed to prevent destruction of the joints.

What are the other treatments?
The aim of physical therapy is to prevent destruction and deformity of joints and maintain a normal joint position and function. This is done by a combination of rest and exercise.

It is necessary to rest an acutely inflamed joint simply to damp down the inflammation and this is achieved by the use of splints which are worn around the joint during the day and all through the night. The splints hold the joint in the position of optimum function.

If joints are immobilized for any length of time, the muscles become

RHEUMATOID ARTHRITIS

EXERCISES FOR ARTHRITIS

Make sure that you put your joints through a full range of movement every day, but don't overdo it – between five and 20 repeats daily is the number to aim for. These exercises will help to maintain muscle strength and keep your joints moving properly.

Wrist joint
Rest your arm on a flat surface without supporting the hand. Bend your hand downwards and then lift it up.

Still supporting your arm move your hand to the left and then the right. Don't let your hand droop, keep it in line with your arm.

Hand and finger joints
Bend your fingers and make a tight fist.

Stretch and spread your fingers outwards in a star shape.

Touch the tip of each finger in turn with your thumb.

---

thin and weak. In rheumatoid arthritis this is prevented with very gentle exercises, taught and performed by physical therapists. There are various methods of physical therapy used to keep the joints in good working order such as exercises in warm wax baths, gentle swimming in warm swimming pools, ultrasonic treatment, massage and exercise. These are usually taught to the patient during a stay in hospital or on an out-patient basis.

Rheumatoid arthritis may burn out after several years, but usually only after a fair degree of joint and organ destruction.

What is the surgical treatment?
When the condition burns out and is no longer active, a joint which has been destroyed and is deformed can be replaced with an artificial joint. Artificial knees, wrists and even elbows can now be fitted.

What can I do?
Rest as much as you can. Fatigue quite often causes the disease to flare up.

As the small joints of the fingers, toes, ankles and wrists are most commonly affected in rheumatoid arthritis, the ability to walk and grip things is severely impaired. There are many gadgets available, particularly for use in the home to make life easier.

◆ There is kitchen equipment for turning on taps, opening screw jars, special cutlery designed to be used by people whose joints are deformed.
◆ Special handles can be fitted to doors and drawers.
◆ Safety devices like rails alongside lavatories, baths and showers improve safety.
◆ Non-skid surfaces should be used where slipping is a danger.
◆ One or two stairs can be replaced by ramps.
◆ A household elevator can be fitted to a staircase to save having to climb stairs.

SEE ALSO:

ARTHRITIS
AUTOIMMUNE DISEASE
HIP REPLACEMENT
OSTEOARTHRITIS
SYSTEMIC LUPUS

RHINOPLASTY

This is colloquially known as a nose job. It is fairly complicated surgery and is not always undertaken for purely cosmetic reasons. The two most commonly performed operations are for reduction of the nose size or augmentation if the bridge of the nose has collapsed. Rhinoplasty for purely cosmetic reasons depends on the shape and size of nose that the patient wants.

Why is it done?

This surgical procedure is usually done because you have problems with breathing. This may be the result of a broken nose, or a sporting injury that has caused the bridge of the nose to collapse, or you have a deviated septum (the central cartilage that runs between the nostrils). Because the septum is made of flexible cartilage it can be easily bent by injury and narrow the air passage on one side.

Few surgeons will attempt to do this operation unless you are more than 18 years old when the skull bones are mature and the face fully formed.

How is it done?

Whether you have a local or general anesthetic will depend on the extent of the operation. You will be interviewed by the ear, nose and throat specialist or the cosmetic surgeon about what you hope to achieve with the operation and what nose shape or what imperfections you want removed.

The surgery is performed within the nose to avoid visible scarring. The nasal bones are fractured during the operation and then repositioned to the desired shape. To shorten a nose that is too long or to alter the curvature, cartilage which forms the bridge of the nose is cut away. If your nose is to be augmented or tilted, small pieces of cartilage are transplanted from elsewhere in your body into your nose. Any pieces of bone or cartilage are removed or inserted through your nostrils. Silicone implants are sometimes used. There is no stitching in this operation.

Your nose will be packed with gauze and probably have a plaster of Paris cast or splint put onto it to prevent movement while it heals. This takes approximately 10 days.

What are the results?

Your nose will be sore and there will be a lot of swelling and bruising under your eyes. Ice packs will limit this. You will not be allowed to blow your nose for about three weeks and then the stuffiness should disappear. There may be numbness for two months and it will be six months before your nose feels fully recovered.

The results are usually excellent. A possible but rare complication is recurrent nosebleeds due to persistent crusting at the incision sites.

SEE ALSO:

COSMETIC SURGERY
DERMABRASION
FACE LIFT

RUBELLA

German measles or rubella is a common childhood viral illness. It has no serious side effects in adults or children. However, if a pregnant woman is infected with the virus, this can interfere with the development of her unborn baby.

What is the risk?
The risk is greatest during the first twelve weeks, part of which you may not be aware that you are pregnant. It is in the first eight weeks that your baby's vital organs are forming and developing. As the baby becomes stronger and more highly developed, the risk decreases although the fetus is still sensitive to the virus. A woman who has had German measles or been vaccinated against it has developed antibodies to the virus and an infection cannot harm her baby. An injection of a protective blood protein known as gamma-globulin will provide the antibodies for a pregnant woman who is at risk.

· S y m p t o m s ·

▲ Slight red rash and swollen lymph glands in the neck of the pregnant woman

▲ A baby born with rubella may have malformations which produce deafness, blindness and heart disease

---

Should I see the doctor?
At your first prenatal visit, you will be asked whether or not you have ever had German measles. A blood test will be taken in any event to check that you are immune.

If you think you have been in contact with a case of German measles during your pregnancy – either during the disease itself, or up to one week before the rash appears, consult your doctor immediately.

If you are thinking about trying to conceive and you have not had German measles as a child and have never been vaccinated against the disease, consult your doctor and ask for a blood test to see if you are immune.

What will the doctor do?
Your doctor will take a blood sample to check for rubella antibodies. If you are not immune and you are pregnant, your doctor may offer you a booster injection of gammaglobulin, which will protect you if you have not yet been infected. If you have been infected, you may be advised to consider termination of your pregnancy because the risk of malformation is so high.

If you have not yet become pregnant, your doctor will vaccinate you against the disease and advise you to wait three months before attempting to conceive.

What can I do?
If you are aware of a case of German measles, try to avoid all contact with the sufferer.

Make sure your daughters have the vaccination against rubella at puberty. In many countries schools offer the vaccine to pubescent girls as a matter of course.

SEE ALSO:

PRENATAL CARE
TERMINATION OF
  PREGNANCY

SEX DIFFERENTIATION

Sex differentiation is the natural process by which the physical differences between males and females develop. This process starts early in embryonic life and continues until the end of puberty.

Unfortunately, in a small minority, sex differentiation does not proceed smoothly, and the result may be a child with ambiguous external sex organs at birth, or who fails to develop the full physical characteristics of one sex or the other, or whose outward appearance is not in accord with his or her gonadal sex (presence of testes or ovaries). These problems are usually noticed at birth and can be tackled straight away, but in some cases they do not become apparent until later in childhood.

What are they caused by?
The majority of people possess, in each of their body cells, two sex chromosomes. The normal female chromosome complement is XX, and the male complement XY. These chromosomes are acquired at conception, one coming from each parent. The mother's egg always carries the X chromosome and the father contributes either X or Y in his sperm, determining the sex – XX is a girl and XY a boy.

The original components of the internal and external sex organs in the two sexes are identical, that is they can develop in either the female or male direction. In male fetuses the presence of the Y chromosome leads to the formation of testes; these then produce hormones, some of which suppress the development of female internal sex organs, while others stimulate the development of the male reproductive tract and organs. In the female embryo, the two X chromosomes stimulate the development of ovaries. The other female organs develop automatically, without any specific hormonal stimulation from the ovaries; in other words there is an innate tendency towards femaleness. At puberty, the surge of hormones produced by the testes or ovaries leads to the development of further, secondary sex characteristics.

Defects or disturbances arise in two ways: there may be a fundamental problem at the level of the sex chromosomes – usually an abnormal complement. Alternatively, the sex chromosomes may be normal but there is a disturbance or defect at hormonal level.

How do abnormalities arise?
This usually occurs through a fault during egg or sperm cell formation. A few sperm or egg cells, instead of receiving one sex chromosome (X or Y), may receive none or two (XY, XX or YY), and when these combine with a normal egg or sperm, this can give rise to unusual sex chromosome complements such as X, XXY, XXX or XYY. Alternatively, during the first few divisions of a fertilized egg, the sex chromosomes divide up unequally, so that some cells in the embryo receive one set of sex chromosomes and other cells get a different set – for example, X in some cells and XXX or XYY in others. Such individuals are termed "mosaics" and may show any of a wide range of characteristics intermediate between male and female.

One of the most common sex chromosome abnormalities is the presence of just a single X chromosome – sometimes denoted XO. This is the usual cause of a condition called gonadal dysgenesis. Because no Y chromosome is present, those affected are essentially female, with vulva and vagina at birth. However, as they lack one of the X chromosomes, these girls have only rudimentary ovaries, and at puberty do not menstruate or develop secondary sex characteristics such as breasts.

When gonadal dysgenesis is caused by the XO chromosome pattern, it is called Turner's syndrome. Gonadal dysgenesis can also be caused by mosaicism where there is a mixture of XO and XX, XY or XXX chromosomes complements.

Girls with the XXX chromosome complement ("super females") usually develop normally, although a proportion with this pattern suffer mental retardation.

The chromosome patterns XXY and XYY give rise to males due to the presence of a Y chromosome. XYY individuals are physically near normal but the XXY pattern causes a variety of abnormalities in the male; this is known as Klinefelter's syndrome.

HORMONAL DISTURBANCES

A number of girls are born who have a normal female sex chromosome pattern (XX) and normal ovaries and internal sex organs, but their external genitals are masculinized.

In an extreme case, the labia may be fused together to look like a scrotum and the clitoris enlarged to look like a penis. These girls are sometimes called pseudohermaphrodites. The cause is a high level of certain male hormones in the fetus which masculinize the external genitals while leaving the internal organs untouched. The condition is sometimes caused by the mother taking hormones during pregnancy, or if she develops a hormone-secreting tumor. The most common cause, however, is a disorder of the baby girl's adrenal glands, called congenital adrenal hyperplasia. In this condition the glands inappropriately pump out large amounts of male hormones.

Another specific, though rare, condition is the testicular feminizing syndrome. There are male chromosomes and testes in the abdomen. These produce normal amounts of male hormones which, however, fail to bring about masculinization in the fetus, although they do suppress the development of some internal female organs. The result is a girl who at puberty develops a full female outward appearance but has a blind-ending vagina, no uterus and does not menstruate.

SEX DIFFERENTIATION

What problems can arise?

One general problem is that even with the best therapy it may not be possible to establish fertility in an affected individual, although it can be established in some cases.

Girls with Turner's syndrome, in addition to poorly developed sex characteristics, usually have other physical abnormalities such as a shield-like chest, webbing of the neck, short stature, elbows which turn out from the side and fore-shortened bones in the foot. Quite often there is color blindness and abnormalities of some of the blood vessels. Girls with forms of gonadal dysgenesis other than Turner's syndrome do not usually have these associated abnormalities.

In patients with testicular feminizing syndrome the problem usually first comes to light at puberty when menstruation fails to occur, and on examination by a physician, testes instead of ovaries are found in the abdomen and the uterus is absent. There are no associated abnormalities except for sparse pubic hair.

In a girl whose masculinized external genitals are not recognized and treated early, there may also be absence of, or an incompletely formed, vagina; a membrane obstructing the passage of menstrual blood which then collects causing lower abdominal discomfort (this can occur as an isolated abnormality – in an otherwise entirely normal girl); and possibly the appearance of male features at puberty such as deepening of the voice, enlargement of the clitoris, abnormal hair growth.

What tests are carried out?

It is usually important for the doctor to find out the underlying chromosomal sex of the affected person. This can be done simply by taking a scrape from the inside of the mouth and looking at the cells under a microscope after they have been specially stained. The appearance of the cells gives important clues to the chromosome complement.

A full physical examination is carried out to establish exactly what features of female or male anatomy are present. Hormone analysis from a 24-hour sample of urine can give an idea of the functioning of the ovaries or testes, adrenal glands and of other glands such as the pituitary. All these tests help to build up a profile of the essential femaleness or maleness of the patient.

What is the medical treatment?

Patients with Turner's syndrome and other types of gonadal dysgenesis, who have no ovarian tissue, can be treated with estrogens to produce secondary sexual development at puberty and a withdrawal bleed from the uterus each month. Most can live a normal married life but are infertile.

The testicular feminizing syndrome patient cannot be made to menstruate for she has no uterus. The testes are usually removed after full secondary sexual development has occurred because they have a potential to develop cancer. These patients are entirely female in their lifestyle and psychosexual identity, but are infertile.

In the case of ambiguous genitals, the appropriate treatment will often depend on what age the child has attained when the problem is first recognized. In a girl with masculinized genitals at birth, appropriate hormonal and later surgical treatment can be given, including construction or reconstruction of the vagina if this is absent or poorly formed. Such girls can then usually lead normal lives as females, and in some cases will be fertile. However, if the genitals are markedly masculinized and as a result the child has been reared for some years as a boy, it may be considered inappropriate to attempt gender reassignment as the child will have formed a male gender identity. In that case, ovarian tissue and uterus may be removed and the child given male hormones. It is impossible to establish male fertility without testes.

All cases of this type are difficult and have to be considered carefully according to the individual circumstances; the aim always being to give the child the best chance for a reasonably normal and happy life.

SEX THERAPY

Sex therapy is usually carried out at a specialist clinic where trained therapists conduct physical and psychological tests. The types of problems that would be dealt with by a therapist are nearly always looked upon as something couples have to explore together, requiring frank discussion. There are instances where women can be treated on their own, or more usually in groups of other women.

If you feel that sex therapy will be useful for you, the first step you have to take is to admit that you have a problem, and this will mean you have to overcome many inhibitions.

SEX THERAPY PROGRAMS

Most programs are slow, gentle and exploratory. They nearly always start with a long discussion about possible problems and then define the problems clearly. Your counselor will help you to talk openly and without embarrassment to your partner about all aspects of the problem and to air any feelings and sentiments that you may have held back.

The program will be mapped out for you over several weeks. The therapist will set out a series of exercises for you and your partner. You'll be told what's going to happen and what is expected of you. You will be encouraged to think positively. In joining a sex program you are entering into a contract with your partner and your therapist.

Techniques

Depending on the particular problem, you will be:

◆ Given advice about relaxing and losing your anxieties
◆ Encouraged to go back to the beginning and find out how your body responds to sexual contact
◆ Asked to return to the simplest exploration of your partner's body through touch without sexual response
◆ Taught to concentrate on feelings, experiences and enjoying every sensation felt by your body
◆ Told to forget about orgasm for the time being
◆ Asked to refrain from sexual intercourse for a few days or weeks.

You may be given exercises to practice, such as the pelvic floor exercises, or the squeeze technique to inhibit your partner's urge to ejaculate.

Later you can go on to enjoy lying with your partner, touching, fondling and caressing each other. As your program progresses, you will be counseled to experiment with different ways of bringing yourself and your partner to orgasm – at first this will be without penetration – and then gradually graduate to orgasm during intercourse.

What responds to therapy?

If a couple cannot enjoy intercourse, or can't manage intercourse at all, whether for physical or emotional reasons, there are many problems, but they can be overcome. Some of the more common problems that can be helped with sex therapy, as opposed to those which may require medical treatment are:

Dyspareunia – this is painful intercourse and the reasons can be physical or psychological. They will need to be explored and treated accordingly.

Impotence – this inability to maintain an erection can result from anxiety about sexual performance.

Loss of libido – this can result from some physical cause, such as at menopause when the vagina is drier and penetration may be uncomfortable. If this or any emotional problem is untreated, a lack of interest in sex will result.

Premature ejaculation – this is the most common male problem. If a man ejaculates before or immediately upon entering the vagina, this can lead to loss of interest for both partners. Sometimes the cause is an infection, but usually it is psychological, resulting in anxiety and an inability to control the timing of an orgasm, much as we control our bladder and bowel.

Vaginismus – this is the involuntary spasm of the vaginal muscle so that the penis can't enter.

Other reasons may include poor sexual technique and you may have to accept that you are not attracted by your partner any more.

SEE ALSO:

ANXIETY
MENOPAUSAL PROBLEMS
PAINFUL INTERCOURSE
PRURITIS VULVAE
SEXUAL PROBLEMS
VAGINISMUS
VAGINITIS

SEXUAL PROBLEMS

Frigidity is a pejorative term that is used loosely. It is used variously to mean not wanting to have sex, not liking sex, feeling repelled by sex, not getting excited and failing to reach orgasm. (About 10% of women fail to reach orgasm at all, even with masturbation.) All these things are normal if you don't want to have sex; they only become a problem if you wish to become aroused, enjoy sex and reach climax. There is no reason to suppose that life without sex is in any way inferior.

Problems with intercourse and lack of interest can stem from both physical and emotional factors. It can become a chronic problem and failure to disclose it will have an effect on your relationships, and your image of yourself as a woman.

Physical causes of lack of desire include *depression*, stress (see *Anxiety*), *diabetes mellitus*, pain during intercourse (see *Painful intercourse*), taking certain drugs such as alcohol, barbiturates, a contraceptive pill high in estrogens or *hormone replacement therapy*. Removal of the ovaries in a *hysterectomy* depletes the supply of testosterone, which is believed to be the hormone that affects libido. An underactive thyroid gland, hypothyroidism (see *Hyperthyroidism*), reduces energy and sex drive. *Menopause* is, however, not a time when you should experience loss of interest. This is more likely a result of other symptoms such as insomnia and dryness of the vagina.

Some symptoms that make sex uncomfortable and painful relate to *sexually transmitted diseases*. You should check whether your partner has had sex with anyone else recently, and if that is so, you should insist that he wear a condom. The onus is now on men to take precautions against transmitting diseases such as *genital herpes* and *chlamydia*. There is also the threat of *AIDS* where women need to be assertive to protect themselves.

The physical cause could lie with your partner. He may have problems with premature ejaculation and impotence. However, failing to achieve orgasm and enjoy sex in the long term, is almost always due to psychological not physical factors, even if a physical problem was the initial cause.

Fear is the commonest cause of loss of desire. A woman may be fearful of letting herself go both physically and emotionally. She may have ambivalent feelings about intercourse, stemming from some incident in early life. These feelings will inevitably be transferred onto her partners. She may use her reluctance to punish herself; wanting to enjoy sex but punishing herself for doing so. She may be angry with her partner or lovemaking may be rather predictable. Pregnancy is often a fear if *contraception* isn't discussed and practiced.

Total sexual inhibition, which is very rare, can arise from many causes, often being a combination of factors such as family upbringing, religious teaching, and childhood trauma. These problems are difficult to solve even by a loving partner.

Sexual disappointment between two people can always be cured by better information and greater openness. Professional counseling is often the answer particularly if there is friction in a relationship. A trained sex therapist will try to uncover the reasons for your fear, although if your relationship is no longer a loving one, sex counseling will not help. A broken relationship cannot be helped with sex and this should be admitted from the outset of any *sex therapy*.

Many women prefer to attend sex clinics where women are treated on their own by counseling, followed by masturbation training. The view is that a woman must be able to excite herself before she can be excited by anyone else. This treatment involves a degree of honesty which many women find difficult. If a woman cannot reach orgasm through penile penetration, she has to be honest and consider other ways of stimulating herself. She should concentrate on her own pleasure – simultaneous orgasm is hard to achieve anyway. Even when aroused and desiring sex, unless there is sufficient clitoral stimulation and the vagina lubricates enough to make penetration easy and comfortable, there won't be good sex. This is where aids such as lubricating jelly and vibrators can be useful.

SEXUALLY TRANSMITTED DISEASES

These are diseases that are transmitted by close sexual contact, whether genital, anal or oral. Chronologically, STDs can be divided into two types: the "old" ones which have been around for many years – *syphilis* has been around for centuries – and the "modern" types such as *chlamydia, genital herpes* and *AIDS*. Some of the newer STDs are difficult to treat and the chance of eradication and cure is not very great. *Gonorrhea* and syphilis, once correctly diagnosed, are eminently treatable with simple antibiotics such as penicillin. Genital warts (see *Warts*) can be treated topically with various simple agents.

The most common STD is referred to sometimes as non-specific urethritis, though this is misleading because in women the cervix is more likely to be affected. Chlamydia is the one bacteria that has been positively identified. All these comparatively symptomless STDs in women require culturing; a *pelvic examination* will not give a reliable diagnosis. The absence of symptoms means that the infection can get a strong hold and be difficult to eradicate when treatment is begun. It also means that an unwitting carrier can spread the infection to many partners if she is sexually promiscuous.

The incidence of STDs with obvious symptoms in women such as *trichomoniasis*, has increased with the advent of the permissive society and the transference of STDs to an ever-increasing population.

Infestations
Pubic lice or crabs, a variety of body lice, are found in the pubic hair where they bite and suck blood, causing intense itchiness. They are easily spread by genital contact but can be treated with a special shampoo and fine combing, like head lice.

Scabies, a tiny mite that is highly contagious, burrows under the skin and lays its eggs. This results in an itchy rash. If it appears near the genitals, this rash can be mistaken for syphilis so a blood test may be necessary for sexually active women. Treatment is simple and effective by applying a lotion all over the body. The whole family should be treated as well as clothing and bed linen.

Along with many other viral conditions, we have no ideal way of treating genital herpes. Most sufferers feel that their sexual life is seriously curtailed and some even opt for celibacy. The shock-waves from the AIDS epidemic will ripple through society for decades to come and has also resulted in a return to a more circumscribed sex life – interpreted as a return to moral behavior by some – throughout the whole of society.

Symptoms of an STD may not necessarily be refer- rable to the genital organs. Others have genital signs you should be on the look-out for, such as sores and burning during urination. If you find any of them, you should report to your family doctor or to an STD clinic. There are several reasons for prompt action. One of them is that untreated, any STD could cause *pelvic inflammatory disease* resulting in sterility. The second reason is that contacts should be traced, warned and tested, so that the spread of the disease can be contained.

By far the best source for advice and treatment is the local STD clinic. These clinics are not mysterious, they operate just like any other hospital clinic, except that total confidentiality is a matter of principle. You may not even have to disclose your name or home address to have sympathetic support and therapy. Most clinics have a counselor who can advise you about future actions and also help you come to terms with the fact that you have an STD. The importance of contacting all your sexual partners will be stressed and you should be assiduous about doing so, so that they can be treated. If you prefer, the clinic will get in touch with contacts, thus relieving you of that res- ponsibilty.

The advent of AIDS and the increase in STDs has resulted in a more responsible attitude to sex in the community at large. The statisticians will tell you that people are taking fewer sexual partners than before which has resulted in a 70% decrease in STDs. More and more people are practicing safe sex by using spermicides and condoms (see *Contraception*) and if this practice spreads, the downward trend in the spread of STDs will continue.

SKIN CANCER

The majority of skin cancers are slow growing and non-invasive and therefore don't present problems of treatment or anxiety about spread. There are three main types of skin cancer: the basal cell carcinoma, squamous cell carcinoma and malignant melanoma. Malignant melanoma is much more serious because, unlike the other two, it spreads quickly throughout the body (metastasizes).

All of these cancers can be recognized while still small and they go through quite long pre-malignant phases. With basal cell carcinoma and squamous cell carcinoma complete eradication and cure is possible in 100% of cases – in 95% by a single, simple surgical procedure.

· S y m p t o m s ·

▲ White or flesh colored ulcer
▲ Hard lump, which may resemble a wart, that grows larger
▲ Rough, red patch of skin
▲ Usually these signs appear on those parts of the body that are exposed to the sun such as the face, ears and hands.

Should I see the doctor?
See your doctor immediately if you notice any change in your skin pigment or an existing mole or freckle. Don't wait for any possible spread. Before a benign melanoma undergoes malignant change, there are certain signs and if you note them and act quickly the lesion can be excised before it ever spreads. Pay attention to any of the following changes to an existing mole or freckle anywhere on the body even on the soles of the feet. Pay particular attention to any new mole that grows after puberty.
Things to watch for include:
◆ A darkening in color
◆ Variation in color
◆ Growth in size
◆ Spread of pigment from the border, giving an uneven edge

◆ Weeping, bleeding or ulceration

What will the doctor do?
Your doctor will almost certainly arrange for you to have a biopsy of the suspect lump, ulcer or mole. A sample of the growth will be removed for laboratory analysis.

BASAL CELL CARCINOMA

This is the most common skin cancer and it results from longterm exposure to sunlight. The cells change and ulcerate so the lump appears white or flesh colored and develops very slowly over many years.

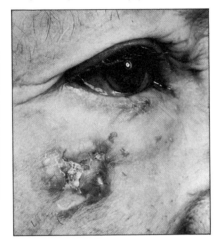

If a basal cell bleeds and scabs over, it still never heals. In some cases the ulcer looks more like a patch of red flaky skin.

The ulcers usually appear on those parts of the body exposed to the sun, such as the face. This cancer does not spread to the rest of the body.

SQUAMOUS CELL CARCINOMA

This usually starts as a lump of malignant cells and is also probably due to exposure to the sunlight, therefore it tends to occur on those parts of the body that are exposed to the sun, such as the face and hands. It may arise from a pre-malignant lesion, solar keratosis, which is a

small, scaling red area of skin that has been exposed to sunlight. This cancer can spread to other parts of the body at an advanced stage.

Both basal cell and squamous cell carcinomas are therefore encouraged by sun tanning which, in this context, is to be avoided. They are both more commonly found in fair-skinned people with years of exposure to hot sun. They are rarely found in dark-skinned people.

MALIGNANT MELANOMA

This is the skin cancer which causes most concern. It can arise from a pigmented patch in the skin, often a freckle or a mole. It is one of the most malignant tumors, spreading at an enormously fast rate to distant parts of the body.

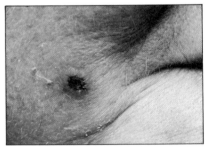

A malignant melanoma tends to develop from an existing mole and slowly enlarge or darken.

Unless it is treated at an early stage it is nearly always fatal. Although sun tanning plays some part in this cancer, it is not such a positive cause.

What is the medical treatment?
If the biopsy showed some cancerous growth, it will be treated in a number of ways depending on its size and the stage it is at. The microscopic examination will also reveal if there are malignant changes.

Carcinomas are usually easily treated with minor surgery. They are either excised, frozen (cryosurgery), scooped out with a curette, or destroyed by radiation therapy. You will need to go back for checkups in case there is any recurrence and possible further treatment.

If a melanoma is deemed benign then it will be simply excised to the wide border of normal skin. This is a minor operation but if the area is large, you may need a skin graft. Surgical treatment for a malignant melanoma is always radical.

Any surgery is nearly always followed by radiation therapy and/or chemotherapy.

What can I do?
I believe that all moles which are subject to friction in the skin should be excised before they become troublesome. These would include moles under bra straps or fastenings around the waist, in the soles of the feet, on the tops of the feet where straps may rub, etc. If your own family doctor is unwilling to excise such a mole, ask for a referral to a dermatologist who will examine you and probably understand immediately and comply with your wishes.

CARE OF THE SKIN

Nearly all the effects of aging, with the exception of the downward pull of gravity, are related to exposure to the sun. Sunbathing is one of the most harmful things you can do to your skin. Excessive exposure to ultraviolet radiation stimulates development of skin cancer and ages your skin. The sun splinters and cracks the subtle architecture of the skin, the collagen. When collagen bundles are broken, the skin loses its elasticity and the force of gravity is able to pull the sagging skin into wrinkles, pits and hollows.

Despite this, many people actively chase the sun and if you must go out in the sun take these precautions: Wear a sunscreen with a high protection factor; the higher the number, the greater the protection.

If you have fair skin, never expose your skin to the sun for longer than 10 minutes on the first day and build up with 10 minutes a day thereafter.

SUN SAFETY CHART			
Sun protection factor	4	8	15
Skin type	Safe exposure time		
Fair	10 mins	40-80 mins	1½-2 hrs
Medium	50-80 mins	2-2½ hrs	5-5½ hrs
Dark	1½-2 hrs	3½-4 hrs	All day
Black	4 hrs	All day	All day

Don't forget that every time you are sunburnt, you reduce the resistance of your skin to cancerous agents. A sunscreen needs replacing after swimming. Moisturize your skin as many times during the day as you remember.

SEE ALSO:

BIOPSY
BIRTHMARKS
CANCER
FACIAL TREATMENTS
MOLES
RADIATION THERAPY
SKIN PROBLEMS

SKIN PROBLEMS

These days the skin has to withstand several modern onslaughts which are extremely deleterious to its health. Modern detergents are hard on the hands; central heating, with its demoisturized air and changes in temperatures, encourages skin vessels to dilate, then contract, which is not good for retaining moisture in the skin.

Because of our passion for the outdoors, we expose our skin to inclement weather, thereby cooling it down, only to heat it up again when we come indoors to fierce central heating. We chase suntans and that in itself is extremely harmful to the skin. Sunlight has two major damaging effects on the skin. The first is that it encourages malignant change. In the last few years there has been a five-fold increase in *skin cancer* around the globe, even in countries such as Iceland. Secondly, exposure to strong sunlight is aging. It has the effect of disrupting collagen. Collagen is the elastic architecture which gives the skin its suppleness, stretch and spring. In a young skin as yet unexposed to sunlight, the collagen lies in regular parallel bundles – just as in a new piece of elastic. With years of exposure to the sun, the collagen bundles disrupt, break and lie in many different directions, just like a very old piece of elastic which is no longer stretchy and has no rebound (see *Wrinkles*). Therefore getting a suntan every summer of your life will add between five and ten years to your apparent age by the time you are 50. At the very least, always wear a sunblock whenever you are out in direct sunlight or where sunlight may be reflected.

Many allergies show up in the skin in a variety of forms. A measles-like rash which arises about eight to ten days after you have been exposed to the allergen, is characteristic of penicillin sensitivity. Much more dramatic is angioedema, swelling and puffing of the eyes, mouth, lips, cheeks and face, which can arise within minutes of contact with the allergen. Then there are hives which come and go every ten minutes or so. These occur as the result of an allergen, such as food, pollen, insect stings, binding to antibodies formed inside your body. The first time you eat something to which you are going to be allergic you will have no response at all; the body needs one exposure to interpret the foreign protein as allergic and form antibodies.

When the antibody reaction takes place in your body, substances like histamine are released. They cause dilation of the capillaries and loss of fluid into the surrounding tissues, causing swelling, itchiness and possibly blistering.

A variety of unsightly *birthmarks* may occur in the skin. Some will disappear of their own accord if you are patient and wait. Like acne, which can leave severe scarring and pitting, some birthmarks can be removed without surgery by methods such as *dermabrasion* and chemical skin peeling (see *Facial treatments*). Cancers of the skin in later life are not uncommon, but fortunately they are slow growing, fairly benign in nature, radio-sensitive and can be cured simply and easily.

Atopy

Eczema, the commonest form of skin disease, runs in families. Also known as dermatitis, it often shows up in the first year of life. At the root of this condition is what is called "atopy." Atopy means that you are an individual who has an inherited tendency to react to allergens.

Atopic subjects not only suffer from dermatitis, they may also suffer from a family of related conditions such as asthma, hayfever, migraine and travel sickness. Atopic eczema has a predilection for certain sites of the body – the inner sides of the elbows, behind the knees, the hands and the face. It is extremely itchy and you will always need help from a dermatologist so that you can have special anti-inflammatory creams.

Do not wash with water. Water, because of the salts it contains, is dehydrating which encourages cracking and splitting. Stop using soap, it de-fats the skin and makes it drier, more scaly and irritable. Use an emollient ointment and cream. Avoid all woolen or hairy, fluffy garments, use linen or cotton or silk. If you suffer from any of the above problems, always wear gloves when doing household chores.

SPORTS INJURIES

The range of sports injuries suffered by women is in general no different from that of men. Sprains, strains and muscle tears occur in the same places according to the sport or athletic activity being performed. Only in a few areas are sports injuries specific to the female sex. However, the growing interest and involvement in sporting and keep-fit activities by women means that they need to be more knowledgeable about possible ill-effects.

How to prevent injury

There are a number of ways you can prevent sports injuries.
◆ Warm up slowly and thoroughly before any sporting activity.
◆ Don't exercise too soon after eating or drinking.
◆ Invest in well-designed and appropriate equipment, such as proper shoes for jogging or tennis, for example.
◆ Learn how to take your own pulse and don't exert yourself beyond your fitness level.
◆ Stop if you feel pain, this is not normal.
◆ Make sure you are exercising on a good surface; for example, jogging on uneven roads can cause strain.

JOGGING

During jogging, high impact forces are borne by the bones and joints of the legs, hip, pelvis and spine. Running shoes are therefore of crucial importance. No woman should attempt jogging without buying the best designed pair of shoes for jogging that she can afford. It is very unwise to embark on an ambitious program of jogging without toning up your body and improving the strength of your legs and spine by preliminary walking and easy running exercises. If you do, you are asking for trouble.

The commonest injuries seen in women joggers are ligament and tendon sprains in the ankle, knee and hip. These may be caused by wearing shoes that are badly fitting or that are excessively worn, running on uneven ground, or by an abnormal foot posture (so that the foot is tilted each time it strikes the ground.)

Continual jarring can cause back or knee pain, which may be improved by running on softer surfaces or having an insole fitted in your shoe. Jarring occasionally causes a stress fracture of a bone in the foot or lower leg. This shows up as a hairline fracture on X-ray, and means that you will have to give up jogging for several weeks to allow time for healing. Your doctor may advise you to avoid jogging altogether in the future. Experts agree that you can exercise the body just as efficiently by walking briskly rather than running.

You should not jog if you have any joint disorder such as osteoarthritis or rheumatoid arthritis; this puts pressure on your weightbearing joints, and could damage them further. Gentle exercise, such as swimming, is more appropriate here.

KNEE PAIN

The angle made by the long axis of the femur, the thigh bone, and the tibia, the leg bone, is known as the Q-angle. Because the pelvis of women is wider than that of men to allow for childbirth, the upper end of the femur is set more apart and the Q-angle is greater. This has a weakening effect on the knee and athletes such as hurdlers and marathon runners who put great strains on the knee may develop an inflammation called chondromalacia patellae or runner's knee which causes severe pain at the front of the knee sufficient to prevent walking. Additionally, the patella or knee-cap may slip to the outside of the knee.

What is the treatment?

At the first indication of pain, apply ice packs and rest your injured joint. You should stop your sporting activity and rest until the inflammation subsides. Supportive strapping has to be worn so that the patella is held in the correct position. Weights to strengthen the quadracep muscles can help you to regain fitness again.

OSTEOCHONDRITIS OF THE SPINE

Young girl gymnasts in heavy training can put enormous strain on the rather primitive spinal column which is still growing and developing. A fairly common sports injury in these girls is osteochondritis of the epiphyses of the spinal bones. The epiphyses are those parts of the vertebrae which are still growing, and with over-use they become inflamed. If the stresses and strains continue there may be distortion of the vertebral bone itself, giving rise to spondylosis in later life when the spinal column stiffens and becomes less flexible.

The condition gives rise to pain in the back and the only advice to the gymnast is to stop exercising completely so that the inflammation can subside and bone growth proceed normally.

SPORT AND PREGNANCY

Physical activity during pregnancy is highly recommended but this is not a good time to take up a new sport. However, as long as you avoid water skiing and diving, when water could be forced into your vagina, and contact sports such as volleyball, where you could receive a knock on your abdomen, you will be fit throughout your pregnancy and recover quickly from the birth. Remember though that if you exercise until you are out of breath, your baby will also be deprived of oxygen in the uterus.

OVER TRAINING

Women athletes who train very hard, particularly long distance and marathon runners, are nearly always lean to the point of thinness. Anorexia nervosa is quite common.

Over-training is also a cause of secondary amenorrhea and sub-fertility. With over training, the ratio of body fat to lean muscle mass diminishes. The body interprets this as a threat to survival. To keep a woman's body alive, it becomes sub-fertile because biologically her body is not strong enough to carry a pregnancy. The first sign of this is amenorrhea.

What is the treatment?
The treatment for osteochondritis and over training is to give up strict athletic training. In nearly all athletes menstruation returns when they stop training and most who want to, can start a family.

TENOSYNOVITIS OF THE WRIST

The synovial membrane keeps joints lubricated to allow freedom of movement. This membrane may become inflamed and swollen because of overuse of the joint. (Typists can get this condition in their fingers.) Women tennis players, rowers and canoeing experts quite often develop a tenosynovitis of the wrist where the sheaths covering the tendons on the front of the wrist become inflamed, swollen and exquisitely painful so they have to discontinue their sport.

What is the treatment?
A modern surgical treatment hardly short of miraculous involves opening up the synovial sheaths and decompressing them. Many sportswomen can then return to their sport even before the stitches have been taken out. There are records of sportswomen having won events with the stitches still intact.

SPRAINED ANKLE

A sprained ankle with rupture of the lateral ligament on the outer side of the ankle is quite common, but in a woman who is active, a sprained ankle can recur once the lateral ligament has been weakened, leading to a chronically unstable ankle joint.

What is the treatment?
A sprained ankle is usually treated by applying an ice pack to reduce swelling, wrapping the joint with a bandage, and resting it in a raised position until pain and swelling subside.

A chronically unstable ankle joint can sometimes be treated surgically. A new type of operation, which has been tried out on Olympic athletes, stabilizes the joint by shifting a small muscle attachment. The tendon is simply moved slightly forward on the bone to which it is attached and this holds the outer side of the joint in a stable position.

When the operation was first devised, the ankle was put in a cast for six weeks, now, with more experience, only two weeks in a cast is necessary and then the ankle is strapped and given intensive physical therapy. This allows the athlete to return to training and reach match fitness quickly.

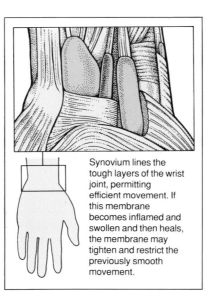

Synovium lines the tough layers of the wrist joint, permitting efficient movement. If this membrane becomes inflamed and swollen and then heals, the membrane may tighten and restrict the previously smooth movement.

TENNIS ELBOW

Tennis elbow is so called because the backhand movement, if performed incorrectly, can put enormous strain on the tendon that attached to the elbow, causing pain on the outer most tip. But tennis elbow is not only found in tennis players; anyone who does anything involving the backhand movement can get the same injury with the same symptoms. Spring-cleaning or hanging curtains can lead to tennis elbow.

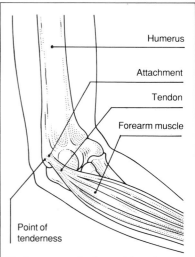

Humerus

Attachment

Tendon

Forearm muscle

Point of tenderness

The forearm muscles that straighten the wrist and fingers are attached by a tendon to a bony prominence on the outer side of the elbow. If these muscles are overused, the area around the tendon may become inflamed and painful as a result of the constant tugging of the tendon on its point of attachment.

What is the treatment?
The treatments for tennis elbow include resting the elbow, ultrasound treatment to the inflamed tendon and hydrocortisone injections into the inflamed tendon.

SPORTS INJURIES

PHYSICAL THERAPY

This employs all sorts of methods to help restore your body to fitness. It originated with massage which enhances circulation and increases your muscle flexibility by speeding blood flow to the muscle. This also removes waste products from your system and relieves soreness. You can look upon it as feeding the muscles with fresh blood more frequently. This is vital if you are unable to train when your muscles can waste from under use. Ultrasound, the same as is used in pregnancy, sends sound waves to the blood vessels, breaking up swelling in the tissues by increasing the absorption of the blood vessels so there is less swelling.

Various forms of superficial and deep heat treatments help to relieve pain and reduce muscle spasm. This also increases blood flow to the area. Superficial methods include hot packs, bathing and infra-red lamps. Deep heat methods apply high frequency electric currents; this is known as short-wave cautery.

SEE ALSO:

AMENORRHEA
ANOREXIA NERVOSA
FITNESS TESTING
MENSTRUAL PROBLEMS
OSTEOARTHRITIS
RHEUMATOID ARTHRITIS
ULTRASOUND

STERILIZATION

This is a permanent surgical means of birth control which makes it impossible for an egg to be fertilized and conception to take place. The simplest procedure is carried out on men and involves tying the tubes that connect the testicles to the penis. Ejaculate is still emitted during orgasm, but it contains no sperm and therefore is not capable of fertilizing an ovum. This operation is called a vasectomy and it is done under local anesthetic in about 20 minutes.

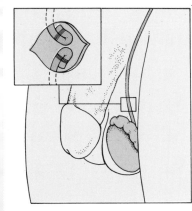

Vasectomy
Male sterilization consists simply of dividing and tying back each vas deferens – the tubes which conduct sperm from the testes. The procedure is normally performed in an out-patient department under local anesthesia. A very small incision is made in the scrotum.

In women the usual method is tubal ligation or cauterization which closes off the fallopian tubes, resulting in an obstruction which is impenetrable to the ovum in its passage to the uterus.

Why is it done?
This is usually only performed on men or women who have already had children and do not want to have more. As it is essentially a permanent operation which cannot be reversed (some few procedures have been reversed but the patient should not count on the possibility),

doctors are anxious to emphasize that there will be no possibility of starting another family should anything happen in the future. For this reason, they are loath to sterilize childless women or women under 30.

For some women the decision is a difficult one. While they may be freed from the fear of having an unwanted pregnancy, they need to come to terms with their feelings about taking the irrevocable step of having no more children, and possibly of having to accept their partners' refusals to take the step and have a vasectomy.

How is it done?
There are five different methods of female sterilization which use either the abdominal or vaginal

approach. All are carried out under general anesthetic or occasionally an epidural. Carbon dioxide gas may be introduced into the abdomen to inflate it so that the internal organs can be more clearly seen. While all the procedures describe tying or closing the tubes in some way, a small portion of the tube itself is almost invariably removed. Other forms of surgery, such as hysterectomy, result in sterilization but should not be used solely for this purpose.

Tubal ligation is the commonest method and is treated separately.

In cauterization, the fallopian tubes are burned with an instrument. Different instruments are used to locate the tubes and view them during the operation and the individual procedures bear their

FEMALE STERILIZATION

The simplest methods of female sterilization involve interrupting the connection between the fallopian tubes and the uterus. The

separation is brought about by two principal methods – cauterization and rings or clips.

Cauterization
Under direct visualization via a laparoscope, the surgeon applies an electrically heated forceps to each tube. The current coagulates the tubes, destroying much of their lengths.

Rings or clips
Rather than cauterizing the tubes, a surgeon may choose to close them off by applying clips or elastic rings.

STERILIZATION

names. The cauterization instrument is inserted through an incision just above the pubic line.

In laparoscopy, a laparoscope is inserted through an incision in the abdomen, usually in the navel.

In hysteroscopy, an hysteroscope is passed through the vagina into the womb.

In culdoscopy, a culdoscope is passed through a tiny incision in the wall of the vagina.

Laparotomy is the method most commonly used after childbirth; it is particularly appropriate after a Caesarean section. A larger incision is made in the abdomen and the tubes are lifted out and tied before the incision is stitched closed.

What are the after effects?
You will notice no change in your normal menstrual pattern; you will have a normal menopause because your ovaries have not been affected. The ovum produced is absorbed into the body as it would be at any time when fertilization did not occur. Some women have a routine D & C when they are sterilized; this is a check of the uterus for any growths or problems. Usually there is bleeding from the vagina for a day or two and some local discomfort where the incision(s) was made. You may notice pain in your shoulder. This is caused by irritation from the carbon dioxide gas. You may also have a reaction to the general anesthetic. If you've had a reaction to a general anesthetic previously, suggest to your doctor that an epidural might be used.

If you had a vaginal sterilization, you will not be able to have intercourse for a couple of weeks because of the danger of infection. You will have no external scar.

What are the risks?
There are few serious risks or complications with any of the methods of sterilization except those normally expected of any

surgical procedure. Tubal ligation by the vaginal route has a slightly increased risk of infection.

Is it effective?
Sterilization has a higher efficiency rate than any other means of birth control and it is permanent. After the operation no other form of birth control is necessary. The operation is considered irreversible, although microsurgery, in a few cases, has succeeded in sewing the tubes together. There will be no effect on your libido or sex life. Men often feel their potency has been interfered with after vasectomy; this is only in the mind and has no physical reality.

SEE ALSO:

CONTRACEPTION
DILATATION AND
  CURETTAGE
EPIDURAL ANESTHETIC
LAPAROSCOPY
TUBAL LIGATION

SYPHILIS

Two or three hundred years ago syphilis was the medical scourge of the time in very much the same way that AIDS is now. It is a venereal disease that infected large numbers of both sexes. Syphilis has a very long life-history and produces severe symptoms; to many it was fatal. With the advent of penicillin, syphilis declined at a steady rate. However, following a sharp increase in cases in 1987, syphilis has been on the rise.

Syphilis is caused by a bacterium Treponema pallidum and can be transmitted from person to person through sexual contact.

· S y m p t o m s ·

▲ A chancre or sore on the vulva
▲ Swollen glands in the groin
▲ Rash, especially on the palms of the hands

Should I see the doctor?

Primary and secondary syphilis can be treated and cured completely with a single course of penicillin. It is therefore a great tragedy if the disease goes undiagnosed. If you suspect that you may have contracted syphilis, seek confidential medical attention immediately. Once the disease has destroyed certain tissues such as joints, it is impossible to cure.

What will the doctor do?

The diagnosis will be made after taking samples from the sore or rash and a blood test.

Treatment involves a course of antibiotic injections. You should also

FOUR STAGES OF THE DISEASE

Syphilis has four stages:

Primary stage: this is when the condition is first contracted, the only visible sign being a small sore or chancre, which is highly infectious, where the bacteria entered the body. This is usually through an abrasion on the vulva or through the cervix. The lymph glands nearby become enlarged.

Secondary stage: quite often the body responds to the invasion with a rash which covers most of the body. The rash develops about 14-28 days after contracting the infection. The rash can form pimples which may persist for some weeks before they fade.

Tertiary stage: this stage is much rarer these days because of anti-biotic treatment. After several years many organs in the body have been affected and some of the most dramatic changes take place. For example, syphilitic disease of the joints completely destroys them, rendering them swollen, mis-shapen and immobile. Syphilis can affect almost any part of the body, including the heart.

Quaternary stage: the fourth, and terminal part of the disease, is when it attacks and destroys the brain. This is called general paralysis of the insane when social and intellectual functions are gradually destroyed.

have regular blood tests for at least two years to ensure the disease has been eradicated.

What can I do?

◆ Avoid casual sexual contacts.
◆ If you discover a genital or any other kind of sore which you can't account for, have a medical check-up.
◆ If you suspect that you may have caught a venereal disease, go to your doctor or sexually transmitted diseases clinic for a blood test.
◆ You can help eradicate the disease if you give your doctor or the clinic the names of all your sexual partners so that they can be traced and treated. Because the disease can be cured, it is imperative that all partners are treated, otherwise the risks remain. This information is always kept confidential.

SYPHILIS AND PREGNANCY

The disease can pass the placental barrier. A woman who has syphilis will therefore infect her developing child who will be born with congenital syphilis. The classical signs are heart, skull and brain defects. Few of these children survive.

It is for this reason that every pregnant woman is given a blood test during her prenatal treatment to screen her for the disease. This is known as a VDRL (Venereal Disease Research Lab) or Wasserman or Kahn test. The test will be done at the first visit.

SEE ALSO:

AIDS
CHLAMYDIA
GONORRHEA
PRENATAL CARE
SEXUALLY TRANSMITTED
  DISEASES

SYSTEMIC LUPUS

Systemic lupus erythematosus (SLE) is one of the autoimmune diseases that is worthy of special mention because 90% of sufferers are women. The peak age for onset of first symptoms is between ages 15 and 25. The mean age at the time of diagnosis is 30 years.

All the autoimmune diseases are caused by the same underlying process. Because of an allergic reaction in the collagen, a protein that is the principal component in the body's connective tissue, chemical substances are released which cause inflammation and destruction; the collagen swells and disintegrates. The basic change in systemic lupus is in the arteries' collagen with resultant damage to the skin, kidneys, heart, joints and lungs. In severe cases, there are signs that all of these organs are involved. Characteristically, the disease spares no tissue or organ. The joints are commonly involved and symptoms resembling rheumatoid arthritis to mild joint pain may result. Muscle weakness and wasting may be severe.

How serious is it?
SLE is an uncommon but serious condition which affects about 7.6 women per 100,000 annually. While the disease affects individuals of all races, the incidence in black females is higher than in white females in the U.S.

The onset of SLE is usually insidious with a history of vague ill-health, weight loss, flitting joint pains and increased sensitivity to sunlight. The disease is usually chronic with remissions and exacerbations. Rarely, death can occur after only a few weeks.

Should I see the doctor?
In the initial stages patients are very ill and severe forms of SLE may be life threatening.

What is the medical treatment?
The diagnosis of systemic lupus will be made from blood tests. The hall-

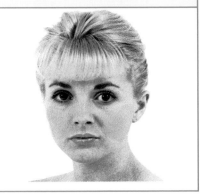

· Symptoms ·

▲ Skin rash with the characteristic "butterfly" redness over the nose and cheeks; it may spread to the upper part of the body when exposed to sunlight
▲ Joint swelling and pain; this could be mistaken for rheumatoid arthritis
▲ Breathlessness and chest pain
▲ Swelling of glands
▲ Kidney failure
▲ If the brain is involved there may be convulsions

mark of the disease is the finding of a particular protein, the antinuclear factor, in the blood. This is an antibody and is probably responsible for kidney damage which results from deposits of antigen/antibody complex in the fine filaments of the kidney.

The mainstay of treatment in the acute phase is anti-inflammatory drugs such as corticosteroids and immunosuppressants. Anti-cancer drugs may also be helpful.

After the initial serious phase of the disease, you may be given physical therapy to help bring mobility back to affected joints.

You will need regular check-ups so that your medical advisers can monitor the disease.

One of the essential parts of treatment is to avoid undue exposure to strong sunlight. Anti-malarial drugs are useful in protecting against the effects of sunlight.

What is the prognosis?
The prognosis of the disease is variable and depends mainly on the extent of damage to the kidneys and the response to treatment with corticosteroids. Renal involvement is one of the most serious complications. If this is absent one or two years after diagnosis, it is unlikely to develop later and the prognosis is greatly improved. When renal involvement occurs, it may start as a mild form and then progress to renal failure

with very high blood pressure; there is nearly always anemia.

Treatment can stop or slow down the progress of the disease but because the autoimmune system is damaged, the patient will eventually succumb to infection. It will be necessary to get medical attention for the slightest problem.

SEE ALSO:

ANEMIA
AUTOIMMUNE DISEASE
HYPERTENSION
RHEUMATOID ARTHRITIS

TERMINATION OF PREGNANCY

This is also known as a medically induced abortion. With changes in attitudes, this is now legally performed in the U.S. up to the 12th week. Individual states may legally enact certain restrictions on abortions between the 12th and 24th weeks and may prohibit abortions beyond the 24th week. (You should check with Planned Parenthood for the laws applicable in your state.) In some countries, abortion is illegal, and even in countries where it is allowed, the terms under which it is performed and the time of gestation differ considerably. Even in America, some religious groups and anti-abortionists feel that abortion at any time constitutes murder – this includes the abortion of a badly deformed fetus as well as an abortion carried out for the victim of a rape.

What are my options?

The venue and procedure chosen for an abortion depends upon many factors, most important of which is the week of pregnancy. The choices available to a woman after the 12th week are limited according to state legislation.

Despite the accusation that abortion is used lightly as a means of controling fertility, the choice is always a difficult one for women to make, and rarely taken with murderous intent. Many women feel that they should have the final say about what happens to their bodies, and that abortion is their choice. The choice should not be made by others who may never even have to face the fact of an unwanted pregnancy, and the child it brings. If abortion were non-exploitative and non-traumatic, the procedure would be less riddled with guilt, leaving less aftermath of misery.

The alternatives to abortion are bringing up the child on your own if you have no partner, putting the child up for adoption or bearing the financial and emotional strain within your existing family.

What are the risks?

Legally induced abortion is a relatively safe surgical procedure, especially when performed during the first 2 months of pregnancy. For example, the risk of death from abortion by dilation and evacuation performed during the first two months is about 0.6 per 100,000 procedures. The relative risk of dying as the consequence of abortion is approximately doubled for each 2 weeks of delay after 8 weeks of gestation. Medically induced abortion, whether legal or illegal, brings the following risks:

- Infection of the uterus.
- Infection of the Fallopian tubes.
- Blockage of the Fallopian tubes leading to sub-fertility or infertility.
- Increased likelihood of an ectopic pregnancy.
- The cervix is so stretched that it becomes incompetent.
- Perforation of the uterus.
- Retained placenta leading to hemorrhage and risk of death.

Why is it done?

The reasons a woman seeks an abortion are many and varied and include an unwanted pregnancy for personal or financial reasons because of failed contraception, and as the result of medical tests which show that the fetus is abnormal. With more sophisticated prenatal tests, more damaged babies are being picked up during early pregnancy. The problems may arise because of maternal illness, such as rubella or syphilis, or because of some congenital or chromosomal disorder. When the results of the tests are known, the parents of the unborn child are usually offered termination and they must then make the difficult decision to abort a wanted baby who may be damaged.

There are many important questions to consider in such a case. You should determine that:

- Continuing the pregnancy involves greater risk to your life than the abortion.
- Continuing the pregnancy involves a greater risk of injury to the physical and mental health of your living children than the abortion.
- There is a substantial risk that the child will be born seriously deformed or suffering from a life-threatening disorder such as hemophilia.
- Trauma and unnecessary misery would result from the birth of a child conceived in rape.

What should I do?

You should go to your own doctor. If you feel you can't approach your doctor, consult a Planned Parenthood or any other family planning clinic.

How will I feel?

No matter how well prepared you are, an abortion always causes

HOME TRUTHS ABOUT ABORTION

- There is nothing you can take by mouth which will safely and efficiently result in abortion.
- Hot baths, bottles of gin and jumping from a great height will not bring about abortion if the baby and placenta are healthy.
- A sharp instrument inserted into the vagina may induce abortion, and it may also kill you or cause you to become sterile.
- An abortion which results in heavy bleeding should be treated immediately. There may be some retained placenta or an infection which should be treated as an emergency.

TERMINATION OF PREGNANCY

psychological and mental trauma. Just making the decision to go ahead with the abortion means considering the opposite, going ahead with the pregnancy and bringing up the child or offering it for adoption. Once you start to think about the baby and its life, it is very difficult to face up to. The choices are painful and you will need counseling and support from your family, partner or trained counselors.

Most women feel fearful, anxious, guilty and ashamed. There are many decisions to make and there are many questions you will be asking yourself.

Will it be painful?
Will I be punished?
Will I be sterile?
Will I have regrets?
Will I fear sex?
Will I become frigid?
Will I ever be normal again?

All these fears are normal, but after the abortion be prepared to feel depressed. It is not uncommon to feel withdrawn, tearful and inadequate as well as being unable to cope for several weeks after an abortion. The majority of women do, however, feel relieved after it has happened, although they may feel sad as well.

How is it done?
You certainly must not rush your decision about an abortion but once you have made up your mind, you should make arrangements quickly. It's important to have the abortion performed at the best time. This is before 16 weeks, and preferably before 12. After 16 weeks, it is not only more difficult but also more dangerous because the abortion is induced by a prostaglandin injection which produces the abortion within 12 to 36 hours. It can be very painful.

EARLY VACUUM ABORTION (4–12 WEEKS)

This is a very early termination and may be carried out with no anesthetic if it is early in the pregnancy. A small flexible tube is inserted through the vagina into the uterus. The tube is connected to a syringe or pump which gently sucks out the uterine lining and any fetal material. The technique takes about 5 minutes.

The advantages are that there is little disturbance of the cervix and it can be performed even before a pregnancy test is done. This, of course also presents a disadvantage in that it may be performed unnecessarily. The method is certainly the safest and least traumatic form of termination. It can be done in a doctor's office, clinic or outpatients department.

DILATION AND EVACUATION (D&E) (13–24 WEEKS)

This may be carried out under general anesthetic or with a local paracervical block, depending on the duration of pregnancy. It is often done on an outpatient basis but may involve an overnight hospital stay. Dilating rods are used to widen the cervix until the appropriate sized vacuum tube can be inserted. The tube is connected to a pump machine whose suction action frees the fetal material and the womb lining, and sucks it out into a container. You may be given drugs to help the uterus contract afterwards to reduce bleeding and the possibility of infection. The entire procedure takes about 30 minutes and recovery will involve some painful cramps. Some doctors will perform this procedure up to the 24th week of pregnancy while others feel it is not a recommended form of termination beyond the 20th week.

DILATATION AND CURETTAGE (D&C) (12–16 WEEKS)

This method is used after 12 weeks and before that time by doctors who are less confident about the D & E method (above). The routine is the same as for D & E but a curette and forceps are the instruments used to scrape out the lining of the womb and remove it instead of the suction tube. The factor to remember here is that if it is less than 12 weeks since the first day of your last period, you should request that a D & E be performed as this involves less bleeding, discomfort and possible complications.

AMNIOCENTESIS ABORTION (16–24 WEEKS)

By 16 weeks the walls of the uterus are thinner and can more easily be perforated, and the fetus is larger so an amniocentesis abortion with its attendant emotional and physical pain is necessary. Either a saline solution, prostaglandin hormone or urea are injected into the amniotic sac through your abdomen in the same way as with amniocentesis.

After a local anesthetic, a hollow tube is inserted through your abdominal wall into the uterus. The solution is fed down the tube. This is removed and you will need to wait for labor which may be within a couple of hours or not for perhaps 24 hours. You will experience painful contractions and should be offered painkilling drugs if you want them.

You may be given drugs such as oxytocin to increase contractions or dilating rods to dilate the cervix if the labor isn't progressing quickly enough. The baby and placenta are expelled relatively easily. The fetus will be recognizable and if you had prostaglandins, it may live for a few minutes. (The saline solution and urea kill the fetus in utero.) This is upsetting for everybody.

AFTER AN ABORTION

- You should get treatment immediately if you have any heavy bleeding, severe abdominal pain, vomiting or a smelly vaginal discharge.
- Your periods will probably resume within a month to six weeks.
- Abstain from sexual intercourse for at least three weeks to avoid infection.
- An early abortion should mean you are back to normal physically within a week. For a later termination, give yourself 2–3 weeks. You will find your depression may last for as long as three months.
- Have a check-up a week after the abortion.
- Start using some form of contraception after about a week.
- Don't use internal tampons for about a month.

You may then have a D & C to check that there is nothing left in your uterus. You will probably be in the hospital for about 3 days.

HYSTEROTOMY (16–24 WEEKS)

This is rarely performed because it is a major operation. It is only used for women who cannot have saline or prostaglandin treatment or for whom the other methods have not been successful. It is rather like a Caesarean section with the fetus removed through a cut in the abdominal wall and uterus. You will be given a general anesthetic.

SEE ALSO:

ABORTION
AMNIOCENTESIS
CERVIX PROBLEMS
CHROMOSOMAL PROBLEMS
DILATATION AND
  CURETTAGE
GENETIC COUNSELING
MISCARRIAGE
PELVIC INFLAMMATORY
  DISEASE

TOXEMIA OF PREGNANCY

This is a condition which has two stages. Pre-eclampsia is the first stage and it usually occurs after the twentieth week of pregnancy. You may feel fine but your blood pressure suddenly starts to rise for the first time in the pregnancy. If this is not checked, it will continue to rise and progress to eclampsia or toxemia of pregnancy which is very serious. Both baby and mother are at risk. Eclampsia is now a relatively rare condition because regular prenatal checks have meant that the danger signs of this slowly developing condition are immediately spotted.

The cause of pre-eclampsia is not known but it has been associated with poor nutrition. If you do develop the symptoms, they will be treated. As soon as your baby is born, they will usually disappear.

The risk to the baby develops because the rise in blood pressure causes a strain to be put on the placenta which functions less efficiently. There is then a possibility of a premature labor or death in utero. The risk to the mother occurs with the convulsions which can lead to coma.

· S y m p t o m s ·

▲ Edema; swelling of the fingers so your rings are too tight, swelling of the ankles and puffiness of your face
▲ Any rise in blood pressure
▲ Excess weight gain
▲ Protein in the urine
▲ In advanced stage a dramatic increase in blood pressure, nausea, vomiting, headaches, mental dullness, visual disturbances and convulsions

---

Should I see the doctor?
You may not notice the onset of this condition yourself, except for the puffiness and tightness of rings or shoes. If you do, mention them to your doctor as soon as possible. Pre-eclampsia usually develops slowly.

WOMEN AT RISK

Those in their first pregnancies are most at risk but the following should also take care

 With pre-existing disease or previous history of eclampsia
Both kidney disease and diabetes mellitus predispose you, so does migraine. There is a 1 in 10 chance of it recurring after a previous episode

 Expecting twins or more
Multiple births of all types increase the risk

 With affected relatives
If members of the family have high blood pressure or pre-eclampsia

Hypertensives
Women with blood pressures of at least 140/90

Younger or older women
Girls in their teens or women over 40 have a greater risk

If you are attending your prenatal clinic regularly, any change in your blood pressure or signs of edema or protein in your urine will be noted.

What will the doctor do?
In the early stages of the condition, you will be advised to get plenty of rest and to reduce your salt intake to limit the edema.

If you have developed true eclampsia, you will be admitted to hospital and given bed rest and sedation with constant monitoring of your blood pressure and kidney function. Depending on how advanced your condition is, for example if you are having convulsions, your doctor will prescribe drugs to control your blood pressure.

These measures almost always limit the condition and if your blood pressure falls below a certain level (120/90) and remains constant you should be allowed home as long as you can confidently give an assurance that you will get plenty of rest.

On the rare occasions when symptomatic treatment fails to control pre-eclampsia, your baby will be monitored and may be induced or delivered by Caesarean.

What can I do?
Pre-eclampsia is a common complaint in pregnancy – it affects between five and ten percent of all pregnant women – and hardly ever progresses to true eclampsia but the best treatment is prevention and your medical advisers will be the ones who can help you by monitoring your pregnancy through regular prenatal checks. Don't miss any appointments. You can do a great deal to avoid pre-eclampsia by eating well and having adequate protein, whole grains, fresh fruit and vegetables.

Get as much rest as you can; make special times of the day when you can put your feet up. Never stand when you can sit, never sit when you can lie. This increases the flow of blood to the uterus and your baby.

If your ankles, fingers and face are swelling, you may have to consider giving up your job or getting help at home with your other children.

SEE ALSO:

CAESAREAN SECTION
INDUCTION
PRENATAL CARE

TOXIC SHOCK SYNDROME

This rare condition has been known about for over 50 years but it has only recently been associated with menstruation. It is most often seen in women under 30. Toxic shock syndrome will accompany any overwhelming infection with the bacterium *Staphylococcus aureus* which is a normal inhabitant of the human body (of both men and women). If this bacterium is present in the vagina, and it overgrows because its growth is not contained by other bacteria that are normally present, it produces a powerful toxin. If this toxin enters the bloodstream in sufficient quantity, this can cause cardiac collapse, renal failure, coma and death.

How does it occur?

The association with menstruation was discovered when new, super-absorbent tampons came onto the market. These were designed to be left in the vagina for longer periods – even overnight. By the nature of the syndrome, a number of conditions have to apply before it erupts and therefore it is very, very rare. Not only does the bacterium have to be present in the vagina in large quantities, but the woman must also be susceptible to the toxin. In fact, there needn't even be a tampon in the vagina for the syndrome to occur. It would appear that tampons do help to promote the condition though and in a complicated way. However, the major factor is sensitivity to the bacterium. A few cases of toxic shock syndrome have been reported in users of the contraceptive sponge. Again, this is because sponges were left in too long.

The condition has even been noted in men, children and non-menstruating women.

Should I see the doctor?

If you are menstruating and experience a sudden high fever (38°C/102°F or over) with or without

· **Symptoms** ·
▲ Sudden onset of high fever, vomiting and diarrhea
▲ Headache
▲ Sore throat and aching muscles
▲ Dizziness and faintness
▲ Characteristic rash which looks like suntan and the skin peels on the palms of the hands up to 14 days later
▲ Cardiac collapse and renal failure if left untreated for 24 hours or more

vomiting and diarrhea, you should contact your doctor immediately. If you are using a tampon, remove it.

What will the doctor do?

If toxic shock syndrome is diagnosed, you will be prescribed antibiotics to overcome the infection and any other complications will then be dealt with.

What can I do?

Toxic shock syndrome does tend to recur, but only in about one in three women. If it is going to recur this happens within six months of the first attack, so be vigilant. Never wear tampons again in any case and watch for the signs of fever, vomiting and diarrhea during menstruation.

Even though it is very rare, toxic shock syndrome has taught us some lessons about personal hygiene. Never leave tampons in for more than six hours and except for a very heavy flow, you might be wise to avoid the super-absorbent variety. If you have a heavy flow use a sanitary towel as well. Don't leave tampons in overnight. If using contraceptive sponges, make certain they are removed as directed on the instructions.

SEE ALSO:

MENORRHAGIA
MENSTRUAL PROBLEMS

TRICHOMONIASIS

This is a vaginal infection caused by *Trichomonas vaginalis*, a tiny one-celled organism. The symptoms of trichomoniasis are similar to a yeast infection but the discharge is green and has an offensive smell. It is a contagious condition and nine out of ten sexual partners will be affected too, though the infection can be picked up from damp towels or bathing suits. The most common time of infection is just after a menstrual period. Trichomonas, which causes these symptoms, lives in the vagina, cervix, urethra and bladder and is most common in sexually active women.

· S y m p t o m s ·

▲ Offensive smelling, yellowish green, bubbly vaginal discharge
▲ Itching of the vagina and perineum
▲ Burning sensation when urine is passed
▲ Symptoms of cystitis if the bladder is affected

Should I see the doctor?
If you suspect you may be infected, see the doctor immediately for an accurate diagnosis and refrain from sexual intercourse. Let your sexual partner know that you think you may have a sexually transmitted infection and that treatment might be necessary for him, too.

What is the treatment?
Your doctor will probably take a swab of the discharge for laboratory analysis. This is important because the drugs used to cure trichomoniasis are strong and should not be overprescribed, and because another sexually transmitted disease may be diagnosed too. Give your doctor full details of your medical history. The drug Flagyl (metronidazole) is the normal treatment taken over a period of a week but should not be taken by pregnant or lactating women, for example. Flagyl can have unpleasant side effects. You may experience a strange taste and your tongue may feel furry. You may feel nauseous during the treatment.

What can I do to help?
Take the full course of pills as prescribed. However, do not take alcohol while you are on Flagyl, and if a second course is necessary, you should have a blood count first to check that your blood is normal.

As with other vaginal infections, observe good hygiene; avoid vaginal deodorants, douches and tampons, wear cotton or silk panties and don't have sexual intercourse until you are clear of the infection.

You should provide the names and addresses of your sexual partners for them to have treatment too.

SEE ALSO:

CYSTITIS
SEXUALLY TRANSMITTED
  DISEASES
VAGINAL DISCHARGE
YEAST INFECTION

TUBAL LIGATION

Tubal ligation is the ultimate form of contraception for a woman – the equivalent of a man's vasectomy – because it results in sterility. After tubal ligation a woman cannot conceive and it is best to think of the operation as irreversible. Attempts at reversing the operation can be made using microsurgical techniques but they are frequently unsuccessful.

When is it done?
In the past, the procedure was often carried out directly after childbirth, but complications are less likely if the decision to have the operation is left until a few months later.

How is it done?
The operation is designed to seal off the fallopian tubes so that the sperm cannot reach the ovum. The tubes are either tied and cut, destroyed by electrocautery, clamped with rings or clips, plugged or frozen. There are a number of ways this can be carried out usually under general anesthetic.

LAPAROTOMY

This is an old-fashioned operation largely abandoned because it involves a deep wound. A fairly large abdominal incision is made, the abdominal muscle layers cut and each fallopian tube dissected out. The tubes are then divided into two pieces, the two ends tied off and folded back into the surrounding tissue. This is performed only when another abdominal operation is being carried out at the same time.

MINI-LAPAROTOMY

This is a more common version of the above procedure, though it is not suitable if you are very overweight. Earlier operations, adhesions from infections, tumors or endometriosis may also make this procedure impracticable.

First a slim surgical tool is inserted into the vagina to manipulate the top of the uterus close to the abdominal wall. The surgeon makes a small incision – about 2.5cm (1in) – into the abdomen, near the uterus, lifts out each tube in turn and clips and ties it.

LAPAROSCOPY

A laparoscope, containing a fiber-optic filament, is inserted into the abdomen, often through a tiny incision in the navel, and under direct vision, the fallopian tubes are sought out. If operating instruments are not combined with the scope, another tiny incision is made just above the pubic hair line for the instrument that seals off the tubes.

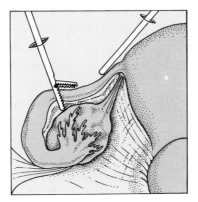

The laparoscope is inserted through one incision while the clamping tool, inserted through another, applies the rings.

Laparoscopy is the most commonly used technique. The stay in hospital should be one day but laparoscopy can be done on an out-patient basis in some clinics. Recovery is usually rapid.

CULDOSCOPY

In this procedure, an incision is made in the vagina just below the cervix. A clamp on the cervix is used to position the uterus so the tubes can be seen. One at a time, the tubes are brought down and cut, tied, clipped or blocked. The instrument is called a culdoscope or colposcope. The abdomen remains free of scars.

The procedure is technically more difficult than laparoscopy and as the vagina contains more bacteria, there is a greater risk of infection.

What are the after-effects?
Before a laparoscope actually passes into the peritoneal cavity, the abdomen is pumped up with air or carbon dioxide so that the surgeon has a clear field of vision. This can occasionally cause a bloating sensation post-operatively, or, very rarely, pain needing painkillers.

Sterilization does not affect ovarian function therefore menstruation continues normally. The sexual response, depending on female hormones, the health of the vagina and clitoral sensitivity are in no way affected, nor is sexual drive. Some women find that libido improves when fear of pregnancy has been removed.

What are the risks and complications?
There may be some pelvic cramps which usually subside spontaneously within 36 hours, though painkillers may be necessary.

There may be some menstrual bleeding; this could be heavy if you had a D & C as a routine check.

There are few serious complications: infection, bleeding and damage to internal organs and the inherent risks of the anesthetic are unlikely to result in complications with this operation.

Rare failures occur if the tissue forms a new channel and the egg or sperm can breach the gap in the tube. Other failures can result if you are already pregnant at the time. A pregnancy test may be done as a precaution.

SEE ALSO:

DILATATION AND
   CURETTAGE
ENDOMETRIOSIS
STERILIZATION

ULTRASOUND

This is a way of producing a photographic picture using sound waves. The picture is formed by the echoes of sound waves bouncing off different parts of the body. The echoes differ in their waves according to the consistency of the part. Ultrasound scanning can give pictures of soft tissue, as well as bone, in detail. If done during pregnancy, it will print out a very accurate picture of the fetus in utero and can therefore be used as a non-invasive means of examining the fetus.

Why is it done?

Ultrasound is used in many areas of medicine as a diagnostic tool particularly to detect the cause of abdominal pain, such as gallstones or hiatus hernia. It can also be used to treat abnormalities. For example, high levels can destroy stones in the bladder. A gynecologist uses ultrasound to detect an ectopic pregnancy or an ovarian cyst. In pregnancy it is used to:

◆ Confirm the pregnancy and determine the age of the fetus by calculating the head circumference and the body measurements.
◆ Determine the estimated date of delivery.
◆ Measure growth and spot possible growth retardation on

AN IMAGE FROM SOUND WAVES

Ultrasound has proved to be an invaluable aid throughout pregnancy. It can help doctors assess the health and growth rate of the fetus and also make certain there are no problems which might hinder delivery.

leg   arm   head

Ultrasound uses sound waves to look within the body. Electric pulses are converted into vibrations that penetrate the body. These sound waves are reflected back and are converted into electric signals. These are processed by a computer to form a video image.

babies who are small for dates. If these scans are taken over a period of time, fetal growth can be accurately monitored.

◆ Find the exact position of the fetus and the placenta prior to an amniocentesis test.

◆ Locate the placenta and its condition in cases of placenta previa and placental insufficiency.

◆ Determine how many babies there are in the uterus.

◆ Pick up any visible malformations and abnormalities of the baby such as a defect of the brain or the kidneys.

◆ Monitor any intrauterine transfusions and surgical procedures.

◆ Identify any growths such as fibroids which might hinder delivery.

How is it done?

The procedure is painless and takes about ten to twenty minutes. You will need to undress from the waist down and to drink plenty of fluids so that your bladder is full and clearly visible on the ultrasonic scan.

Warm oil is poured over your stomach and a receiver, the transducer, is passed over it by the technician. The receiver passes back signals which show up on a black and white monitor.

It is very exciting to see a picture of your baby in the womb, though the shape may be quite difficult to discern. Ask the technician to point out the head, limbs and organs for you. You should be able to see the beating heart.

What are the risks?

There appear to be no risks to the unborn child or the mother. There is no evidence that it is completely safe either. It took 40 years to discover the harmful effects of X-rays. However, most centers have this equipment. Scans are only done during pregnancy if doctors think it advisable. If you are extremely worried about something, such as having twins, then your doctor would probably comply with your request for an ultrasound scan. Older women tend to be scanned more frequently.

SEE ALSO:

AMNIOCENTESIS
ECTOPIC PREGNANCY
FIBROIDS
GALLBLADDER DISEASE
MULTIPLE PREGNANCY
OVARIAN CYSTS
PLACENTA PREVIA
PREGNANCY PROBLEMS

URINARY PROBLEMS

Because of the female pelvic anatomy very few of us manage to escape urinary problems completely. Women have several more organs than men which have to fit in the pelvic space – the uterus, the cervix, the fallopian tubes, the ovaries and the vagina. Because of the proximity of other pelvic organs, the bladder tends to reflect the health of the pelvis and responds more sensitively to changes in the pelvis than does the male bladder. In addition, the female urethra is considerably shorter than the male one. This short distance from the skin of the perineum to the entrance to the bladder means that infecting organisms can quickly ascend and take root if there are predisposing factors. Under ordinary circumstances, however, bacteria do not ascend that readily. A good flow of urine maintained by drinking plenty of water and other fluids is the best safeguard.

Cystitis, inflammation of the bladder, is the most common female urinary complaint. Infections all along the urinary tract are quite common in pregnancy, during the climacteric (see *Menopausal problems*) and in the presence of a *prolapse*.

Frequency of urination is common in pregnancy and should not be confused with *incontinence*. Many women may suffer from a degree of incontinence for transient periods from their middle twenties onwards, particularly if they have borne children. The best way to combat this is to keep up the pelvic floor exercises.

Pyelonephritis

Probably the most serious urinary problem is pyelonephritis – a severe kidney infection. This usually starts as an infection in the bladder which ascends up the ureters. The symptoms are quite different from those of cystitis even though one may lead to the other. Pyelonephritis is nearly always accompanied by a high fever, nausea, vomiting and pain in the flanks, possibly radiating round to the front of the abdomen and into the groin. Pyelonephritis is a serious condition, requiring rigorous antibiotic treatment. Since it may arise from cystitis, it has a tendency to become chronic in women. This should be prevented by always completing the full dose of antibiotics and by treating recurrent symptoms promptly.

UTERINE CANCER

This rare cancer results from a malignant growth on the wall of the uterus, the endometrium. It is sometimes known as endometrial cancer. Sometimes, cervical cancer is mistakenly referred to as uterine cancer as the cervix is part of the uterus.

Pre-cancerous forms of the disease may exist for years before the condition becomes malignant. This cancer is more common in older women – less than 5% are under 40; in those who used DES during pregnancy (or whose mothers did), and those of the higher socio-economic groups.

There has been much controversy about the incidence of uterine cancer amongst women who take hormone therapy for menopausal symptoms. There is, however, still no evidence to show that estrogen therapy will result in this cancer developing.

WOMEN AT RISK

The women at risk from endometrial cancer are almost the reverse side of the coin to those who contract cervical cancer. The high risk group includes

 Overweight women especially those who are grossly overweight

With menstrual irregularities such as disturbed menstrual patterns, long intervals between periods, failure to ovulate, or women who have few or no pregnancies

 With affected relatives A family history predisposes you

 With pre-existing disease such as high blood pressure, diabetes, fibroids, estrogen-dependent tumors of the ovaries

 Older women 75% of patients are over 50

· S y m p t o m s ·

▲ Abnormal vaginal bleeding, between periods or after intercourse
▲ Heavy or prolonged periods
▲ Post-menopausal bleeding
▲ Cramping pain in the lower abdomen
▲ Pressure in the lower abdomen
▲ Frequency of urination due to pressure of the tumor on the bladder

---

Should I see the doctor?
If you have any change in your normal menstrual pattern or if you have any post-menopausal vaginal bleeding, consult your doctor immediately.

What will the doctor do?
If your doctor suspects some growth in your uterus, the only effective way to check whether there is any malignancy is to do a D & C. If the uterine lining has some cancerous cells, your doctor will recommend a total hysterectomy with removal of the ovaries and fallopian tubes as well as the uterus. This is nearly always combined with four to six weeks of radiation therapy.

If the growth is advanced, an extended total hysterectomy will be performed to remove the top of the vagina and the glands of the pelvis too.

What is the outlook?
The news is good. The overall cure rate is as high as 90% when the cancer is localized to the lining of the womb itself. If the spread is beyond the lining and the muscles of the uterus, the figure after five years is reduced to a 40% cure rate.

SEE ALSO

BLEEDING
CANCER
CERVICAL CANCER
DES
DIABETES MELLITUS
DILATATION AND
   CURETTAGE
FIBROIDS
HORMONE REPLACEMENT
   THERAPY
HYSTERECTOMY
MENSTRUAL PROBLEMS
RADIATION THERAPY
UTERINE PROBLEMS

UTERINE PROBLEMS

The uterus is a pear-shaped, muscular organ about the size of a small grapefruit and the site for the implantation of the fertilized ovum. To accommodate the growing baby during pregnancy, it increases its volume about 1000 times. Following *menopause*, it shrinks and eventually becomes very small.

The walls of the uterus are solid – about 90% muscle – and enclose a cavity, lined with endometrium, which undergoes changes during menstruation. One of the normal characteristics of uterine muscle is that it undergoes contractions all the time which are hardly felt. During *labor*, however, the upper half of the uterus, which is the most muscular part, contracts to push the baby out. The lower half of the uterus, which contains a strong, tight band of fibrous tissue, contains the neck or cervix.

The uterus normally lies at an angle of 90° to the vagina. In about 20% of women, however, it bends backwards – it is retroverted. Commonly known as a tipped uterus, this does not prevent conception and pregnancy; neither does it lead to back pain unless another condition, such as *pelvic inflammatory disease*, is present.

The most common symptom indicating a disorder of the uterus is a change in the normal menstrual pattern. The uterus usually refers pain, most commonly to the back. Severe cramping pain, particularly towards the end of the period, could be *endometriosis*. If you have an IUD and experience changes in your normal pattern, see your doctor as soon as possible; this could indicate infection of the uterus (see *Contraception*).

Pelvic examination and *Pap smears* pick up growths such as *ovarian cysts*, *fibroids* and *cervical cancer*. However, uterine tumors, because they are contained within the cavity of the uterus, are only detected in about 50% of cases. *Uterine cancer* is rare before the age of 40 but it has been found in the female children of women who took *DES*.

The uterus is the most likely organ to prolapse into the vaginal canal. If the prolapse is severe and the uterus protrudes from the vaginal entrance, surgical removal of the uterus may be be necessary.

VACUUM EXTRACTION

The name, vacuum extraction, conjures up a picture of what this is – an alternative method of assisted delivery to forceps.

Why is it done?
It is used if the mother has had a local or epidural anesthetic and there is some delay in the second or final stage of labor; in some cases, an epidural will limit the mother's ability to push. The baby should be presenting normally, that is head first, and the birth canal needs to be big enough to accommodate him or her easily.

How is it done?
A cup made of soft silicone rubber, which is connected to a vacuum apparatus, is passed into the vagina and applied to the baby's head. This may take about 15 minutes and can be applied before the cervix is fully dilated, unlike forceps. When the vacuum is created, the cup sticks to the baby's head and with very gentle pulling, and the mother pushing, the baby's head is brought into the birth canal and delivered gradually.

What are the risks?
There are few problems with this method of assisted birth. There may be a slight swelling on the baby's head where the cup was applied but this will settle down within a day or two after delivery. There is some disquiet about the use of vacuum extraction and forceps as soon as something goes wrong rather than allowing the delivery to progress normally but slowly. Originally U.S. doctors questioned the safety of vacuum extraction when metal, instead of silicone rubber cups were used in this procedure. High risks of scalp lacerations and hematomas were associated with the attachment of metal caps to the baby's head. As a result, vacuum extraction has not attained in the U.S. the popularity it enjoys in Europe.

PROCEDURE FOR A VACUUM EXTRACTION

Used most widely in Europe, vacuum extraction can be used when the cervix is not fully dilated, unlike forceps. It is employed when there is a delay in an otherwise easy delivery.

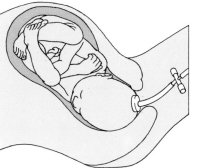

The small silicone rubber cup, connected to a vacuum apparatus, is passed into the vagina and applied to the baby's head.

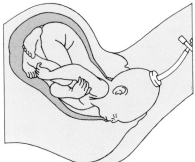

The cup sticks to the head when a vacuum is created. Gentle pulling, combined with the mother's pushes, brings the baby's head down the pelvis.

SEE ALSO:

EPIDURAL
FORCEPS DELIVERY
INDUCTION OF LABOR
LABOR

VAGINAL DISCHARGE

The vagina is kept clean and moist by the secretions of its lining. These change in character during the month due to hormonal factors. During the first half of the cycle, under the influence of estrogen, the mucus is thin, transparent and very elastic almost to the point of being runny. After ovulation, when progesterone is produced, the mucus changes character completely and becomes thick, opaque and jelly-like. By examining the discharge you can tell when ovulation takes place; the change in the cervical mucus, both to the naked eye and under a microscope (the fern test), is so marked that it is used as a test of ovulation.

During pregnancy the discharge is thick and white. The discharge increases with sexual excitement to lubricate the vagina for intercourse. Abnormal discharge is usually noticeable because there may be other symptoms such as an unpleasant smell.

In general terms, any other symptoms that accompany abnormal vaginal discharge, such as itchiness, bleeding or a rash should be investigated promptly.

If you are unable to make a diagnosis from this information, consult your doctor.

NATURE OF THE DISCHARGE	PROBABLE CAUSE
There is an increase in your normal secretions	You may be pregnant, or you have just started taking the contraceptive pill, or have recently had an IUD fitted. This is normal and nothing to worry about (see *Contraception*).
It is thick and white and your vulva is itchy	This could be *yeast infection*, a candida infection of the vagina. This is more common during pregnancy and if you are taking antibiotic medication for any reason.
The discharge is greenish/yellow and has an unpleasant smell	This could be *trichomoniasis*, a sexually transmitted disease, or perhaps you have forgotten to remove a tampon or your diaphragm and infection has resulted.
You have low back or abdominal pain and you feel sick	You could have an infection of the pelvic organs, such as the fallopian tubes (see *Pelvic inflammatory disease*).
You notice a slight discharge, and your sexual partner has sores on his genitals	This could be an infection of the cervix, possibly due to a *sexually transmitted disease* such as *gonorrhea*.
The discharge is brown, like blood, and usually follows intercourse	This is probably cervical erosion (see *Cervix problems*).
The discharge is spotted with blood, either mid-period or following intercourse	This could be a polyp on the cervix (see *Cervix problems*).

VAGINAL PROBLEMS

Vaginal problems are nearly always signified by a discharge which is different from usual. During child-bearing years, the vagina is kept clean and moist by a fluid which maintains a balance of bacteria in a weak acid environment. The fluid increases during inter-course, pregnancy and at the time of ovulation. This balance can be changed if you are under stress, diabetic, taking the contraceptive pill or antibiotic medication. In these circumstances, certain infections which may or may not be sexually transmitted can be picked up.

Urine and semen both being sterile present no threat to the vagina, but bowel movements do. A woman should always wipe her anus from front to back. Vaginal infections will not always be felt as there are few nerve endings in the vagina. It won't be until the infection reaches the vulva or you notice a discharge and there are symptoms such as burning when passing urine that you realize you have a problem.

Chronic forms of vaginal infection can in severe cases spread to the pelvic organs and lead to subfer-tility or even *infertility*. It is therefore vital that any vaginal infection is diagnosed promptly to prevent infertility and to exclude the possibility of sexually transmitted disease.

The most common vaginal infections are *yeast infection* or moniliasis, caused by the fungus candida albicans, and *trichomoniasis*, caused by the single-celled organism trichomonas. Occasionally the discharge may be the symptom of a *sexually transmitted disease*, such as *gonorrhea*, though unfortunately many STDs are symptomless in women.

Other problems relating to the vagina are usually sexual in their cause. The connection can be quite complicated, however. Many women feel a fear or disinclination for sexual intercourse and this can manifest itself by symptoms such as involuntarily closing the vagina to prevent penetration (*vaginismus*), and dryness of the vagina making penetration very painful (*vaginitis*).

VAGINISMUS

This is an involuntary spasm of the muscles around the entrance to the vagina causing the opening almost to close whenever an attempt is made to insert something into the vagina, such as a speculum, tampon or penis. The spasm can be so great that it prevents intercourse or means that penetration is extremely painful. A pelvic examination may have to be carried out under anesthesia.

Sexual drive and arousal are normal until penetration itself is attempted. The pelvic floor muscles then tighten up, virtually closing the vaginal entrance, and a sufferer will arch her back, and her legs will straighten and close together.

What is it caused by?

Vaginismus usually occurs in anxiety-prone individuals who have never been able to insert a tampon or a finger into the vagina because of the anticipation that this will be painful. In some women, a contributing factor may be underlying guilt or fear associated with the sexual act due to a restrictive upbringing or an inadequate sex education.

Vaginismus can occur also when a woman is in sexual disharmony with her partner. Disharmony is often the result of a partner liking the idea of something by which the other is repelled. There can also be difficulty if the role a woman wants to play with her partner – active or passive – is at odds with his likes and dislikes.

Vaginismus may also result after a shocking experience, such as rape.

· S y m p t o m s ·

▲ Involuntary closing of the vagina; the thighs often close tightly too

---

Should I see the doctor?

If you find you are unable to enjoy sex and you are unable to resolve it with your partner, see your doctor and talk it over so that you at least share your problem. Don't let this situation continue because it may cause disenchantment with the sex act altogether.

What will the doctor do?

Your doctor will first examine you to rule out the possibility of anatomical abnormalities that might be causing pain resulting in spasm.

Your doctor may then put you in touch with a sex therapist or marriage guidance clinic where counseling for this kind of problem is undertaken. You may also like to make contact with a self-help group.

Treatment for vaginismus usually involves the use of a series of graded dilators which the sufferer introduces into her vagina. Starting with the smallest size, she practices inserting and removing it and also learns to relax and tighten her vaginal muscles with the dilator in place. Over the course of a number of sessions, the size of the dilator is gradually increased until she is quite comfortable with the largest size – about that of the average erect penis.

Many women who experience vaginismus are not familiar with their sex organs. Some therapists work by helping you to familiarize yourself with your genitalia. By learning that the insertion of your own finger or a speculum is not painful, you may gain confidence about allowing penetration by your partner's penis.

What can I do?

Vaginismus is an uncommon result of sexual problems but be reassured, most problems don't stem from you or your inadequacy. You are not abnormal. You need to look at the problems in your sexual relationship and see where the disharmony lies and discuss it with your partner. The commonest problem is when you feel something is distasteful.

Perhaps you don't like any position other than the male lying on top. Perhaps oral sex, anal intercourse, too frequent lovemaking or different than "normal" upsets you.

The best thing is to talk about your likes and dislikes with your partner.

If he understands, you should both acknowledge that either of you is not abnormal for wanting it, or for not wanting it, and that it is not selfishness to refuse, though it is somewhat selfish to insist on something that either partner finds upsetting and distasteful.

SEE ALSO:

PAINFUL INTERCOURSE
PRURITIS VULVAE
RAPE
SEX THERAPY
SEXUAL PROBLEMS

VAGINITIS

With menopause, levels of the female hormone, estrogen, diminish in the blood. Estrogen is instrumental in stimulating the secretion of vaginal fluid which keeps the vaginal wall healthy and well lubricated. If the vaginal cells stop secreting this fluid, the walls of the vagina and the skin of the vulval area dry out. Known medically as atrophic vaginitis, this can lead to itchiness and pain with sexual intercourse. Infections are more easily picked up and if the itchiness becomes chronic, the skin will harden.

Other reasons for vaginitis which are not related to menopause are vaginal infections such as yeast infection or trichomoniasis and Sjögren's Syndrome (see box). Here I am concerned with vaginitis relating to menopause.

· S y m p t o m s ·

▲ Reduction of normal vaginal discharge
▲ Tingling, itching and scratching of the vulva
▲ Increased incidence of vaginal infections
▲ Painful intercourse (dyspareunia)

Should I see the doctor?

If, as menopause approaches, or when an artificial menopause has been induced by surgical removal of your ovaries, you notice dryness and scaling of the linings and the skin of the genitalia or pain during intercourse, see your doctor.

What will the doctor do?

Your doctor will question you about your medical history and give you an internal examination. If a drop in your circulating hormones is the likely cause of the problem, your doctor may first prescribe a hormonal cream to apply to the area. If this is not successful, he or she may prescribe hormone replacement therapy.

SJÖGREN'S SYNDROME

Certain autoimmune disorders such as rheumatoid arthritis and systemic lupus erythematosus can be accompanied by a condition in which the eyes, mouth and vagina become excessively dry. The exact cause is unknown but because the body's defense system is upset, it begins to destroy the glands that normally produce lubricating secretions.

Ninety percent of sufferers are women, mostly middle-aged and often post-menopausal. Therefore, it is essential that these more serious disorders are ruled out as the cause of vaginal dryness rather than it being assumed that it is a normal post-menopausal event.

What can I do?

There are commercial vaginal lubricants which will make intercourse less painful if your problem is a mild one. However, don't hesitate to seek medical help before your sexual relationships and family life suffer.

SEE ALSO:

HORMONE REPLACEMENT
  THERAPY
ITCHING
MENOPAUSE
PAINFUL INTERCOURSE
TRICHOMONIASIS
YEAST INFECTION

VARICOSE VEINS

Valves in the veins normally prevent the backflow of blood down the legs back into the feet. However, when these veins are damaged, usually by a past deep-vein thrombosis, the resulting back pressure causes the walls of the veins to balloon, become soft, thin and irregular. This is seen in the skin as soft, irregular swellings. The veins affected are nearly always those running down the backs of the legs and thighs. Sometimes women have varicose veins in the vulva, particularly during pregnancy when they are caused by the weight of the baby.

Pregnancy is often an exacerbating factor, partly due to the increased back pressure on the veins due to the enlarging uterus, but also because all blood vessels relax during pregnancy under the influence of the pregnancy hormones.

Hemorrhoids is another name for varicose veins of the anus. There is a tendency for varicose veins to run in families.

· S y m p t o m s ·

▲ Prominent varicosities mainly around the calves and lower thighs
▲ Tired aching legs after standing for a long time
▲ Swelling of the ankles
▲ Dermatitis on the inner side of the ankles where the circulation is most sluggish
▲ Swollen vulva

Should I see the doctor?

Even if you have very few varicose veins consult your doctor early about treatment as it's much easier to remedy mild varicose veins than severe ones.

What will the doctor do?

There are two main types of treatment for varicose veins and both require surgical intervention. A small number of superficial varicosities can be treated very successfully by injection with sclerosing agents. These substances cause the blood to clot, then shrink and then be completely reabsorbed. As this happens, the varicosities diminish in size, flatten out and the skin looks perfectly normal. There is no danger in this technique as the clot cannot move elsewhere in the body and there are plenty of alternative venous channels which open up to take the place of the old obstructed ones.

Stripping is a radical operation that takes quite a long time. It is performed under general anesthetic and you will have to be in the hospital. Prior to surgery, your surgeon will ascertain which of the veins are thrombosed and which need stripping. During surgery incisions are made at various points down the leg and burrs inserted as far as possible down the veins which are then pulled out through the incision. New venous channels open up to take the place of those veins which have been removed. These veins are, however, healthy and patent valves and varicosities should not recur.

After the operation, heavy supportive bandages are bound around the leg to help the incisions heal and prevent any swelling. While early mobilization after the operation is to be encouraged, it will take six to eight weeks before you can walk without discomfort so don't expect a too rapid return to normal.

You may find that wearing light support hose, even long after the operation, helps. If you notice any swelling of the ankles after the operation, consult your doctor as there is the possibility of developing varicose ulcers around the inner sides of the ankles if ankle swelling is not prevented.

Varicose ulcers are best prevented but should they occur they can be treated with drainage, the application of healing dressings and supportive bandaging.

What can I do?

◆ Wear support hose. These will have a two-fold effect; they will support the veins, prevent the varicosities becoming very big, and keep the venous pump going so that blood does not stagnate in the lower legs. They will also help to relieve aching and discomfort. Put them on first thing in the morning. They need not be thick and unsightly; there are some very fine modern hose and stockings available including fashion support hose.
◆ Avoid standing on your feet for long periods of time.
◆ Whenever you sit down try to put your feet on a stool and if you're stretched out, your feet are at the same level as your heart, when fluid can drain back naturally into the system.
◆ If you really want to give your feet a treat, lie flat on the floor and rest them against the wall.
◆ When the fluid has drained out of your feet, this is the time to put on support hose. They will help to prevent further collection of fluid in the feet and ankles.

SEE ALSO:

DEEP-VEIN THROMBOSIS
HEMORRHOIDS
PREGNANCY PROBLEMS

WARTS

Warts are small, benign lumps of skin made up of dead cells that protrude above the surface of the skin. They are less common in adults although as many as 1 in 20 school children have them. If you have children you are more at risk because the virus may infect several members of the same family.

What are they caused by?

They are caused by a common viral infection of the skin which can take many forms. The most common is the small, round, raised lesion with its rough, cauliflower-like surface. If warts appear on pressure sites, such as the soles of the feet, they will hardly raise above the surface of the skin and may be painful. These common warts are also known as verrucae. In moist areas of the body, around the anus and genitalia, for example, the tiny genital warts spread more easily and tend to be itchy. These are also known as venereal warts. Flat plane warts are more common in children.

It takes the body about two years to build up resistance to the wart virus, at which time the warts may disappear overnight. As they are spread by direct contact, they are most commonly found on the hands and feet or on the genitals where they are spread by sexual contact or from your own hands.

The virus may take a varied course. A single wart may appear and persist relatively unchanged for many years. Another single wart may be followed by the development of many satellite ones. Sometimes the mode of transmission is obvious; warts may develop on the lips if you bite the lesions on your hands, for example.

Should I see the doctor?

Even though warts are harmless and disappear on their own, if they appear on your genitals or on the soles of your feet or on your face, you should seek medical help. Recently an association between genital warts and the development of cancer of

---

· Symptoms ·

- ▲ Small, round raised lesions that appear spontaneously
- ▲ White or brown flat lump on the sole of the foot or underside of the toes
- ▲ Tiny, itchy lumps on the perineal skin, the labia or in the vagina

---

the cervix has been established. Cancer of the cervix is more common in women who suffer from genital warts than in the rest of the population. The role of the wart virus in causing cervical cancer is, however, not entirely clear.

For all other warts, see the self-help treatment below.

What will the doctor do?

There are many methods for treating warts, all of them successful if properly done. One of the principal problems is to avoid scarring which is worse than the wart itself.

For warts on the genitals, each wart is touched with podophyllin suspension. The surrounding skin is first protected, the solution applied and then left for a specified number of hours. The vulva should then be washed thoroughly with warm water. This treatment is repeated weekly until the warts disappear. The treatment is often quickly successful and after three or four applications the warts diminish in size and disappear. If the surrounding skin is affected, this may set up an allergic reaction, resulting in inflammation and soreness.

If warts on other parts of your body are proving to be recalcitrant or they are in your vagina, they can be burned out in a dermatology clinic with carbon dioxide snow, liquid nitrogen or electrocautery.

Verrucae are usually frozen, burnt off with strong nitric acid or scraped out with a curette after the area is first numbed with a local anesthetic.

What can I do?

Psychotherapy or placebo therapy should be the first line of treatment for warts on the hands, fingers or legs. This is because about one third of warts disappear after suggestion therapy, so it is worth a try, especially with children.

If you aren't prepared to wait for two years, try patent wart cures from your pharmacist. These work by the application on a daily basis of a weak acid solution, and gentle removal of the burnt skin. It is a laborious process and the surrounding healthy skin should be protected from the medication with vaseline or a corn plaster. Apply a dressing over the wart until the next treatment.

If you have a verruca, you should be meticulous about foot hygiene and take care in public swimming pools and gymnasia. Cover the verruca with a waterproof Band-aid or sock. Over-the-counter medications can often cure these successfully .

If the warts are on your fingers, don't nibble at the skin around your nails. If you are prone to do so, see your doctor to have them removed. You may pass them to your lips. Any shed skin from a wart spreads the infection.

If you have genital warts, avoid sexual contacts until they have been treated. If you have an outbreak of genital warts, be extra vigilant about having regular Pap smears.

SEE ALSO:

CERVICAL CANCER
GENITAL PROBLEMS
PAP SMEAR
SEXUALLY TRANSMITTED
 DISEASES

WRINKLES

Wrinkles come to us all and have two basic causes: the unavoidable force of gravity pulling the skin downwards, and a loss of elasticity in the skin. The latter is almost entirely due to exposure to sunlight.

There is, therefore, absolutely nothing anyone or anything can do to prevent aging of the skin and stop wrinkles from appearing.

What are they caused by?

Elastic tissue in the skin, collagen, loses its suppleness, bounce and rebound after years of exposure to ultraviolet light. This causes loss of plumpness and stretchiness of the skin and the formation of wrinkles. The next most important factor is heredity. The age at which wrinkles appear depends on the kind of skin you inherited from your parents. In our society, wrinkles are regarded as a sign of decline in the cult of youth and beauty. There has been a recent trend towards the return of age and experience, but women tend to suffer most at the hands of youthful advertisements and fashion magazines and so their self-images are constantly being eroded. The best thing to do is to see wrinkles as a badge of maturity, and don't give up but maintain good health and fitness.

What can I do?

The suppleness of your skin is dependent on its water content. The best you can do for your skin throughout your life is to moisturize it efficiently as often as you can – at least morning and night and much more often if you live in a hot climate or spend a lot of time in hot sunlight. If you don't want to encourage wrinkles, you should avoid suntanning yourself.

The effect of any moisturizer, no matter what the claims of its manufacturers, cannot last more than a few hours and must be reapplied. This is because moisture is constantly lost from the skin into the atmosphere. The drier the air, the faster the water is evaporated. This applies not only to a hot, windswept

MOISTURIZERS

Whatever moisturizer you prefer, don't imagine that the most expensive is the best. Whatever the claims by the manufacturers, there is no evidence to support the efficacy of hormone creams and skin foods to nourish the skin. Hormone creams (containing estrogen) do retain water in the skin, giving it a youthful puffy appearance, but they need to be applied daily to maintain this effect and as they can be absorbed by the body, there will be less desirable

beach, but to a stuffy heated room.

Makeup is another excellent barrier to water loss. If you are going out in the sun, wear makeup with a sun block in it or use a sunblock with a protection factor according to the strength of the sun. The sensible approach is to avoid strong sunlight. Wear a hat and sit in the shade.

When you cleanse your skin, avoid soaps and harsh cleansers as they de-fat the skin and encourage dryness.

It is possible to camouflage wrinkles with makeup if you wish to lessen their effect. Take a little color from a pale stick of a solid base with an eyeliner brush and paint a fine line in the crease formed by the wrinkle. Working from the top to the bottom, gently roll the brush inside the wrinkle to blend in the color. Set with powder.

What is the medical treatment?

Although they can't be avoided, wrinkles can be removed altogether – for as long as six to eight years. Cosmetic surgery, or face lift, can pull, tighten or nip the skin and iron out the wrinkles. The aging process continues inexorably, however, and the wrinkles do return.

Skin treatments such as dermabrasion and chemical skin peeling can make wrinkles and fine lines less obvious. The effect is transient and

side effects in the longterm.

There are two kinds of moisturizer you can use. One is a light, fluffy type of cream or lotion which disappears into your skin immediately. This keeps the skin moisturized for about 15 minutes, so obviously you will need regular applications.

Another type is heavier, oilier and encourages the natural sebum and prevents water loss. This lasts two hours or so.

usually doesn't last more than a year.

For any of these surgical methods, you will need to be referred to a qualified cosmetic surgeon for advice and treatment.

Recently, a drug, Retin-A, used in the treatment of acne, has been shown to be effective for wrinkles. It works by loosening the outer layers of skin thus speeding up the process of skin renewal. However, like all prescription drugs, it does have side effects, and more research will have to be done before it will be widely available.

SEE ALSO:

COSMETIC SURGERY
DERMABRASION
FACE LIFT
FACIAL TREATMENTS
SKIN PROBLEMS

YEAST INFECTION

This is a common infection caused by a fungus, *Candida albicans,* that normally lives along the digestive tract and is kept under control by other bacteria. If it appears in the mouth, most commonly in children, the elderly and those adults suffering from infection or who are on antibiotics, it is known as oral thrush. If you attempt to wipe it away, red sore patches are left. The presence of Candida albicans in the vagina causes a discharge and itchiness, and is referred to as a vaginal yeast infection.

For a yeast infection to infect a woman the conditions in her vagina need to be unbalanced so the fungus can thrive. Candida albicans prefers a mildly acidic balance and the vagina is usually too acidic. However, in some circumstances, the acid levels may be lowered. For example, vaginal deodorants and douches can destroy the natural bacteria that prevent the overgrowth of the fungus. A course of antibiotics also alters the natural balance and resistance is low after illness anyway. Diabetics are commonly affected as are women with altered hormonal levels (during pregnancy and pre-menstrually) and women who are on the contraceptive pill.

Should I see the doctor?
See your doctor immediately you notice the symptoms and refrain from sexual intercourse until you have received treatment. There is no self-help treatment that works for an established infection.

What will the doctor do?
Your doctor may take a swab of discharge to check that the initial diagnosis is accurate and that the treatment is appropriate. However, in most cases of yeast infection your doctor will prescribe antifungal vaginal suppositories and soothing ointment immediately to give you relief from the irritating symptoms. Treatment can take from three days to two weeks.

· S y m p t o m s ·

▲ Thick white curdy discharge with soreness and irritation of the vulva.
▲ The red rash can extend down to the thighs
▲ Creamy yellow or white patches inside the mouth that adhere to the mucous membrane
▲ Red rash around the anus and extending to the thighs
▲ Urine may burn or irritate the area
▲ Pain during sexual intercourse (dyspareunia)

What can I do?
Take the complete course of treatment and return to your doctor if the infection recurs. You may be reinfected by your partner during sexual intercourse so it is a wise precaution to apply the cream to his penis.

If possible, don't scratch because the fungus can be spread by hand. It may get under your nails and spread to your mouth or to your children. Any constant scratching can cause toughening of the skin.

Some women gain short-term relief with natural yogurt or gentian violet applied to the genital area. You can insert it on a tampon. Don't apply anything containing a local anesthetic. It may bring instant relief but it may cause a local allergy too.

Because the fungus likes warm, moist conditions, folds of fat around your groin may be a reason for recurrent infections. You may be able to reduce the incidence of these infections by taking off weight.

Always wipe your anus from the front to the back to prevent infection from stools entering your vagina.

Wear natural fibers – cotton or silk – next to your genital area. Avoid nylon panty hose and panties as they don't "breathe" and allow the fungus warm moist conditions for growth.

SEE ALSO:

GENITAL PROBLEMS
ITCHING
PAINFUL INTERCOURSE
PAINFUL URINATION
PRURITIS VULVAE
TRICHOMONIASIS
VAGINAL DISCHARGE

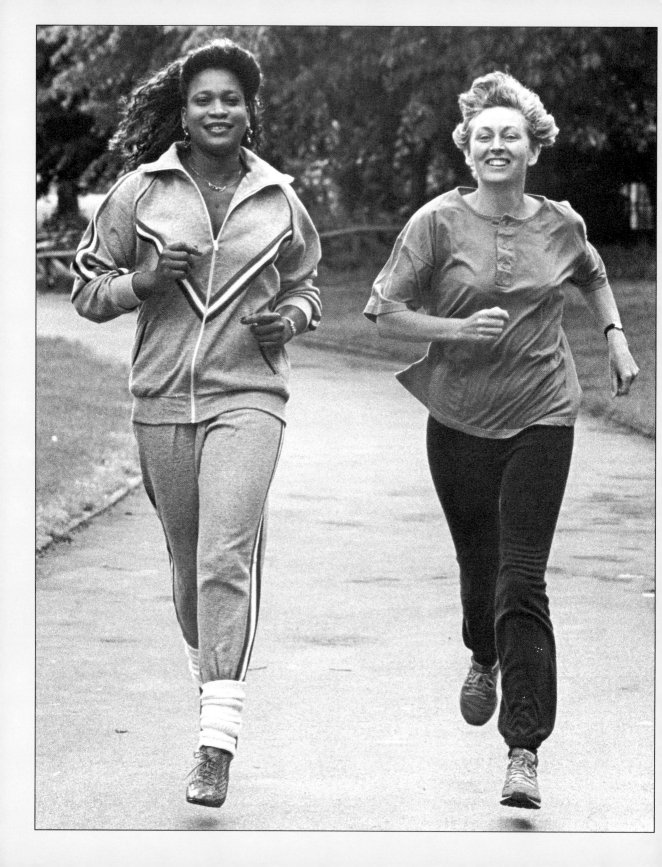

Women
and
Medicine

THE TREATMENT OF WOMEN

Quite a lot of what follows is critical of the medical profession, but I feel many medical practices involving women are less than fair and I think this needs saying – by a doctor, by a female doctor. I include myself in these criticisms. While as a patient, I have suffered at the hands of other doctors, as a practitioner, I was guilty of some of the following male-orientated prejudices passed on to me by my teachers.

Women as second-class patients
In the past, women have had a notoriously bad relationship with doctors. There is no question that male domination of the medical profession is at the root of women's dissatisfaction. For years, bona fide medical complaints such as pre-menstrual syndrome and dysmenorrhea were looked upon by male doctors as neurotic complaints. Many were described as "all in the head" or a woman's "natural inheritance" and therefore to be silently borne and not in need of proper medical attention. Women's complaints were not seen as deserving first-class attention and this sometimes led to women being seen as second-class patients.

Over the years, the medical profession has done women a great disservice. Women have been unjustly made to feel and think, in some instances, that they were neurotic and that their symptoms were not real. They were falsely given the idea that many of their symptoms were a fact of life, simply part of being a woman and therefore untreatable. This meant that women's expectations were extremely low and that for years they suffered treatable symptoms without complaint.

A decade or so ago, however, research showed that there was a real cause for conditions such as dysmenorrhea and pre-menstrual syndrome. Once this was known, researchers were able to come up with specific treatments which enjoy a high degree of success. Even so, a conservative medical profession was reluctant to adopt new remedies for the treatment of women's complaints. Women often met with reluctance, even a rebuff, when they tried to discuss these treatments with their doctors.

The advent of the women's movement and publicity given to new remedies for women's complaints has lead to a loosening up of the medical profession. It is nearly always possible these days to find a doctor in your area who will listen sympathetically to your complaints and give treatments a trial.

Some specific examples
In the treatment of breast cancer, doctors still adopt the radical approach. This usually means mastectomy instead of a simple lumpectomy plus radiation therapy to stop the spread of the cancer. Doctors appear to advise these radical disfiguring operations because they lack the courage to accept research information which shows clearly that in many early cases radiation therapy, lumpectomy or both have better results than mastectomy.

Postpartum depression has not, in the past, been treated as a real and serious illness. Doctors have failed to recognize that when baby blues extends beyond three weeks, this can be a serious mental disorder. Baby blues is not normal after three weeks; it needs radical treatment. If your doctor isn't alerted to the fact that the depression has gone on far too long, the consequences can be extremely serious. Many young women take their own lives during this period when they should be enjoying the pleasures of parenthood.

Menopausal symptoms such as hot flashes, night sweats, depression, irritability, tearfulness, loss of libido, lack of desire and pruritus vulvae have traditionally been given a low priority by doctors and there are still a few who think that women must grin and bear it. If your doctor takes this attitude, move to another one.

Every women has the right to have menopausal symptoms taken seriously and treated properly. It is also her right to be the beneficiary of effective treatment. Modern approaches, particularly with hormone replacement therapy (HRT), can bring relief of menopausal symptoms in something like 90% of women. Don't allow yourself to be fobbed off with tranquilizers and sleeping pills. Even a symptom such as depression can benefit from HRT, though a combination of hormones and anti-depressants may eventually be necessary.

I believe that every healthy woman should be given a four-month trial of HRT for her symptoms, so shop around until you find a sympathetic

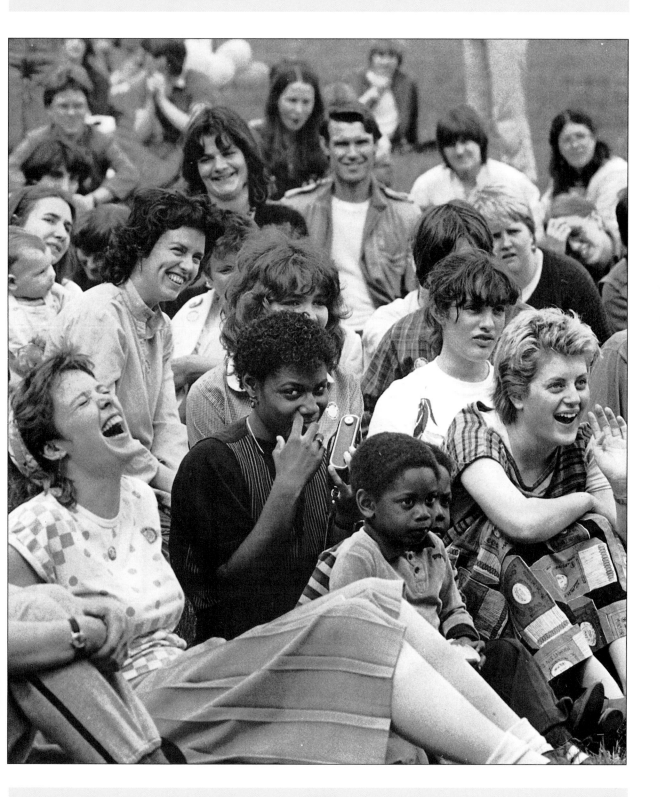

doctor or ask your doctor to refer you to a gynecologist who sees these symptoms more often and is up to date on the latest methods of treatment. The treatment will be with estrogen and progesterone supplements; the doses are much lower than those in the contraceptive pill.

In other areas of health concern, your doctor may show little interest in treating you. One such example is sexual problems. Find out about self-help groups or ask to be referred to a sex therapist. Psycho-sexual problems is an area where doctors should be particularly helpful. Inarticulate women should be encouraged to talk about their problems for which they may not realize there is a simple remedy. You may need to take your health into your own hands if you feel that you aren't being treated seriously or thoroughly enough.

Doctors' offices, with their long waits and speedy consultation, are not the sort of places where some unhappiness can be teased out of someone in need. This is perhaps a reason why tranquilizers are so heavily prescribed; they are seen by the harassed medical profession as an easy way to treat a patient who may only be suffering some personal or financial crisis.

If you are going to change your doctor because he or she is unsympathetic to your medical or health problems, make sure that you tell them so. Like any other person who performs a service for you, your doctor should have the opportunity to put things right if you are dissatisfied and to agree to a change if your differences are irreconcilable.

Women's groups

Since the sixties women have taken a much firmer role in matters relating to their health. Women's groups now exist to cover every aspect of women's lives, such as study groups, consciousness-raising groups and discussion groups on subjects like childcare, health and working.

Making the first step to go along to a women's group may be the most difficult if you feel nervous of what you may perceive as aggressive, confident women. This is in large part a myth, encouraged by the media. Women are of all kinds and backgrounds and the women you meet at a group may be in much the same situation as you find yourself and their comments may help you to

realize what you're feeling and thinking. You can pool your experience and use the group as a starting point to explore problems you face.

Many such groups have started up in response to intractable health matters as a means of support. Women who find themselves without a breast after mastectomy needn't feel isolated if they join a support group which can help them to return to normal life. They can then share their experience with those who come later on.

There are many self-help groups which uphold the interest of patients with women's complaints such as endometriosis, dysmenorrhea, menstrual problems, ectopic pregnancies etc. Self-help groups often become a life-line for some women because they realize that they are not alone and this can bring enormous comfort to women who felt isolated.

The National Health Information Clearinghouse (see *Health Directory*) should have a list of addresses and telephone numbers of women's self-help groups. You may also be able to get this information from your own doctor or from the local public health department or Chamber of Commerce. Your local hospital probably also has the same information. Don't forget that local Women's Health Centers and Planned Parenthood can also be a source of support and comfort and may be able to put you in touch with people who have similar complaints to yours. You will hear many success stories when you go along to self-help groups, but be prepared to hear about the odd failure and try and keep things in perspective.

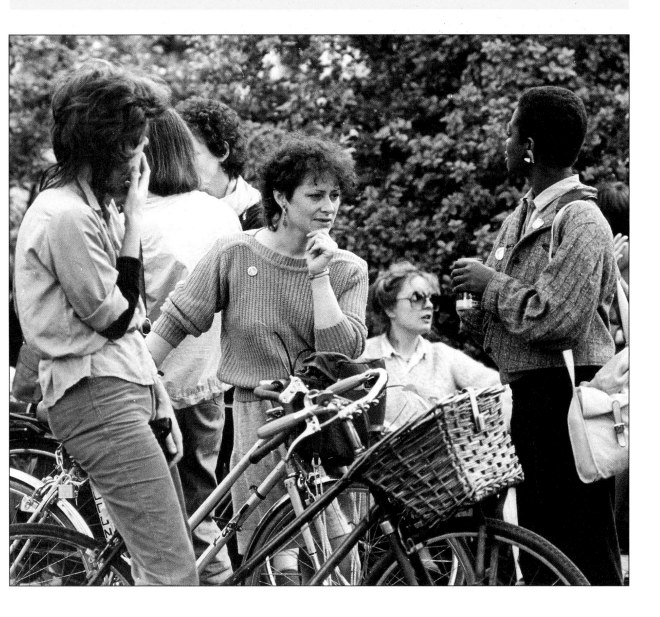

PREGNANCY AND CHILDBIRTH

It is only in the last decade or so that women have taken a more active line on their rights in childbirth. It is one of the most important experiences of our lives. Long before you become pregnant, give a little thought about your preferences for pregnancy, labor and childbirth. Read as many books as you can and find out exactly what your options are and then do a bit of research in your area to find out what kind of facilities are provided for pregnant mothers. Then, with as much flexibility as you can muster, select an option which matches as closely as possible your preference for prenatal treatment. The two important elements in your choice are whether you want a medically-managed or a natural childbirth and whether you want the birth at home or in a teaching or private hospital.

Home birth

Current medical opinion is almost totally opposed to out of hospital birth and many doctors are unwilling to act as birth attendants or to provide back-up for midwives at a home birth.

For women having a normal pregnancy and expecting a normal delivery, home confinement is ideal. Unfortunately many women who could successfully have their babies at home, don't do so because they feel the negative pressure from their general practitioners, consultants and some hospital midwives.

Most pregnant women are healthy, and should be treated as such; pregnancy is not a disease. If everything is going well there should be no reason why you can't have your baby at home with a midwife in attendance. The "but if" argument doesn't stand up because hospital births with their high technology and overworked staff can just as easily result in mistakes. At one time research showed that hospital deliveries were safer, but that women who delivered at home were much happier. It has now been proven that it is just as safe to have your baby at home, providing you are well and there are no reasons for concern.

Birth centers

Special birth centers aim to provide a compromise between a hospital and a home birth. Centers provide a home-like environment and allow family and friends to share in the labor experiences.

Mother, baby and family are not separated during the 12 to 24 hours after birth that they spend in the center. Centers are designed to handle normal, uncomplicated pregnancies and births but are equipped to handle most emergencies other than Caesarean section. During labor, provisions can be made to transfer the mother to a hospital should complications arise. Birth centers are only available in some areas.

There are a number of alternative methods of giving birth naturally which have gained recognition and popularity. One is based on the philosophy of Dr Frederick Leboyer. Many centers offer a Leboyer-based birth with the central elements of darkened room, immersion in water and minimum stimulus for the baby.

Dr Michel Odent is an obstetrician who has established at his clinic in France an environment where the woman giving birth is able to return to a more primitive biological state. This reduces the need for pain relief and other interventions such as episiotomies and forceps. Women are encouraged to give birth in a squatting position with support from their partners or the staff. There is a warm bath, cushions and dim lighting.

Hospitals

Your medical care in the labor ward of a hospital will be the responsibility of the resident doctors on duty. Most of your care is by nursing staff, both trained and student. For a first baby it is assumed that you will stay in hospital for between three to five days.

Some hospitals may be teaching hospitals in which case you must be prepared for much of your prenatal care to come from strangers who you never see more than once. On academic obstetric units care is provided for those women who have a condition that could cause complications during pregnancy and birth or where tests have shown a possible problem with the baby. This is where the most modern medical and technological interventions and procedures are practiced. If yours is a normal pregnancy and labor, you may be disappointed by the level of technology.

The revolution in childbirth in the last two decades has meant greater control over problems in labor. All these medical interventions offer

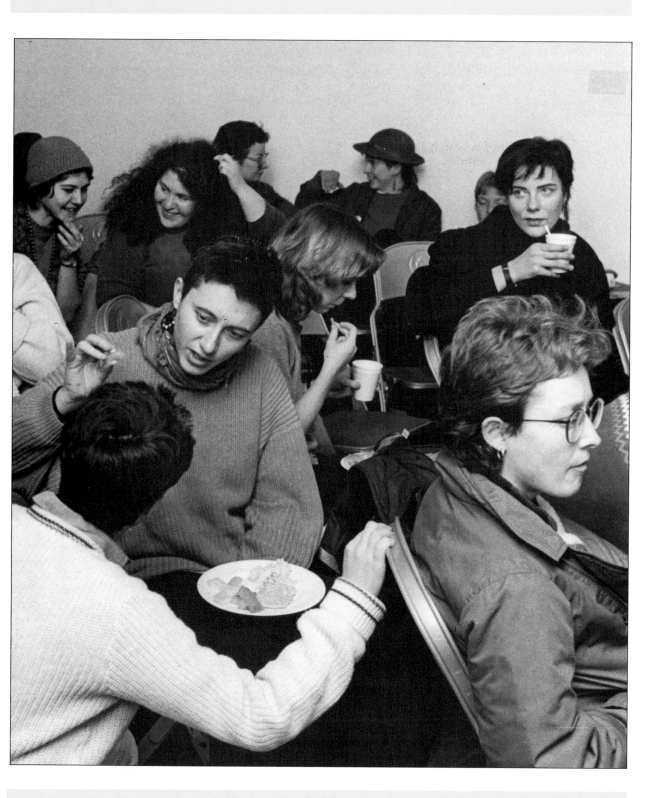

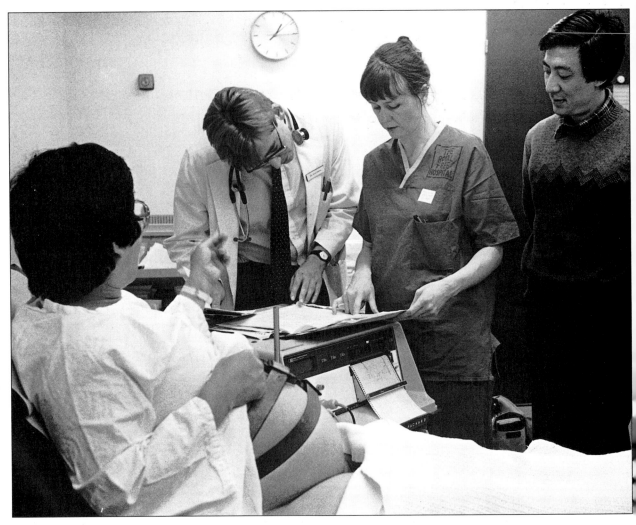

advantages, with only a few risks. None of them should be used unless there is a good medical reason for doing so. For example, induction should never be seen as a convenience. If you are advised to accept something you're not sure about, make sure in your own mind that the arguments are for the baby's well being and not yours or the hospital staff.

If you know you are having a hospital delivery, you can do something to make it what you hope for. Ask questions at your prenatal clinic and make sure your preferences are noted on the records. For example, you may want to avoid having an enema, or being shaved prior to delivery. You may want to try to deliver the baby without an episiotomy if possible. Many hospitals cut your perineum routinely with a first baby.

If you want to walk about during the first stage, make sure that any fetal monitoring is the sort that is strapped to your thigh and not around your abdomen. Refusing monitoring in labor is one of the most difficult arguments you can have with medical staff. So often it means the difference between lying down throughout your labor or walking about and speeding up the process, not to mention the variety of different positions you can find to ease the pain of the contractions.

If you have a supportive partner or friend who

will be with you at the birth, they may be able to negotiate on your behalf. It is important that you know what you want, that you convey this to the hospital staff in a pleasant way and that you know enough about what is happening to you to accept intervention if it is advised.

There are many questions you should put to the hospital staff to find out more about what to expect during your labor and delivery. Some examples are: Can my partner stay with me if I have to have a Caesarean section? Can I hold the baby immediately after the birth? May I walk around during labor if everything is okay? Do I have to be shaved and given an enema? What percentage of women does this hospital induce? Can the baby stay with me all the time? Will my partner be allowed to help with bathing and changing?

Reasons for a hospital delivery

Whatever your feelings, if there are good reasons for a monitored hospital delivery, you should take your doctor's advice and be admitted to hospital for your own and the baby's sake.
Medical background: If you suffer from heart or kidney disease, diabetes mellitus, anemia, epilepsy, obesity or you have high blood pressure.
Previous record: If other deliveries have included a stillbirth, premature labor, problems with the placenta, or difficult lie (breech, transverse).
Obstetric reasons: If you are carrying twins, suffering from toxemia of pregnancy, Rhesus incompatibility, the baby is too big to pass through your pelvis (disproportion), the baby is overdue, you are an elderly primigravida, or the placenta is lying in the lower part of the uterus (placenta previa).

Termination of pregnancy

Abortion is a legally established right up to the 12th week. A woman may choose whether she wants to have a baby or not. There are fairly regular efforts by anti-abortion groups to repeal these laws that protect women and the people who help with abortions. Any restriction on the laws only serves to establish what went before when wealthier women could pay, and those most in economic and social need were forced to the back street abortionists with the inherent legal and physical risks.

If you are contemplating having an abortion, you should immediately consult either your family physician or your local family planning clinic. They will help you come to terms with making a decision and suggest the proper procedure should you decide to carry through with an abortion. While you certainly must not rush your decision, you do not want to delay too much. The further on you are in pregnancy, the greater the risk and the more reluctant doctors are to perform an abortion. After about 16 weeks, you will need to have an amniocentesis abortion which is like a normal labor.

YOU AND YOUR DOCTOR

Every woman and her family have individual needs. If you have young children, for instance, you will want a doctor who takes an interest in pediatrics as well as in women's diseases. It may be that you would prefer to see a woman doctor and your immediate area may not have one. My advice would be to shop around, contact the National Health Information Clearinghouse (see *Health Directory*) or contact your local Chamber of Commerce for a list of all the practices within a suitable radius of your home and find out something about each one. This is not always easy and you may have to collect information from neighbors and friends. Local people and shops may be able to give you helpful tips.

You may feel that you want to go along and see one of the doctor's offices to give you some idea of what the practice's special interests are and whether they coincide with your own. There is absolutely no reason why you should not ask to schedule an appointment and "interview" your prospective doctors. Try and find a doctor with whom you have immediate rapport. If you feel the relationship is strained on the first meeting, imagine how strained it may become if a crisis occurs and you need to agree.

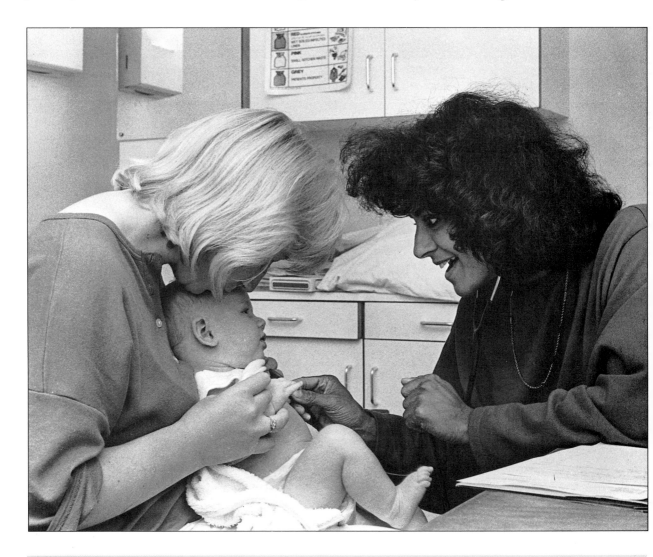

Prescription drugs

If you object to taking drugs or a particular form of treatment, ask your doctor what alternatives are available. The onus may be on you to suggest forms of alternative medicine such as homeopathy or naturopathy. Unfortunately, few doctors will be entirely happy to recommend a form of alternative medicine but it is your right to try it and if you intend to, make sure that your doctor is aware of this. The next time you go to see your doctor you should mention what kind of medicine was prescribed for you by the alternative practitioner.

Whenever you are given drugs ask your doctor to list side-effects, and if you should refrain from taking any special foods, medicines or alcohol with the drugs. Be clear before you leave the office about how often the drugs should be taken, and whether on a full stomach or before meals.

How to handle your doctor

With a sick child under two years old alert your doctor if you are worried. Do not wait until an emergency.

Do not consult another doctor without telling your own doctor first. This is not just professional courtesy, it is in your own interests because your own doctor may have medical information that a second doctor would wish to have while assessing your case.

Some women find it difficult to discuss female complaints with a man. In this instance the initiative lies with women. Male doctors are never embarrassed by such conversations but will appreciate a woman's reticence. You'll be avoiding your responsibility if you're not honest with your doctor so do not lose your nerve and mislead with a minor or fictitious complaint.

Do not be over-fussy about yourself or your family. It is not the best way to gain co-operation from anyone and you may cry wolf once too often.

Ask your doctor for information about yourself, your illness and your treatment. Your questions will almost certainly be welcomed. As a bright-eyed junior doctor, most willing to fulfil a patient's right to have things explained, I quickly became disillusioned with the small number who reciprocated my interest.

Do not always expect a prescription from your doctor. Not all complaints need medicine and quite often medical advice is sufficient.

Do not expect your doctor to be infallible. Your doctor is human and your expectations should be realistic, not only in terms of their fallibility but also their pre-occupations and moods.

Changing your doctor

If you find that you have an unsatisfactory relationship with your doctor there is no reason why you should stay with him. You can move on to another but be sure to talk things over with your doctor before you move. Give your doctor a chance to improve matters, don't leave secretly or in a huff. If you do, you could be doing other patients who feel the same as you a disservice. When you go to a new doctor, you must say which practice you have left and you should be prepared to give your reasons for leaving that practice. Don't try to make these changes furtively; word quickly gets about between doctors and you may find yourself with a bad name for no reason.

PATIENT'S RIGHTS

Every patient has the right to:
- be listened to
- a sympathetic hearing
- participation in decisions which affect her health
- an equal relationship with her doctor
- a full discussion of treatments, instructions and side-effects
- a second opinion
- change her doctor
- refuse treatment if her concerns cannot be allayed
- take advantage of alternative medical practice as well as mainstream medical practice
- see a specialist
- have the most modern treatments available
- be informed about potentially fatal conditions such as cancer – if she wants to be.

RESPONSIBILITY FOR YOURSELF

You should go into your doctor/patient relationship thinking of yourself as an equal. This is not always easy as doctors can be intimidating figures. To bolster your confidence, ask your partner or an assertive friend to go with you. If you feel an equal to your doctor you will find it easier to face up to difficult situations, to discuss them openly and find mutually acceptable solutions. You may for instance be prescribed drugs which you would prefer not to take; you may find that you lose confidence in your doctor's diagnosis and would like a second opinion; you may feel that your doctor is fobbing you off without getting to the root cause of your problem. All of these situations require frank, candid discussions on your part and you should do this.

Before you go to see the doctor, go over in your mind what your dissatisfactions are, list your questions and decide what you'd like to get out of the discussion. If necessary write everything down on a piece of paper and don't leave the doctor's office until a solution has been agreed.

It's understandable that a doctor may view the request for a second opinion or for alternative treatment as a criticism of his or her ability. Try and be a little sympathetic to this professional pride by approaching the subject frankly and diplomatically. If you express your concerns honestly, most doctors will be more than happy to reassure you by arranging an appointment with another doctor, perhaps a partner. If your doctor will not do this, it's probable that your relationship is not a good one and you'd both welcome a change anyway.

If you express your wish to see a specialist in a way such as I've just described, you'll probably find that your doctor is co-operative. If you go to see a specialist without telling your doctor then that in itself suggests that you and your doctor are not getting on too well and you should consider terminating your association.

With greater awareness in the community at large about the significance of health education and the removal of barriers to open discussion about emotive health concerns such as drug dependence, abortion and sexually transmitted diseases, you need to keep yourself informed about the latest research and changes in treatment.

Television, magazines and newspapers regularly join in the debate. Don't worry about mentioning something you've heard to your doctor; effective treatment should involve a dialogue between you.

A positive approach

Your health lies in your hands; you are the guardian of your health and you should call in doctors only when you need medical advice and medical services. The maintenance of body health and fitness is your responsibility so you should make sure that you observe your body, read and respond to its messages. Where you can, examine your body yourself as a health check, for example monthly breast self-examination. You should take advantage of regular health checks such as dental and ophthalmic; even pay visits to the podiatrist.

Whenever you have any consultation about your health, it is important that you let the medical practitioner know about your previous medical history and that of your family. You should also tell the doctor or dentist about any drugs you are taking, and that includes the contraceptive pill and hayfever treatments.

Specific medical check-ups like mammography and Pap smears should be written into your calendar well ahead of schedule so that none of them goes unheeded. Your health is important for yourself, and for many women it's important for their children and their families. You have a dual responsibility to yourself and them to make sure that you do everything within your power to maintain health and fitness.

Recently I had a check-up and I was relieved to find all aspects of it clear and that I had as healthy a body as the tests could reveal. What surprised me was the psychological benefit of a clean bill of health and feeling a sense of self worth and that my body was worth taking care of, at 50.

Your body is worth taking care of, be proud of it, keep it in the best condition that you can, pay attention to a balanced diet and make sure that your lifestyle includes some exercise. If necessary, change your lifestyle to accommodate these essential aspects of health and fitness. You may have to give yourself a higher priority. Forget what you ought to do; do what you have to do.

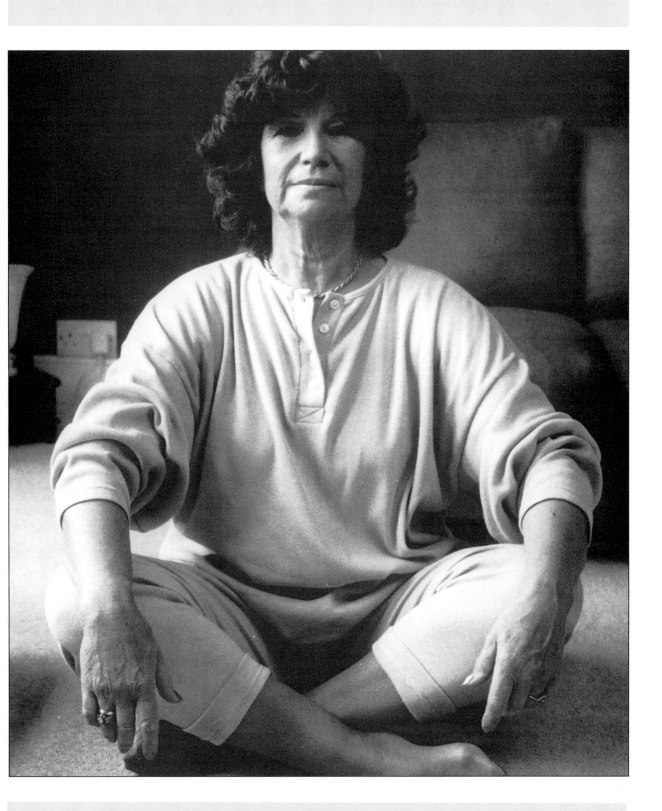

MEDICAL CHECKS

CHECK AND PURPOSE	OCCASION AND FREQUENCY	WHERE TO GO
Blood pressure A check on the state of the heart and arteries.	Annual checks if you are on the pill; if you have a family history of hypertension, heart or kidney disease, diabetes mellitus, if you are overweight. Regular checks during pregnancy.	Your doctor, family planning clinic.
Pelvic examination A check on the pelvic floor, perineum and pelvic organs.	Before you start any new contraceptive; if you are pregnant or have a pelvic inflammation. If you have menstrual problems or a persistent complaint of the pelvis, vagina or perineum; if your mother took DES while carrying you.	Your doctor or gynecologist. Further tests might then be indicated.
Pap smear To detect pre-malignant changes in the cervix.	From the age of 18 onwards, or as soon as you are on the pill or sexually active, have this check every 2 to 3 years. If you have intermenstrual bleeding, irregular periods, or a positive family history of risk factors follow with Pap smears as your doctor recommends.	Your doctor, a gynecologist, or a family planning clinic. Further tests may be indicated.
Vaginal smear To detect pre-malignant changes or infections in the vaginal cells.	From the age of 30 onwards you should have this test annually and if your mother took DES while carrying you, or if you have a positive family history.	Your doctor or gynecologist.
Mammography To detect small breast lumps that cannot be felt by self-examination.	A baseline mammogram is recommended between the ages of 35 and 40. Between ages 40 and 50, mammograms should be requested according to the advice of your physician. After age 50, mammogram should be done annually.	You will be referred by your doctor to a mammography unit.
Eye tests To detect defects in vision and glaucoma.	Annually from the age of 40 onwards, or if you have symptoms earlier. If you have pain in the eye and it is red.	Your doctor, ophthalmologist, optometrist or optician.
Dental check ups To check on teeth and gums, detect caries, scale and polish, fill cavities and correct alignment.	Every six months and if you are pregnant, if you have a rare dental disorder such as soft teeth.	Your dentist or dental hygienist.
Chest X-ray To detect recent or current disease of the lungs.	Annually from the age of 40 onwards if you smoke, if you have chest pains, blood in your sputum, work in a dusty environment. Discuss frequency with your doctor.	Go to your doctor for an X-ray or for referral to a clinic or hospital.

DRUGS LISTING

Many of the drugs in common use 20 years ago have been superseded by newer, safer compounds with broader applications. In the past, many drugs were known by their commercial names. These days the generic name is more commonly used. Where Valium was once an almost universal name for a minor tranquilizer, these drugs are now prescribed by their generic names.

I have included in this index the major groups of drugs, their uses and possible side-effects. It is a selective list and should not be used as a manual of self-prescription for you or your family. Some groups are large and use very different methods to achieve the same result. For example, many drugs have an antihypertensive effect such as diuretics, beta blockers and vasodilators. Ask your doctor how the prescribed drug works for you.

Over-the-counter medicines

There are many commercial products available at pharmacies. They come in pills, capsules, liquids, drops, sprays, creams, ointments and inhalers. These seldom have a direct effect on the cause of a condition but they may relieve painful or uncomfortable symptoms. For instance, some of the remedies for coughs and colds are soothing, and mild analgesics such as aspirin and acetaminophen relieve pain.

However, in most cases, the speed of your recovery depends more on your age and general health than on any such treatment. Nevertheless, if such "cures" make you feel better, they are unlikely to be harmful if you follow the instructions on the container. In some cases your doctor may actually recommend a commercial preparation. If you are unsure about any aspect of an over-the-counter medication, consult your pharmacist or doctor.

Drugs in pregnancy

During pregnancy it is important to avoid any substances that could put the development of the fetus at risk. Most drugs pass from the mother's circulation to the fetus. While some are known to be harmless, there are others that can, in certain instances and at certain times during pregnancy, threaten the health of the fetus, Therefore, if you are pregnant or are contemplating pregnancy, you

GUIDELINES
When taking any medicine you should ensure the drug's effectiveness and safe use.

◆ Never exceed the stated dosage.
◆ Always check with your doctor or pharmacist if you are unsure when or how frequently the medicine should be taken (for example, some drugs work most efficiently when taken with a meal).
◆ Check with your doctor whether it is advisable to abstain from drinking alcohol while taking your medication. The effects of some drugs may be altered by alcohol.
◆ Even if you think it unnecessary and you feel better and have no more symptoms, complete the prescribed course of medicine. Failure to complete a course of antibiotics may prevent complete recovery.
◆ Keep all drugs locked in a medicine cabinet.
◆ Some drugs affect your co-ordination and you may be advised not to operate potentially dangerous machinery or drive a car.
◆ In general, the fewer drugs you take, the better. Except for minor symptoms such as occasional cough or headache, discuss with your doctor all the medicines you could need. You and your doctor can balance the potential benefits of medicine against the side effects.

will need to ask your doctor for advice before taking any drugs, including those available over the counter. If you suffer from a chronic condition for which you are receiving medication, your doctor will advise you on the best treatment while you are pregnant. Both alcohol and smoking are known to have harmful effects on the developing fetus. It is common practice during pregnancy to be prescribed iron tablets and vitamin supplements to prevent anemia. These will be supplied to you at your prenatal clinics.

Drugs and breastfeeding

You should only take drugs while breastfeeding on the advice of your doctor. Some drugs can pass into the breast milk in insignificant quantities and others are known to be safe. If you need to take those that present a risk to the baby, you can switch to bottlefeeding while you take the drugs. If you want to resume breastfeeding later, you will need to express and discard your milk to maintain the supply.

DRUGS LISTING

ANALGESICS

For the relief of pain; many also reduce inflammation and fever. There are 3 main types: simple analgesics – usually containing aspirin or acetaminophen – for mild pain; nonsteroidal anti-inflammatory drugs, often given for muscular aches and pains, rheumatoid arthritis, osteoarthritis and gout; narcotic analgesics – usually chemically related to morphine – for severe pain, especially in terminal illness.
Possible side-effects: Nausea, constipation, dizziness, dependence and development of tolerance to the drug (narcotic analgesics only).

ANTACIDS

Neutralize stomach acid, relieving heartburn and similar conditions. They contain simple chemicals such as sodium bicarbonate, calcium carbonate, aluminum hydroxide and/or magnesium trisilicate.
Possible side-effects: Belching (sodium bicarbonate preparations), constipation (aluminum or calcium preparations) and diarrhea (magnesium preparations).
Warning: Seek medical advice if you are taking other drugs. Antacids should not be taken by anyone with a kidney disorder without medical advice.

ANTI-ANXIETY DRUGS

Sometimes called anxiolytics, sedatives or minor tranquilizers. They reduce feelings of anxiety and relax muscles. May also be used as sleeping drugs and to relieve symptoms of premenstrual syndrome.
Possible side-effects: Drowsiness, dizziness, confusion, unsteadiness and lack of coordination.
Warning: They can be habit-forming and should not be used for more than a few weeks. After prolonged use, withdrawal symptoms may occur if treatment is halted abruptly.

ANTI-ARRHYTHMICS

Control irregularities of the heartbeat. Oldest examples are digitalis and quinidine – both extracted from plants.

ANTIBIOTICS

Substances often derived from living organisms, such as molds or bacteria, that kill or inhibit the growth of bacteria in the body. Some of the newer antibiotics are synthetic versions of naturally occurring substances. Any one type of antibiotic is effective only against certain strains of bacteria, although some antibiotics combat a wide range of bacterial infections. These are called broad-spectrum antibiotics.

Sometimes a strain of bacteria becomes resistant to a particular antibiotic and an alternative is chosen on the basis of laboratory tests. Antibiotics are not effective against viruses.
Possible side-effects: Nausea, vomiting and diarrhea. Some people may be allergic to certain antibiotics and may experience symptoms such as rashes, fever, joint pain, swelling and wheezing. Following treatment with broad-spectrum antibiotics, secondary fungal infection (yeast infection) – for example of the mouth or vagina – may sometimes occur.
Warning: Always complete a prescribed course of antibiotics. Failure to do so, even when symptoms have cleared, may lead to a recurrence of the infection and it will be more difficult to treat due to resistance of the bacteria to the antibiotic.

ANTICOAGULANTS AND THROMBOLYTICS

Anticoagulants prevent blood from clotting and thrombolytics dissolve and disperse blood clots.
Possible side-effects: Increased tendency to bleed from the nose or gums or under the skin (bruising). Blood may also appear in the urine or stools.
Warning: Anticoagulants may react with other drugs, including aspirin. Consult your doctor before taking any other medicine so that the effectiveness of the anticoagulant is not altered. If you are on regular anticoagulant treatment, you will be advised to carry a warning card.

ANTICONVULSANTS

Used to prevent and treat epileptic seizures. These are usually given at least twice a day. Careful calculation of the best dose for the individual is necessary to minimize side-effects. Blood or saliva tests are usually given to monitor drug concentrations in the blood. The drug is given over a prolonged period until the person has gone 2 to 4 years without a seizure.
Possible side-effects: Drowsiness, rashes, dizziness, headache, nausea and thickening of the gums. Abrupt withdrawal of treatment may result in a convulsion.

ANTIDEPRESSANTS

Drugs that counter depression. These fall into two main groups: tricyclics and their derivatives, and monoamine oxidase inhibitors (MAO inhibitors). Because their side effects are likely to be more serious, MAO inhibitors are usually only prescribed for those types of severe depression that are less likely to respond to treatment with tricyclics. The effects of all antidepressants can take up to 4 weeks to be felt.
Possible side-effects: Drowsiness, dry mouth, blurred vision, constipation, difficulty urinating, faintness, sweating, trembling, rashes, palpitations and headaches.
Warning: MAO inhibitors react adversely at once with a number of foods and drugs, possibly leading to a serious rise in blood pressure. Your doctor will advise you and may recommend that you carry a warning card.

ANTIDIARRHEALS

For the control and treatment of diarrhea. There are two main types – those that absorb excess water and toxins in the bowel (kaolin, chalk or charcoal mixtures) and those that reduce the contractions of the bowel, thus decreasing the frequency with which stools are passed (codeine, morphine and opium mixtures).
Possible side-effects: Constipation if taken for prolonged periods.

Warning: Antidiarrheals do not treat the underlying cause of diarrhea. They should not be taken for more than a day or so before seeking medical advice. When treating diarrhea, always drink plenty of fluids.

ANTI-EMETICS

Used to suppress nausea and vomiting. The main groups of drugs in this category include certain antihistamines (especially for nausea caused by motion sickness or by ear disorders) and certain tranquilizers. Such drugs are not usually prescribed when the cause of vomiting is unknown, when vomiting is unlikely to persist for longer than a day or so, as in gastroenteritis. They are useful for nausea caused by drug or radiation treatment. Anti-emetics are prescribed in pregnancy only when symptoms are severe.
Possible side-effects: These vary according to the drug group prescribed – antihistamines cause drowsiness. Prolonged treatment with certain tranquilizers may cause involuntary movement of the facial muscles. These drugs are not usually taken for more than a few days at a time.

ANTIFUNGALS

Treat fungal infections such as ringworm, athlete's foot and yeast infections. They may be applied directly to the skin or vagina in the form of suppositories and a cream, or administered orally over a prolonged period.
Possible side-effects: Oral antifungals may cause nausea, vomiting, diarrhea and/or headaches; locally applied (topical) preparations may cause irritation.
Warning: Always finish a course of antifungal treatment as prescribed; the infection may recur. Some infections, especially of the nails, may require treatment with oral antifungals for many months.

ANTIHISTAMINES

Counteract allergic symptoms produced by the release of a substance called histamine in the body. Such symptoms may include runny nose and watering eyes (allergic rhinitis), itching and urticaria (hives). Antihistamines may be given orally or applied to skin rashes in the form of creams or sprays. Antihistamine drugs also act on the organs of balance in the middle ear and therefore are often used to prevent motion sickness. Their sedative effect may be prescribed to treat sleeplessness. They are also given as a premedication to induce a relaxed, drowsy state prior to going into the operating room. Another class of antihistamine interferes with gastric acid secretion and is used to treat peptic ulcers.
Possible side-effects: Drowsiness, dry mouth and blurred vision.

ANTI-INFLAMMATORIES

To reduce inflammation. This is the redness, heat, swelling, pain and increased blood flow that is found in infections and in many chronic non-infective diseases such as rheumatoid arthritis and gout. Three main types of drugs are used: aspirin and related drugs, corticosteroids and non-steroidal anti-inflammatory drugs such as indomethacin (Indocin) which is used especially in the treatment of arthritis and muscle disorders.
Possible side-effects: These depend on the type of drug. Non-steroidal drugs have fewer side-effects. Rashes and stomach irritation and occasionally bleeding, disturbances in hearing and wheezing.

ANTIPSYCHOTICS

Sometimes called major tranquilizers, these are used to treat severe psychiatric disorders.
Possible side-effects: Jaundice, tremor, abnormal face and body movements, low temperature.

ANTIPYRETICS

To reduce fever and pain. The most commonly used are aspirin and acetaminophen, which are both analgesics. This double action makes them particularly effective for relieving the symptoms of an illness such as flu.

Possible side-effects: Rashes and stomach irritation and occasionally bleeding, disturbances in hearing, and wheezing.

ANTISPASMODICS

Reduction of spasm of the bowel in conditions such as irritable colon or diverticular disease.
Possible side-effects: Dry mouth, palpitations, difficulty urinating, constipation and blurred vision.

ANTIVIRALS

Effective drug treatment is not yet available to combat the majority of viral infections such as cold and flu. However, severe cold sores caused by the herpes simplex virus can be treated by the application of idoxuridine ointment – also used to treat shingles – to the skin as soon as symptoms appear. Another antiviral drug, acyclovir, may be given orally or by injection or applied directly to the skin in the form of a cream to treat most severe types of herpes infection. Research continues into effective treatment for AIDS. Zidovudine may prolong life in some cases.
Possible side-effects: Antivirals used to treat cold sores, herpes genitalis and shingles may cause a stinging sensation, rashes and occasionally loss of sensation in the skin.

BETA-ADRENERGIC BLOCKING AGENTS

Beta-blockers for short, reduce oxygen needs of the heart by reducing heartbeat rate. They are used as antihypertensives and antiarrhythmics, for treating angina due to exertion, and for easing symptoms such as palpitations and tremors during anxiety attacks. Beta-blockers may be taken as tablets or given by injection.
Possible side-effects: Nausea, insomnia, physical weariness, diarrhea.
Warning: Overdose can cause dizziness, and fainting spells. Discontinuance of treatment should be gradual, not abrupt.

DRUGS LISTING

BRONCHODILATORS

For opening up bronchial tubes that have become narrowed by muscle spasm. They ease breathing in diseases such as asthma and they are most often taken as aerosol sprays; also available in tablet, liquid, or suppository form. In emergencies – for instance, severe attacks of asthma – they may be given by injection. Effects usually last for 3 to 5 hours.
Possible side-effects: Rapid heartbeat, palpitations, tremor, headache, dizziness.
Warning: Because of possible effects on the heart, prescribed doses should never be exceeded; when asthma does not respond to the prescribed doses, emergency medical treatment is needed.

COLD REMEDIES

No drug can cure a cold but symptoms can be relieved by aspirin or acetaminophen, taken with plenty of fluid. For drying up nasal secretions and unblocking nasal passages, many preparations contain antihistamines and decongestants. However, these drugs are unlikely to be effective when taken by mouth unless swallowed in doses high enough to produce side-effects which outweigh any benefits.
Possible side-effects: Drowsiness, giddiness, headache, nausea, vomiting, sweating, thirst, palpitations, difficulty in passing urine, weakness, trembling, anxiety, insomnia.
Warning: Cold remedies should be avoided by people suffering from angina, high blood pressure, diabetes, or thyroid disorders, and by anyone taking monoamine oxidase inhibitors.

CORTICOSTEROIDS

A group of anti-inflammatory drugs that are chemically similar to certain hormones naturally produced from the adrenal glands. Often simply called steroids, they are used primarily for their anti-inflammatory effect. They may be applied topically for skin disorders (they relieve itching by preventing the release of the chemicals that trigger the symptoms); injected directly into the joint; or systemically if the other methods aren't efficient.

Corticosteroids such as hydrocortisone or prednisone given orally or by injection are used for acute conditions (e.g. shock, severe allergic reactions or severe asthma). They are used in the long-term treatment of a wide variety of inflammatory conditions. They are not curative but do reduce inflammation, which sometimes enables the body to repair itself.

Corticosteroids may also be useful as immunosuppressants.
Possible side-effects: Weight gain, redness of the face, stomach irritation, mental disturbances and increase in body hair, reduced resistance to infection.

COUGH SUPPRESSANTS

There are many over-the-counter products that relieve coughing, including lozenges and syrups, which contain soothing substances such as honey and glycerin to act on the surface of the throat, pleasant-tasting flavorings and minute doses of antiseptic chemicals. They may give temporary relief to a tickly throat and the taste may be comforting, but it is doubtful whether such products are any more effective than a home-made honey drink. Lozenges are more effective as they stay in the mouth longer. Drugs such as codeine are used to suppress coughs; these should not be used with a productive cough.

CYTOTOXICS

To kill or damage multiplying cells. Cytotoxics are used in the treatment of cancer and as immunosuppressants. They are taken as tablets or given by injection or intravenously, and several cytotoxics, with different types of action, may be used in combination. Also referred to as chemotherapy.
Possible side-effects: Nausea, vomiting, loss of hair.

Warning: Because cytotoxic action can affect healthy as well as cancerous cells, these drugs may also have dangerous side-effects. For example, they can damage bone marrow and affect the production of blood cells, causing anemia, increased susceptibility to infection, and hemorrhage. Frequent blood counts are therefore advisable for anyone having treatment.

DECONGESTANTS

Act on the blood vessels in the lining of the nose to reduce mucus production and so relieve a runny or a blocked-up nose resulting from the common cold or an allergy. These drugs can be applied directly in the form of nosedrops or spray or may to taken orally, though they are less effective this way.

DIURETICS

These increase the quantity of urine produced by the kidneys and passed out of the body, thus ridding the body of excess fluid. Diuretics reduce excess fluid that has collected in the tissues as a result of any disorder of the heart, kidneys and liver. They are useful in treating mildly raised blood pressure. They are also used to reduce fluid pressure in the eye in glaucoma.
Possible side-effects: Rashes, dizziness, weakness, numbness, tingling in the hands and feet and excessive loss of potassium.

HYPOGLYCEMICS

To lower the level of glucose in the blood. Oral hypoglycemic drugs are used in the treatment of diabetes mellitus if it cannot be controlled by diet alone, and does not require treatment with injections of insulin.
Possible side-effects: Loss of appetite, nausea, indigestion, tingling in the skin, fever and rashes.
Warning: If the glucose level falls too low, weakness, dizziness, pallor, sweating, increased saliva flow, palpitations, irritability and trembling may result. If such symptoms occur several hours after

eating, this may indicate that the dose is too high.

IMMUNOSUPPRESSANTS

To prevent or reduce the body's response to infection or foreign tissues. Immunosuppressants are used to treat autoimmune diseases and to help prevent rejection of organ transplants.

Possible side-effects: Susceptibility to infection is increased. Some immunosuppressants may damage the bone marrow, causing anemia.

LAXATIVES

Drugs that increase the frequency and ease of bowel movements. They work either by stimulating the bowel wall (stimulant laxatives), by increasing the bulk of bowel contents (bulk-forming laxatives), or by increasing the fluid content of the stool (lubricants). Taken in tablet, suppository or liquid form.

Possible side-effects: Can cause diarrhea in overdose and constipation if over-used.

Warning: Laxatives are not to be taken regularly; the bowel may become lazy.

REHYDRATING TREATMENTS

These are especially formulated powders and solutions containing glucose and essential mineral salts in measured quantities. When added to water they prevent and treat dehydration resulting from diarrhea or vomiting.

SEX HORMONES

The hormones responsible for the development of secondary sexual characteristics and regulation of the menstrual cycle. There are two main types of female hormone drugs: estrogen and progestogen. They are used in synthetic form to treat menstrual and menopausal disorders and in oral contraceptives. Progestogens may be used for treating endometriosis. Sex hormones may be taken as tablets, given by injection or implanted in muscle tissue.

Possible side-effects: Nausea, weight gain, headache, depression, breast enlargement and tenderness, rashes and skin pigmentation changes, alteration in sexual drive, abnormal blood-clotting causing heart disorder.

Warning: Estrogens are not prescribed for anyone with circulatory or liver trouble, and estrogen treatment must be carefully controlled for people who have had jaundice, diabetes, epilepsy, or kidney or heart disease.

Progestogen treatment is not prescribed for people with liver trouble and must be carefully controlled for anyone who has asthma, epilepsy, or heart or kidney disease.

SLEEPING DRUGS

There are two main groups of drugs used for inducing sleep – benzodiazepines and barbiturates. Benzodiazepines are used more widely than barbiturates because they are safer, have fewer side-effects and there is less risk of physical and psychological dependence.

Possible side-effects: "Hangover" dizziness, dry mouth, and clumsiness and confusion in the elderly.

Warning: Sleeping drugs are habit-forming and should be taken for short periods only, and discontinued gradually. Broken, restless sleep and vivid dreams may follow withdrawal and may persist for weeks.

VASODILATORS

These dilate blood vessels. Most widely used in prevention and treatment of angina, for treating heart failure and circulatory disorders and as antihypertensives.

Possibly side-effects: Headache, palpitations, flushing, faintness, nausea, vomiting, diarrhea and stuffy nose.

GLOSSARY

A

Acid reflux
The welling up of acidic stomach juices into the lower part of the esophagus. Acid reflux irritates the lining of the esophagus and causes heartburn.

Acupuncture
A system of treatment in which needles are inserted into the skin and either left or manipulated for several minutes. Acupuncturists are not usually medical doctors.

Acute
A term applied to an illness or pain that comes on suddenly. Acute attacks of illness tend to be brief but usually more severe.

Addiction
Habitual and irresistible use of a drug or other substance.

Allergen
Any substance, e.g. food, animal fur, pollen grain, speck of dust, that is normally harmless but provokes an allergic reaction in susceptible individuals.

Allergy
A reaction to an allergen to which previous exposure has made the body sensitive. Allergies occur as the result of a misdirected response by the immune system which usually involves production of antibodies against an otherwise harmless substance.

Amnesia
Partial or complete loss of memory.

Analgesic
A painkilling drug.

Anaphylaxis
A generalized allergic reaction, producing symptoms ranging from urticaria and breathing difficulty to collapse due to shock.

Anesthetic
Drugs for inducing loss of sensation and hence pain in many medical and surgical procedures. Local anesthetics, used for deadening pain in only one part of the body, may be either given as injections or rubbed or sprayed onto a limited area. General anesthetics produce unconsciousness and are normally administered by anesthesiologists.

Anesthesiologist
A doctor who specializes in administering anesthetics and caring for patients during a surgical operation and immediately afterwards.

Aneurysm
A swelling that occurs if a blood vessel or the heart wall becomes weakened and balloons outwards as a result of pressure of the blood within it.

Angiography
A technique for examining the interior of blood vessels by the injection – usually through a catheter – of a solution visible on X-ray. The blood vessels can be viewed on a television screen simultaneously with a recording on film of a progression of pictures (angiograms).

Antibiotic
A drug, usually derived from living organisms, that combats bacterial infection.

Antibodies
Complex substances formed by special cells to neutralize or destroy antigens. Antibodies recognize only the antigen that provokes their formation. Their activity fights infection but can be damaging, as in allergies and autoimmune disease.

Anticoagulant
A drug that prevents the formation of blood clots.

Anticonvulsant
A drug for prevention or relief of epileptic fits.

Antidepressant
A drug used to treat depressive illness.

Antifungal
A drug that combats fungal infections such as yeast infection and athlete's foot.

Antigen
Any substance that can be detected by the body's immune system. Detection usually stimulates production of antibodies.

Antihistamine
A drug used to relieve certain allergic symptoms.

Antiseptic
Any substance for killing microbes that is too powerful to be swallowed or injected into the body.

Antitoxin
A substance that neutralizes the effects of a toxin (poison).

Arteriography
Angiography of an artery. The pictures are known as arteriograms.

Artificial insemination
A procedure in which seminal fluid is injected into the vagina in order to accomplish conception without sexual intercourse.

Aspiration
A diagnostic or treatment procedure in which fluid is sucked from a body cavity by means of an instrument such as a syringe. The cavity may be a natural one (abdominal) or one formed as a result of disease (a kidney cyst).

Atheroma
Fatty tissue that develops in an arterial wall and forms a patch or a plaque that narrows the artery and disrupts blood flow.

Atrium
One of the 2 smaller chambers of the heart.

Audiometry
A test of hearing ability.

Autoimmune
A term used to describe a condition in which the body manufactures antibodies against itself, causing damage to tissues that the antibodies attack.

B

Barium enema
An enema containing the metallic chemical barium, which shows up on X-ray pictures. A series of pictures taken while the enema is retained in the bowel reveals the lining of the colon and rectum.

Barium swallow
A liquid containing the metallic chemical barium, which is visible on X-ray. The liquid is drunk and its progress down the esophagus recorded on a series of X-ray pictures. Used for detecting esophageal disease, where there is no need to follow the passage of barium through the rest of the digestive tract.

Behavior therapy
A form of psychotherapy in which, by means of various techniques, patients are trained to replace undesirable by more desirable habits of behavior. Behavior therapists do not normally try to analyze probable reasons for the original development of undesirable behavior patterns.

Benign
A term applied to an abnormal growth, indicating that it will neither spread to surrounding tissues nor recur after removal.

Beta-blocker
A drug that slows heart activity and thus lowers blood pressure.

Biliary colic
Colic in the upper right part of the abdomen, often accompanied by nausea and vomiting. Biliary colic is due to spasm in the muscles of the gallbladder or bile duct.

Biopsy
A small piece of tissue removed from anywhere in the body for microscopic analysis. Biopsies are usually done in order to determine whether or not an abnormal growth is malignant.

Blood count
A diagnostic test of a specimen of blood in order to determine the numbers of the various cells (red, white and platelets) within a standard volume. Also known as a cell count.

Bronchodilator
A drug for widening bronchial passages.

Bronchoscopy
A procedure in which a flexible endoscope is passed down the throat in order to examine the air passages (bronchi).

Bypass
Surgical construction of a diversion to allow a body fluid such as blood to flow round an obstruction.

C

Calculus
Hard, white, creamish or brown deposit formed on the teeth surfaces. Composed of plaque that has become hardened by deposits of calcium compounds.

Carcinogen
A cancer-causing substance.

Carcinoma
A malignant growth composed of abnormally multiplying surface or gland tissue of any organ.

Catheter
A flexible tube for withdrawing liquid or air from or squirting liquid into a part of the body such as the bladder or blood vessel.

CAT scan
Computerized axial tomography is a painless scanning procedure in which hundreds of X-ray pictures are taken to reveal structures within the skull. Scans can also be used to look at other parts of the body such as the lungs.

Cauterization
The destruction of tissue (e.g. growths such as warts) by burning away with caustic chemical or a red-hot instrument.

Chancre
An ulcerated, swollen, painless lump. Can be an early symptom of syphilis.

Chiropractic
System of treatment involving forceful manipulation of joints to effect a cure. Chiropractors are not usually qualified doctors.

Cholesterol
A chemical present in some foods, such as animal fats. An over-high level of cholesterol in the body is associated with atherosclerosis.

Chromosomes
Thread-like structures in a living cell that contain the cell's genetic information. Each chromosome is composed of thousands of genes.

Chronic
A term applied to a condition that has been present for some time. Such conditions tend to improve or worsen slowly.

Climacteric
Another word for the menopause.

Colic
Abdominal pain that comes in waves separated by relatively pain-free intervals.

Colposcope
An instrument used to examine the interior of the vagina, useful for the detection of cervical conditions.

Congenital
A term used for a disease or condition present at birth.

Contagious
A term applied to disease spread by personal contact.

Coronary
Applying to or associated with the structure or functions of the arteries that supply blood to the heart muscle.

GLOSSARY

Cryosurgery
The use of extreme cold to destroy tissue, e.g. cervical erosion, hemorrhoids.

Culture
Growing microbes or living cells on a growth medium to identify disease-producing organisms, and for testing drugs.

Curettage
Removal of a thin layer of skin or internal lining with a curette (e.g. the lining of the uterus) to obtain a sample for analysis.

Cyst
1. Any cavity enclosed by a protective wall of cells or fibrous tissue, containing liquid material.
2. Prefix cyst refers to the bladder (cystitis).

Cystography
A diagnostic procedure in which an X-ray of the bladder (cystogram) is obtained by passing a solution visible on X-ray into the bladder.

Cystoscopy
A cystoscope is passed through the urethra to investigate the bladder.

Cytotoxic
A drug for destroying body cells, particularly cancerous ones.

D

Dependence
The need for regular doses of a drug to maintain a sense of well-being.

Desensitization
1. A process by which sufferers from allergies are repeatedly given small doses of causative substances so that they can build up resistance to allergic reaction.
2. Similar treatment for phobic people by repeatedly exposing them to things they fear so they eventually tolerate them.

Diathermy
The use of high-frequency electric current to heat body tissues. Current passed through a small electrode can burn away the tissues it touches as a form of bloodless surgery. Applied over a large area, the warmth of diathermy relieves pain.

Dilation (Dilatation)
The widening of a passageway or body orifice.

Diuretic
Any substance that increases urine production, thus reducing fluid content of the body.

Douche
A stream of fluid or gas projected onto part of the body or into a cavity in order to cleanse or provide superficial treatment. Doctors do not generally recommend douching or flushing out the vagina for hygienic or contraceptive purposes.

Drip
The common name for an intravenous infusion. A fluid substance is injected into the body by letting it flow down into a vein from an elevated, sterile container. The rate of flow is measured by counting the rate of dripping through a transparent chamber, also commonly referred to as IV.

Dys-
A prefix meaning painful, difficult, and/or abnormal, for example dysmenorrhea (painful periods).

E

Edema
The swelling of body tissue due to excess water content. The ankles are a common site. The swollen tissue may "pit" (remain indented) when you press it with your finger.

Electrocardiography (ECG)
A painless procedure for making a graphic recording of the electrical impulses that pass through the heart to initiate and control its activity. Small changes occur as the heart beats, and the normal form of these is altered by heart disease. Electrocardiography is done by means of metal plates that, when placed on body surfaces, pick up and record the electrical changes.

Electrocautery
Cauterization by means of an apparatus heated to burning points by electricity.

Electrolysis
The passing of an electric current through a small area of body tissue. Electrolysis is used for removing unwanted body hair.

Electroshock therapy (EST)
A treatment for depression in which under a general anesthetic an electric current is passed through the brain. Such therapy is repeated several times at weekly intervals.

Embolism
The sudden blockage of a blood vessel caused by an impacted embolus (the name for a blood clot or other foreign matter carried along in the blood).

Endoscope
An instrument that enables a doctor to look into a body cavity, photograph the interior, and take a sample of tissue or remove a small growth. The basic instrument is a tube equipped with a lighting and lens systems. A claw-like attachment can be passed through the tube for cutting. Endoscopes designed for use in certain parts of the body have special names (cystoscope, laparoscope).

Endoscopy
Any procedure involving the use of an endoscope. The term is most generally used to refer to internal examination of the esophagus, stomach, or duodenum. Special names are usually given to endoscopic procedures involving other parts of the body.

Enema
A liquid drained into the rectum through a tube or syringe and held for a set time before release by

defecation or by being drained away. Enemas are used either for treatment or for diagnostic purposes.

Enzymes
Substances in the body necessary for accomplishing chemical changes (e.g. in the burning up of sugar to produce energy or in breaking down food within the intestinal tract). An example of an enzyme is pepsin, contained in digestive juices.

Estrogen
One of the main sex hormones responsible for female sexual characteristics. In women, estrogen is produced in the ovaries. In men, small amounts of this hormone are produced in the testes. Artificial estrogens are an ingredient of many types of contraceptive pill and are also used in hormone replacement therapy.

Excision biopsy
Surgical removal of an entire lump or patch of skin that may be malignant. If microscopic analysis of the excised tissue shows that it is malignant, further treatment in the form of anti-cancer drugs or radiation therapy may be given.

Excretion
The removal of waste matter from the body by normal processes such as defecation and urination.

G

Gammaglobulin
A type of blood protein that includes antibodies. Extracted from donated blood, it may be used to prevent or treat infections such as hepatitis.

Gene
The smallest unit of inherited information, carrying the code for manufacture of a single protein. Since proteins lead, whether directly or indirectly, to the construction of all body parts and metabolic activities, genes transmit all necessary information for the physical and mental characteristics of every living thing.

Genetic engineering
The manipulation of genetic material in an organism so as to alter the normal pattern of inherited characteristics. By means of such engineering, bacteria can now be reprogrammed to produce artificial human hormones such as insulin.

Gingivectomy
A dental procedure which involves removal of diseased areas of gum.

Gynecologist
A doctor who specializes in conditions affecting female reproductive organs. Gynecologists do not treat problems such as breast cancer, but they are usually specialists in obstetrics as well as gynecology.

H

Hard drugs
Drugs, such as heroin and morphine, whose frequent use is likely to lead to self-destructive addiction.

Heartburn
A burning pain felt behind the breast bone, often beginning at its base and moving upwards. Heartburn is usually due to acid reflux in conditions such as hiatus hernia or during pregnancy.

Hematologist
A specialist in the treatment of diseases of the blood, bone marrow and lymph glands.

Hematuria
The medical term for blood in the urine.

Hemoglobin
A protein compound in the blood. Hemoglobin carries oxygen from the lungs to body tissues; it is present only in red blood cells and gives blood its characteristic color.

Hemorrhage
A medical term for bleeding, which may be either internal (within a body cavity) or external (from the skin or an orifice).

Hernia
A bulge of tissue, such as a portion of the intestines, that protrudes through an abnormal opening between muscles. The opening may be due to a congenital weakness of muscular tissue or to weakness resulting from an external force such as an injury.

Hirsutism
Abnormal hairiness, particularly in women.

Histamine
A chemical that is released into the body, causing a variety of symptoms, when an allergic reaction occurs. A common symptom is dilatation and leakage of small blood vessels, as a result of which the surrounding tissues become swollen and ooze fluid. Another common symptom is itching.

Homeopathy
Treatment of disease by means of extremely small amounts of specially prepared drugs that would, in larger quantities given to a healthy person, produce symptoms of the disease.

Hormone
A chemical in the blood stream that controls the activities of certain body organs or tissues. Hormonal effects and parts of the body affected differ according to the type of hormone involved. Most hormones are produced by special glands known as endocrine glands, and the higher the concentration of a specific hormone, the more active the function or functions it controls.

Hormone replacement therapy
The giving of hormones, in drug form, to replace those which are no longer made naturally. Hormone replacements may be given by implants, injection or in tablet form. The most familiar examples of hormone replacement therapy are the treatment of diabetes with insulin

and the treatment of menopausal symptoms with estrogen and progestogen.

Hyper-
A prefix meaning "above" or "high" as in hypertension (high blood pressure).

Hypo-
A prefix meaning "below" or "low" as in hypotension (low blood pressure).

Hypoglycemia
The condition of having an abnormally low level of sugar in the blood. A hypoglycemic drug, used to treat diabetes mellitus, is one that lowers the level of blood sugar.

I

Immune system
A natural bodily mechanism for recognizing and destroying invading microbes or foreign tissues. White blood cells are the basis of the immune system. Different types of white blood cell can make antibodies or can attack invaders directly. The immune system may itself cause trouble (most commonly, allergies, and autoimmune diseases) if it does not work properly; and it also becomes a problem in transplantation of body organs.

Immunity
Resistance developed against a disease. Immunity may be achieved naturally or by artificial means such as vaccination.

Immunosuppressant
A drug that hampers the body's mechanisms for immunity. This is particularly useful in the treatment of autoimmune disease and after organ transplants.

Incompetence
A medical term applied to poor functioning of a valve (e.g. in the circulatory or digestive system).

Incubation period
The time lag between the moment of

infection and the appearance of symptoms. During this period disease-producing microbes are multiplying but are insufficient in number to cause symptoms or infect other people. Incubation periods range from a few days to months (e.g. certain types of hepatitis).

Inflammation
The reaction of body tissue to any form of injury, e.g. as the result of a physical blow, infection, or auto-immune disease. The affected tissues become red, swollen, warm to the touch, and painful because of increased blood supply in response to chemical and nervous stimuli from the injured area. The influx of extra blood provides large quantities of white cells to combat possible infection and to remove dead tissue; it also supplies extra nutrients to encourage repair and rapid healing.

Inoculation
Injection into the body of a vaccine (a solution containing weakened or altered strains of a disease-producing organism). The aim is to procure resistance against a disease by stimulating the production of antibodies without causing severe symptoms. "Vaccination" is often used as a synonym for "inoculation".

Insufflation
The pumping of a substance such as air or vapor into a body cavity. This is useful in investigating causes of infertility; if gas blown into the uterus does not escape into the abdominal cavity, a blockage of fallopian tubes may be preventing passage of eggs into the uterus.

Intravenous
Inserted into or present within a vein. Intravenous feeding is the insertion of nourishment into the blood stream by means of a drip.

Intravenous pyelography (IVP)
A diagnostic procedure involving the injection into a vein of a solution visible on X-rays, for examining the kidneys and urinary tract by means

of a series of pictures known as pyelograms. IVP takes 1–2 hours and is painless, but patients often feel faint after the injection.

Involuntary
A term applied generally to any physical activity not subject to conscious control. In particular muscles not consciously controlled, such as those that propel food through the digestive tract, are known as involuntary muscles.

K

Keratin
A hard or horny substance present in skin, hair, nails and teeth.

Keratosis
A condition in which a patch of skin surface or mucous membrane (within the mouth, for instance) becomes thickened and toughened. Calluses and warts are familiar examples.

L

Lactation
The production and release of milk from the breasts of a woman after giving birth. The period during which suckling continues is also called lactation.

Laparoscopy
Examination of the inside of the abdomen by means of a laparoscope inserted through a small slit usually made near the navel.

Laparotomy
The cutting open of the abdominal wall in order to do exploratory or surgical work within the abdomen.

Laser beam
An intensified, controlled beam of light powerful enough to cut, destroy, or fuse body tissues. Laser beams can be precisely focused for use in delicate operations such as those carried out in eye surgery and in treatment of cervical abnormalities.

Libido
The emotion and drive that underlie sexual desire.

Lymph
A diluted form of plasma that seeps from blood vessels into tissues and delivers nutrients to local cells. Lymph collects in thin-walled vessels (lymph vessels) and eventually drains back into the circulation, carrying with it waste products from the cells. White blood cells in lymph also help to protect tissues from invasion by microbes.

Lymph gland
A bean-shaped organ at the junction of several lymph vessels. Each of the many lymph glands in the human body contains thousands of white blood cells for combating invading organisms in the lymph as it passes through the gland. A lymph gland may swell if the near-by parts of the body are infected.

M

Malignant
A term applied to a cancerous growth indicating it is likely to penetrate the tissues in which it originated and to spread further (metastasize).

Mammography
A procedure for detecting breast cancer by means of X-rays directed through the breast on to an external surface sensitive to changes in strength of X-rays as they pass through breast tissue. The photographic results are known as mammograms.

Massage
Stroking, rubbing, and/or kneading the body in order to relax muscles. Massage sometimes relieves backaches, headaches, and the pain of injuries caused or worsened by muscle tension.

Meconium
A greenish-black, mucus-like substance present in the intestines of newborn babies. Meconium is eliminated in the first bowel movement after birth.

Membrane
A thin layer of tissue that covers and/or lines each of various organs and cavities in the body.

Menarche
The first menstrual period.

Menopause
Technically the end of the final menstrual period. As commonly used, the word denotes the time of life – around the age of 50 – when menopause occurs. Also called change of life or climacteric.

Metabolism
A collective term for all physical and chemical reactions that occur in the body. The adjective "metabolic" may be applied to any such reaction or series of reactions.

Metastasis
A term applied either to a malignant growth that develops in one part of the body as a result of the transfer of abnormal cells from elsewhere, or to the process by which such transfer occurs. Cancer that has spread to a different tissue from that in which it originated is said to have metastasized.

Mini-laparotomy
Laparotomy through a very small incision adequate for minor procedures such as female sterilization.

Motor
A term applied to nerves that relay commands from the brain to muscles. Areas of the brain that control specific muscle movements are known as motor centers.

Mucous membrane
A thin tissue that lines parts of the body such as the mouth or vagina and secretes slimy or watery substances.

Muscle-relaxant
A drug that relaxes tense muscles or muscles in spasm.

N

Narcotic
A drug derived from opium that causes drowsiness and relief of pain.

Naturopathy
A system of treatment that avoids use of conventional medicines and other procedures and concentrates on diet, fresh air, exercise, massage, etc. Naturopaths, who are seldom medically qualified, are most successful at relieving symptoms caused by an unhealthful life style.

Nausea
An unpleasant sensation originating in the upper abdomen, chest or throat, often accompanied with or followed by vomiting.

Neonatal
Newborn. The term "neonatal" is applied to any event or condition directly affecting a baby during its first month after birth.

Neurologist
A doctor who specializes in treating diseases of the brain and nerves as well as nervous-system-related disorders of sense organs and muscles. Neurologists do not do surgery but often work closely with neurosurgeons.

Neurotic
Predisposed to over-reactions to mental and emotional stresses, but unlikely to lose contact with reality.

Nevus
A congenital abnormality of the skin. Nevi are varied in appearance; they may be dark spots, hairy lumps or fleshy nodules.

O

Obstetrician
A doctor who specializes in the care of women during and immediately following pregnancy and childbirth.

Obstruction
Any blockage of the passageway from one part of the body to

another. A common example is blockage of a length of intestine in a hernia. In obstructed labor the fetus cannot pass out of the uterus owing to the disproportion between it and the size of the mother's birth canal.

Occlusion
A term that dentists apply to a patient's "bite", the way in which the upper and lower teeth come together as the mouth closes.

Ophthalmologist
A doctor who specializes in treating eye disease and injuries.

Ophthalmoscope
An instrument for visually examining the tissues of the interior of the eye by shining a light through the pupil.

Optician
A medical or non-medical specialist who examines eyes for visual defects and supplies corrective lenses where necessary. Opticians do not treat eye diseases or injuries.

Orthodontist
A dentist who specializes in correcting teeth irregularities and treating jaw and facial-tissue disorders.

Orthopedic surgeon
A doctor who specializes in surgical conditions and injuries affecting muscles, bones and joints.

Osteopathy
A system of treatment emphasizing massage and manipulation of joints in addition to other kinds of treatment. Osteopaths may or may not be medical doctors.

Otoscope
An instrument for viewing internal parts of the ear from the outer ear canal through the slightly transparent eardrum in order to diagnose ear disease.

Ovum
The female reproductive cell (egg). A human ovum, though so tiny as to be barely visible to the naked eye, is one of the largest of body cells.

P

Papilloma
A wart-like or branching growth projecting from a surface such as the skin, a mucous membrane or the lining of a gland. Papillomas are formed from the over-growth of cells but are rarely malignant.

Paracentesis
A diagnostic or therapeutic procedure for draining fluid from part of the body (especially the abdomen).

Paranoid
Suffering from a mental illness characterized by extreme over sensitivity and a deluded sense of being constantly persecuted.

Patch test
The application of potential allergens to small patches of skin in order to determine whether or not the sufferer is sensitive to them.

Pathologist
A medical specialist in the study and analysis of diseased body organs and cells. Pathologists normally work in laboratories and have little or no contact with patients.

Pediatrician
A doctor who specializes in treating children.

Phototherapy
The treatment of disease by exposure to ultra-violet rays for set periods of time over several days or more. Severe jaundice in the newborn and psoriasis in adults are sometimes treated by phototherapy.

Physical therapy
The use of physical measures such as exercise, heat, and massage for treatment of disease. Such conditions as arthritis, lung disease and the effects of certain types of injury are particularly responsive to physical therapy, which is carried out by trained medical staff known as physical therapists.

Placenta
The plate-shaped organ that nourishes a baby while it is in the womb, and that also produces hormones responsible for many of the changes in the mother's body during pregnancy. When the baby is born, the placenta is expelled, when it is commonly known as the afterbirth.

Plaque (arterial)
A patch of atheroma on the inside lining of an artery.

Plaque (dental)
Coating on the teeth consisting of mucus, food particles, and bacteria. Plaque builds up rapidly without regular brushing, leading to tooth and gum diseases.

Plasma
The fluid (as opposed to cellular) part of blood. Plasma can be separated from the cells and used as a replacement fluid in the treatment of shock.

Polyp
A short-stalked outgrowth of tissue from the skin or a mucous membrane. Polyps are often caused by inflammation and are rarely malignant.

Polyunsaturated
A chemically descriptive term for fats that are thought to be least likely to encourage the production of arterial plaque when eaten in quantity. Polyunsaturated fats are found mainly in vegetable oils.

Postcoital contraception
Prevention of pregnancy by measures taken after intercourse.

Postnatal
After birth. The term is generally applied to events or conditions affecting a baby's family as well as the baby itself during the first weeks after birth.

Prenatal
Before birth, applied to an event or condition that occurs during pregnancy.

Prepuce

Another name for the foreskin – the fold of skin that covers the tip (glans) of the penis.

Primary

A term applied to the original condition, often of a malignant tumor from which further secondary growths (metastases) develop.

Prolapse

Partial or full slipping of a body organ or structure (e.g. the rectum or uterus) from its normal position. Prolapse is usually due to the weakening of surrounding supportive tissues.

Prophylactic

A substance or procedure that helps to prevent disease – for example, an antimalarial drug or an immunization injection.

Psychoanalysis

A method of treating mental disorders by probing into and analyzing both the unconscious and conscious parts of the sufferer's mind.

Psychosomatic

The medical term applied to a physical disorder due to an underlying mental or emotional condition. Indigestion is a psychosomatic illness, for example, if entirely caused by nervous tension which adversely affects the digestive processes.

Psychotherapy

Any form of non-surgical treatment for mental disorders by other means than the giving of drugs – such as discussion, advice, psychoanalysis.

Psychotic

Incapable of reasonable behavior in certain, or in severe cases, all situations. Unlike neurotic people, psychotics actually lose contact with reality when they are mentally ill.

Puberty

The age when children begin to develop adult sexual characteristics, capabilities and feelings. Usually occurs between 10 and 14.

Pus

A thick fluid, usually yellow or greenish, composed of dead white blood cells, decomposed tissue, and bacteria. Pus is a result of the battle against infection.

R

Radiation therapy

Treatment of disease by either radioactivity or X-rays. Radiation therapy is mainly used for destroying malignant growths and stopping the spread of abnormal cells.

Radioactive

A term defining unstable chemical elements that emit electro-magnetic rays and/or charged particles as they decay. These penetrate the body and are used for diagnosis or treatment.

Radioactive fibrinogen

A radioactive chemical that is incorporated into blood clots so that a clot forming in the body – e.g. a deep-vein thrombosis – can be detected on a scan.

Radioactive implant

Treatment of a malignant tumor by means of a pellet of radioactive material (perhaps radium) inserted into the tumor. The pellet, usually implanted under general anesthetic, is left in place for several days and then removed.

Radioactive isotope

A radioactive form of a chemical element, which, when introduced into natural body substances, is detectable by specialized equipment. Radioactive isotopes (commonly known as radio-isotopes) are used for locating blood clots, malfunction of thyroid glands, etc. Findings of radio-isotope scans are recorded either in individual photographs or on a screen.

Referral

Transfer of a patient's care, usually temporarily, from one doctor to another doctor who is for some reason particularly capable of dealing with the current problem.

Rehabilitation

1. Restoration of movement and strength to a limb in which a bone or joint has been immobilized after an injury. Generally carried out by physical therapists.
2. Preparation of a patient recovering from an accident or serious illness for a return to domestic and working life, largely carried out by occupational therapists.

Retention

1. The medical term for a condition in which a substance that should be excreted is retained in the body. Urinary retention, for example, is the inability to pass urine.
2. A term used in dentistry for the maintenance in correct position of a denture or brace.

Rheumatologist

A doctor who specializes in treating diseases that affect the joints. Rheumatologists do not perform operations. Patients who require surgery for joint diseases are referred to orthopedic surgeons.

S

Sarcoma

A malignant tumor composed of diseased connective tissue. Sarcomas originate in bones, cartilage, fibrous or muscular tissues. All types are rare and tend to be difficult to treat.

Saturated

A term applied to fats that are thought to encourage production of arterial plaque when eaten in quantity, e.g. dairy products and vegetable oils such as coconut and palm oils, often used in margarines.

Scan

A diagnostic procedure for viewing a body organ in order to examine some aspect of structure or functioning. Scanning is done by observation of detectable waves – e.g. from ultrasound or X-rays – as they are passed through the appropriate area of the body. Findings may be recorded on a screen or in photographs.

Sclerosant
An irritant substance such as phenol sometimes used for treating hemorrhoids and similar conditions. Sclerosants heal by causing the formation of thick scar tissue as a result of prior inflammation.

Screening
Blanket testing of large groups of apparently healthy people in order to detect disease that might not otherwise be diagnosed early.

Sebum
The oily substance produced by sebaceous glands. Sebum spreads out over the skin, helping to keep it supple and moistened.

Secondary
A term applied to a condition, often a malignant growth that develops as a result of spreading (metastasis) from an earlier (primary) tumor.

Secretion
The production of a substance – e.g. hormones or lubricating fluids – from special glands or cells. Substances so produced are also known as secretions.

Sensory
A term applied to nerves or body organs that relay information about sensations – sight, sound, touch, etc – to the brain. The areas of the brain that receive this information are known as sensory centers.

Serum
The clear fluid content of blood when separated from all blood cells and clotting substances. Most blood tests are done on this portion of the blood. The term is often used loosely as a synonym for antiserum.

Shock
1. Any mental upset, which may or may not cause a physical reaction such as fainting.
2. A medical emergency in which, for some reason such as severe loss of blood, blood pressure falls and circulation suddenly becomes inefficient. Sufferers become cold and clammy, with rapid, feeble heart beats and breathing. Vomiting, thirst, and unconsciousness may also occur.

Smear
A scraping from a body surface, or a drop of fluid such as blood or pus, that has been smeared on a glass slide in preparation for microscopic examination.

Spasm
An uncontrollable contraction of one or more muscles.

Speculum
An instrument for examining the interior of a normally closed body orifice such as the vagina or rectum.

Sphincter
A ring of muscle that narrows or closes off a passage-way by contracting. Obvious examples are those at the anus and at the opening from the bladder to the urethra.

Spider nevus
A skin blemish composed of small red lines that radiate from a central point. Such spider-like blemishes develop because a blood vessel erupts near the surface of the skin and fans out into a circle of blood-filled vessels. Spider nevi appear only on the upper part of the body and their presence often indicates liver disease.

Sterile
1. Infertile – a person of either sex incapable of conceiving children.
2. Free from contamination by living microbes.

Steroid
A name given to a group of hormones normally found in the body. There are two types of steroid given as drugs. Corticosteroids damp down inflammation and immune reactions. Anabolic steroids have a protein-building effect.

Stethoscope
An instrument for monitoring the activity of various organs, especially the lungs and heart.

Streptococcus
A group of bacteria responsible for diseases such as pneumonia, scarlet fever, and rheumatic fever.

Suppository
A soluble medicated tablet inserted into the rectum or vagina to be either absorbed or to act directly on the surrounding area.

Suture
1. Thread for sewing up wounds or surgical incisions. Stitches from the thread are also called sutures, and the stitching process is known as suturing.
2. The interlocking joints that unite the bones of the skull.

Synovectomy
Surgical removal of diseased synovial membrane. Synovectomy relieves pain but is not practical if several joints or tendons are affected.

Synovium
A membrane that lines the tough layers surrounding a joint or tendon. Synovial membranes normally produce small amounts of fluid to lubricate – and probably nourish – adjoining surfaces.

T

Therapy
The technical term for treatment of diseases and disorders. Various types of treatment are identified by appropriate prefixes, e.g. radiation therapy.

Thrombectomy
Surgical removal of a blood clot.

Thrombolytic
A drug that acts to dissolve blood clots.

Thrombosis
Formation of a blood clot (thrombus) on the lining of a blood vessel or the heart. A thrombus that breaks away and is carried along in the bloodstream is one type of embolus.

Thyroxine
A hormone produced by the thyroid gland. Release of thyroxine is controlled by the pituitary gland. Thyroxine is partly composed of iodine and assists growth, repair and efficient functioning of the body and regulates metabolic rate.

Tolerance
A term used medically to characterize a situation in which, because of habitual use of a drug, the body requires increasingly large doses in order to feel the effects.

Toxin
A poisonous substance produced by bacteria, other microbes, and some plants and animals.

Transfusion
The transfer of blood or one of its components such as plasma from a donor to a recipient.

Trauma
Any wound or injury, whether physical or mental.

Tumor
A medical term for any localized swelling; usually swellings due to abnormal multiplication of cells within a tissue.

U

Ulcer
An open sore on any external or internal surface of the body. The tissues of an ulcerous area rot away, and pus is likely to ooze from the sore.

Ultrasound
High-frequency sound waves, which are absorbed and reflected to different degrees by various body tissues. Ultrasound is useful for both diagnostic and treatment procedures. The reflections may be seen as pictures and high-powered doses of ultrasound can be used to destroy abnormalities such as gallbladder stones.

Unsaturated
A chemically descriptive term for fats that are thought not to encourage the production of arterial plaque when eaten in quantity. They include the polyunsaturated fats; they are found in most vegetable oils.

Upper GI series
A series of X-rays taken of the upper gastrointestinal (GI) tract after the patient has drunk a liquid containing the metallic element barium. Barium is visible on X-rays and its progress through the upper part of the digestive tract during the next 2 to 3 hours can be followed, usually on a screen simultaneously with the recording on film of a progressive series of X-ray pictures.

Urologist
A doctor who specializes in treatment of urinary-tract disorders.

V

Vaccine
A solution containing a killed or altered strain of a disease-producing organism. Vaccines, usually given by injection, give resistance against the diseases they cause.

Vaginismus
A rare condition of women in which sexual intercourse or vaginal examination causes painful muscular contractions that prevent penetration.

Vascular
A term applied to activities, functions, tissues etc directly associated with blood vessels.

Vasoconstrictor
Any substance that causes blood vessels to narrow.

Vasodilator
Any substance that causes blood vessels to widen.

Venereal
A term usually applied to disease caused by, or resulting from, some form of sexual contact.

Venography
A technique for viewing the interior of a vein by injecting a solution visible on X-ray. Passage of the solution through the vein is recorded on a series of pictures (venograms).

Ventricle
1. One of the 4 fluid-filled cavities of the brain.
2. One of the heart's 2 larger chambers.

Voiding cystography
A diagnostic procedure for observing bladder activity during urination by recording the working of the urinary system on an X-ray film known as a voiding cystogram. The procedure is often done at the conclusion of an IVP and is painless. Occasionally, however, a solution visible on X-rays is injected into the bladder by means of a catheter passed through the urethra.

Voluntary
A term applied generally to any physical activity subject to conscious control. Muscles that move the arms and legs are known as voluntary muscles.

X

X-rays
Rays with a short wavelength that enables them to pass through body tissues. An X-ray photograph resembles a negative of an ordinary photograph, with dense tissues such as bones showing up as white shapes. X-rays with very short wavelengths, which can penetrate tissues deeply enough to destroy them, are used in radiation therapy.

HEALTH DIRECTORY

GENERAL HEALTH

Black Women's Health Project
Martin Luther King Community
Center, Suite 157
450 Auburn Avenue NE
Atlanta, Georgia 30312
404–659–3854

Centers for Disease Control
Technical Information Services
Bureau of State Services
Atlanta, Georgia 30333
404–639–3286

**Medicaid/Medicare Consumer
Inquiry Office**
Health Care Financing
Administration
Washington D.C.
202–245–0923

**National Health Information
Clearinghouse**
Rosslyn, Virginia
800–336–4797

**National Women's Health
Network**
224 Seventh Street SE
Washington, DC 20003
202–543–9222

TEL-MED
(Recorded medical messages in
250 communities across the U.S.)
22700 Cooley Drive
Colton, California 92324
714–825–6034

AGING-RELATED ISSUES

Gray Panthers – National Office
3635 Chestnut Street
Philadelphia, PA 19104
215–382–3300

**HERS – Hysterectomy
Educational Resources and
Services**
422 Bryn Mawr Avenue
Bala Cynwyd, Pa. 19004

**National Self-Help
Clearinghouse**
33 West 42nd Street, Room 1222

New York, New York 10036
212–840–1259

CANCER

**AFTER – Ask a Friend to Explain
Reconstruction**
99 Park Avenue
New York, New York 10016

American Cancer Society
777 Third Avenue
New York, New York 10017
212–599–8200

National Cancer Institute Hotline
800–422–6237

Reach to Recovery
90 Park Avenue
New York, New York 10016
212–599–8200

DEPENDENCY

Al-Anon and Ala-Teen
New York, New York
212–481–6565

Alcoholics Anonymous (AA)
New York, New York
212–686–1100

**National Clearinghouse for Drug
Abuse Information**
Rockville, Maryland
301–443–6500

Phoenix House
New York, New York
212–787–7900
(They will refer callers in other
areas of the country to resources
that can help with a drug-related
problem)

EATING DISORDERS

**American Anorexia/
Bulimia Assn.**
133 Cedar Lane
Teaneck, N.J. 07666
201–836–1800

**Anorexia Nervosa and Related
Eating Disorders**
P.O. Box 5102
Eugene, Oregon 97405
503–344–2244

**National Association of Anorexia
Nervosa and Associated
Disorders**
P.O. Box 271
Highland Park, Illinois 60035
312–837–3438

FAMILY PLANNING

Birthright
Woodbury, New Jersey
609–848–1818

**National Abortion Information
Hotline**
Oreland, Pennsylvania
800–523–5350

**National Pregnancy Information
Hotline**
Necedah, Wisconsin
800–356–5761

**National Women's Health
Network**
224 7th Street
Washington, D.C. 20003
202–543–9222

**New Hampshire Feminist Health
Center**
38 South Main St.
Concord, New Hampshire 03301
603–225–2739

**Planned Parenthood Federation
of America**
810 Seventh Avenue
New York, New York 10019
212–541–7800

Pregnancy-Risk Hotline
800–532–3749

FERTILITY

American Fertility Society
1608 13th Avenue South, Suite 10
Birmingham, Alabama 35205
205–933–8494

Resolve, Inc.
Belmont, Massachusetts
617–484–2424

RAPE COUNSELLING

Check your telephone directory
for "Rape Crisis Center"

**National Center for Prevention
and Control of Rape**
5600 Fishers Land
Rockville, Maryland 20857

**National Coalition Against
Sexual Assault**
Minnesota Program for Victims of
Sexual Assault
430 Metro Building
Minneapolis, MN 55105

Rape Crisis Center
P.O. Box 21005
Washington, DC 20009

SEXUALLY TRANSMITTED DISEASES

San Francisco AIDS Foundation
333 Valencia Street
San Francisco, California 94103
Information and referrals for
AIDS
415–864–4376

**Santa Cruz Women's Health
Collective**
250 Locust Street
Santa Cruz, California 95060
24-Hour Information Line:
408–427–3500

STD Hotline
American Social Health
Association
Box 100
Palo Alto, California 94302
800–227–8922

VD National Hotline
1–800–227–8922

ALTERNATIVE MEDICINE

**American Association of
Acupuncture and Oriental
Medicine**
50 Maple Place
Manhasset, New York 10030

**American Holistic Medical
Association**
6932 Little River Turnpike
Annandale, Virginia 22005
703–642–5880

Holistic Health Referrals
1 Brattle Circle
Cambridge, Massachusetts 02138
617–661–3732

INDEX

Italicized page numbers indicate illustrations; page numbers in bold indicate a major entry; a small "g" following page numbers refers to a glossary entry.

INDEX

NOTES

ACKNOWLEDGEMENTS

Dorling Kindersley would like to thank the following individuals and organizations for their help in the production of this book: Carole Ash, Helen Clair Young and Sandra Schneider for design assistance; Marian Broderick and Christiane Gunzi for editorial assistance; Angela Thurstan; Fiona Sloman; Dr Patricia Last at BUPA; Maria Storey and Jacqueline Wastell at the Science Photo Library; Clinical Oncology Unit at Guy's Hospital, London.

For the American edition, Ballantine Books would like to thank their two medical consultants: Jeremy Sugarman, M.D., and Jeanne Kassler, M.D.

Editor
Charyn Jones

Managing Editor
Amy Carroll

Art editor
Julia Harris

Designer
Sarah Ponder

Illustrators
David Ashby,
Andrew Macdonald,
Coral Mula,
Sheilagh Noble,
Sue Smith,
Nick Oxtoby (retouching and airbrush),
Jim Robins,
Kevin Marks.

Photography
Antonia Deutsch

Typesetting
Windsor Graphics, The Setting Studio, DMD Ltd

Computer setting
Peter Cooling

Reproduction
Repro Llovett, Barcelona

Printed and bound by Leefung ASCO, Hong Kong

Photographic Sources
page 11: FLEX magazine, The Kobal Collection, Pictor International; page 17: Transworld Feature Syndicate; page 38: Lennart Nilsson from *A Child is Born* (Faber and Faber); pages 35, 43, 47, 352: Nancy Durrell McKenna; pages 47, 55, 63, 347, 349, 351: Sally and Richard Greenhill; page 57: Maggie Murray; pages 58, 357: Anthea Sieveking; page 70: Camilla Jessell; page 104: Donald R. Marshall; page 111: The London Foot Hospital and School of Chiropody; page 140: Austenal; page 344: Brenda Prince; page 354: Jenny Matthews.